Subcortical Dementia

SUBCORTICAL DEMENTIA

Edited by
JEFFREY L. CUMMINGS, M.D.

Director, Dementia Research Program,
Associate Professor of Neurology and Psychiatry &
Biobehavioral Sciences,
UCLA School of Medicine

Director, Neurobehavior Unit, Psychiatry Service,
West Los Angeles Veterans Administration
Medical Center (Brentwood Division),
Los Angeles, California

New York   Oxford
OXFORD UNIVERSITY PRESS
1990

Oxford University Press

Oxford   New York   Toronto
Delhi   Bombay   Calcutta   Madras   Karachi
Petaling Jaya   Singapore   Hong Kong   Tokyo
Nairobi   Dar es Salaam   Cape Town
Melbourne   Auckland

and associated companies in
Berlin   Ibadan

Library of Congress Cataloging-in-Publication Data
Subcortical dementia / edited by Jeffrey L. Cummings.
p. cm.
ISBN 0-19-505716-3
1. Dementia—Pathogenesis.   2. Brain—Diseases.
I. Cummings, Jeffrey L., 1948–
[DNLM: 1. Brain Diseases—pathology.
2. Dementia—pathology.   WM 220-S941]
RC521.S83   1990
616.8'3—dc20
DNLM/DLC for Library of Congress
89-23077   CIP

9 8 7 6 5 4 3 2 1

Printed in the United States of America
on acid-free paper

To Inese and Juliana

Preface

Subcortical dementia is a clinical syndrome characterized by bradyphrenia, memory impairment, diminished executive function, and mood and personality changes. It results from dysfunction of subcortical structures, white matter tracts connecting frontal lobe and subcortical nuclei, or frontal lobe regions projecting to specific subcortical targets. The concept of subcortical dementia has been under development for the past 15 years and no major summary of the current status of the idea, its clinical significance, or its neurobiologic importance has appeared. This volume is intended to fill this information gap.

Most of the contemporary architects of the idea of subcortical dementia have contributed chapters. The book provides information on nearly all diseases associated with subcortical dementia including degenerative disorders, vascular processes, demyelinating conditions, brain infections, and a variety of other less common illnesses. It also summarizes anatomical and neurochemical information pertinent to understanding how subcortical structures play a crucial role in the mediation of cognitive function. A history of the emergence of the idea of subcortical dementia affords insight into the roots of this concept.

This book is intended primarily for a clinical audience. Practitioners engaged in the evaluation and care of intellectually impaired patients are faced with difficult questions of differential diagnosis, treatment, and prognosis. Increased appreciation for the clinical applicability of the concept of subcortical dementia can improve diagnostic accuracy, facilitate the recognition of treatable dementing illnesses, and enhance understanding of the patient's disease and disease-related behavior. This compendium of information should prove useful to neurologists, neuropsychologists, geriatricians, psychiatrists and others caring for dementia victims and their families.

Theoretical advances have also contributed to the emergence of the idea of subcortical dementia and they are reviewed in this volume. There is increased understanding of parallel neural circuits that yoke specific cortical and subcortical structures together into integrated systems. A much larger interface between the limbic system and basal ganglia has also been identified, suggesting that subcortical structures play a considerable role in the emotional and experential life of the individual. Research on transmitters and neuromodulators in subcortical nuclei and their alteration by disease has improved our understanding of the chemical dimension of subcortical dementia. Together, this information gives us greater insight into the relationship between cortical and subcortical function and helps establish a more comprehensive vision of brain function in the service of the intellect.

J.L.C.

Los Angeles, California
September, 1989

Acknowledgments

The concept of subcortical dementia has been controversial since its reintroduction to the scientific literature in 1974. It has challenged traditional views of the role of subcortical structures in human cognition, has stimulated research in humans and animals with basal ganglia pathology, and is leading to an enhanced understanding of the functional relationships between the cerebral cortex and subcortical nuclei. The dialogue that developed between supporters and critics of the idea sharpened and focused studies of relevant diseases and contributed to the growth and evolution of this model of the neurologic mediation of intellectual function. I would like to acknowledge the contributions of both the advocates and the antagonists of the concept of subcortical dementia; it takes both to develop a synoptic understanding of the nervous system.

Each of the authors of this volume sacrificed valuable personal time in graciously contributing to this project and has my wholehearted gratitude. The principal architects of the concept of subcortical dementia are included in the authorship, and together the chapters provide a comprehensive view of the characteristics and etiologies of the syndrome.

A devoted secretarial staff including Norene Hiekel, Bontia Porch, and Kami Peden provided essential support and allowed the smooth preparation of the final manuscript.

Work would be impossible without the loving support of my wife Inese and my daughter Juliana.

Contents

Contributors

Martin L. Albert   Department of Neurology, Boston University School of Medicine, and Veterans Administration Medical Centers, Boston and Bedford, Massachusetts 02130

D. Frank Benson   Departments of Neurology and Psychiatry & Biobehavioral Sciences, UCLA School of Medicine, Los Angeles, California 90024

Jason Brandt   Department of Psychiatry, Johns Hopkins University School of Medicine, Baltimore, Maryland 21205

Eric D. Caine   Department of Psychiatry, University of Rochester School of Medicine and Dentistry, Rochester, New York 14642

Jeffrey L. Cummings   Departments of Neurology and Psychiatry & Biobehavioral Sciences, UCLA School of Medicine, and Neurobehavior Unit, Psychiatry Service, West Los Angeles Veterans Administration Medical Center (Brentwood Division), Los Angeles, California 90024

Valerie B. Domesick   Harvard Medical School, McLean Hospital, Belmont, Massachusetts 02178

Christopher M. Filley   Departments of Neurology and Psychiatry, University of Colorado School of Medicine, Denver, Colorado 80262

Marshal F. Folstein   Department of Psychiatry, Johns Hopkins University School of Medicine, Baltimore, Maryland 21205

Susan E. Folstein   Department of Psychiatry, Johns Hopkins University School of Medicine, Baltimore, Maryland 21205

Morris Freedman   Department of Medicine (Division of Neurology), University of Toronto, and Mount Sinai Hospital Research Institute, Baycrest Centre for Geriatric Care and Rotman Research Institute, Toronto, Canada MGA2E1

Daniel Hier   Department of Neurology, Michael Reese Medical Center, Chicago, Illinois 60616

Steven J. Huber   Department of Neurology, Ohio State University College of Medicine, Columbus, Ohio 43210

James P. Kelly   Department of Neurology, University of Colorado School of Medicine, Denver, Colorado 80262

Deborah A. King   Department of Psychiatry, University of Rochester School of Medicine and Dentistry, Rochester, New York 14642

A.J. Lees   National Hospital for Nervous Diseases, Queen Square, London, England WCIN 3B6

Michael Mahler   Department of Neurology, UCLA School of Medicine, and Neurobehavior Unit, Psychiatry Service, West Los Angeles Veterans Administration Medical Center (Brentwood Division), Los Angeles, California 90024

Alan M. Mandell   Department of Neurology, Boston University School of Medicine, and Veterans Administration Medical Centers, Boston and Bedford, Massachusetts 01730

Keith D. McDaniel   Department of Neurology, University of Rochester School of Medicine and Dentistry, Rochester, New York 14642

Robert Y. Moore   Departments of Neurology and Neurobiology and Behavior, State University of New York at Stony Brook, Stony Brook, New York 11794

Bradford A. Navia   Department of Neurology, Massachusetts General Hospital, Program in Neuroscience, Harvard Medical School, Boston, Massachusetts 02159

Stephen M. Rao   Departments of Neurology and Psychiatry, Medical College of Wisconsin, Milwaukee, Wisconsin 53226

Edwin C. Shuttleworth   Department of Neurology, Ohio State University College of Medicine, Columbus, Ohio 43210

Donald T. Stuss   Departments of Psychology and Medicine, University of Toronto, and Rotman Research Institute of Baycrest Centre, Toronto, Canada M6A2E1

Wilfred G. Van Gorp   Department of Psychiatry and Biobehavioral Sciences, UCLA School of Medicine, and Psychology Service, West Los Angeles Veterans Administration Medical Center, Los Angeles, California 90073

Subcortical Dementia

1

Introduction

JEFFREY L. CUMMINGS

Subcortical dementia is a clinical syndrome whose principal characteristics include bradyphrenia, memory abnormalities, dilapidation of complex intellectual functions, and mood and personality changes. The lesions producing the syndrome involve axial structures of the rostral brain stem, thalamus, basal ganglia, and frontal lobe projections of these subcortical structures. Diseases exhibiting the subcortical dementia syndrome include the degenerative extrapyramidal syndromes, subcortical infarctions, multiple sclerosis, acquired immunodeficiency syndrome (AIDS), thalamic degenerative disorders, and subcortical trauma, inflammatory processes, and neoplasms. The diverse etiologies of the subcortical dementia syndrome are unified by an overlapping pathologic anatomy and a common pattern of neuropsychological dysfunction.

Intellectual impairment has been a recognized part of subcortical disorders for more than a century. In 1861 Charcot and Vulpian (quoted by Boller, 1980) noted that dementia was present in idiopathic Parkinson's disease; in 1912 Wilson called attention to the "narrowing of mental horizons" occurring in progressive lenticular degeneration; von Stockert used the term *subcortical dementia* in 1932 to describe the intellectual deterioration occurring in postencephalitic Parkinson's disease. In more recent times, Albert and colleagues reintroduced the concept of subcortical dementia in a study of progressive supranuclear palsy in 1974, and McHugh and Folstein described a similar pattern of dementia in patients with Huntington's disease in 1975. In the past decade subcortical dementia has been recognized in other extrapyramidal disorders as well as a variety of other conditions affecting deep gray and white matter structures (Cummings and Benson, 1983). The history and evolution of the concept of subcortical dementia is reviewed in Chapter 2 by Mandell and Albert.

There has been an explosive growth of information supporting the concept of subcortical dementia, but the idea remains controversial. The intent of the current volume is to collect the relevant information together in a single source. The observations presented derive from clinical, neuropsychological, neuroanatomic, neurochemical, and neuroimaging investigations.

This introduction will review important theoretical and conceptual issues regarding subcortical dementia and introduce the information presented in the remaining chapters of the book. Terminological controversies as well as criticisms of the concept of subcortical dementia are presented and discussed. Diseases producing subcortical dementia, contrasting characteristics of cortical and subcortical dementias, and the significance of subcortical involvement in dementia of the Alzheimer's type (DAT) will be reviewed. The anatomical and biochemical basis of subcortical dementia, the nature of the cognitive psychological deficits associated with cortical and subcortical dementias, and the importance of the concept of subcortical dementia are also described.

TERMINOLOGY

Diseases producing the syndrome of subcortical dementia may have pathological changes extending beyond the subcortical regions to involve the cerebral cortex. For this reason, the term *subcortical* has been criticized. In most cases, the areas of cerebral cortex involved in patients with "subcortical" dementia syndromes are within the frontal lobes. Extensive connections exist between the frontal lobes and subcortical structures, and lesions confined to the frontal lobes produce syndromes that share many features with subcortical dementias. The terminological shortcomings of subcortical dementia reflect the problems inherent in the anachronistic tendency to emphasize structures rather than functional relationships. The striatum is most closely connected with the frontal lobe, and it is this functional system that is disrupted in subcortical dementia. Alternate terms that avoid this anatomic imprecision acknowledge frontal lobe participation in many putative subcortical syndromes and may be less objectionable include *axial dementia, frontal-subcortical dementia, frontal systems disturbance*, and *fundamental deficits syndrome*. The original term is retained here because it is well established after more than a decade of use, the characteristics of the clinical syndrome referred to by the name are familiar, and the alternative terms are cumbersome. The name *subcortical dementia* does not imply that the pathologic alterations associated with the clinical syndrome are necessarily confined to subcortical structures; on the other hand, subcortical dementia describes a clinical syndrome that *can* be produced by exclusively subcortical dysfunction and is unlike the symptom complexes produced by most disorders of the cerebral cortex.

Another terminological problem relates to use of the word *dementia* to refer to the mental status changes exhibited by many patients with subcortical disorders. Some affected patients are not occupationally disabled and perform normally on screening mental status evaluations; deficits are demonstrable only when specific functional domains are probed with demanding evaluations and the results contrasted with the performance of age-matched controls. Many investigators are reluctant to label such subtle disturbances as dementia, particularly in view of the traditionally nihilistic connotations associated with that term. Patients with these limited abnormalities might not meet the criteria for dementia presented in the *Diagnostic and Statistical Manual of Mental Disorders* (American Psychiatric Association, 1987). Subtle intellectual deficits, however, are included in the definition of dementia proffered by Cummings and Benson (1983). They defined dementia as an acquired persistent disturbance in neuropsychological function involving at least three of the following spheres of mental activity: language, memory, visuospatial function, cognition (abstraction, judgment, mathematics, executive function), and personality or emotion. The magnitude of the deficits need not be severe, and the patient may continue to function acceptably well; the emphasis is on the multiplicity of deficits regardless of severity. Patients with intellectual compromise secondary to subcortical pathology meet criteria for a dementia syndrome when defined in this way. Thus, whether the disturbances associated with subcortical dysfunction should be regarded as a dementia syndrome depends on the definition of dementia applied.

Recognition of the ubiquitous presence of mild neuropsychological deficits in subcortical disorders strengthens the attribution of behavioral deficits to striatal dysfunction. If subcortical structures contribute to intellectual function, then cognitive disturbances should be identifiable in most patients with subcortical disorders. This condition is met when patients are tested with instruments sensitive to the types of abnormalities induced by subcortical diseases and when small but significant deviations from the patient's predicted optimal performance are sought (Cummings, 1988).

DISEASES PRODUCING SUBCORTICAL DEMENTIA

Subcortical dementia has been most intensively studied in the extrapyramidal syndromes (Table 1-1). The typical profile of neuropsychological deficits has been reported in Huntington's disease (Chapter 7), Parkinson's disease (Chapter 8), progressive supranuclear palsy (Chapter 9), idiopathic basal ganglia calcification, thalamic degeneration, and spinocerebellar degenerative syndromes (Chapters 10 and 14). Patients affected by other extrapyramidal syndromes such as Hallervorden-Spatz disease, choreoacanthocytosis, Guamanian parkinsonism-dementia complex, striatonigral degeneration, and the Shy-Dragaer syndrome might be expected to possess a subcortical dementia syndrome, but information regarding the neuropsychological function of these patients is currently inadequate to establish its presence.

Table 1-1 Diseases in which the Syndrome of Subcortical Dementia has been Described

Degenerative disorders
  Parkinson's disease
  Huntington's disease
  Progressive supranuclear palsy
  Idiopathic basal ganglia calcification
  Spinocerebellar degenerative syndromes
  Thalamic degeneration

Vascular disorders
  Lacunar state
  Thalamic infarction

Metabolic disorders
  Binswanger's disease
  Wilson's disease
  Hypoparathyroidism

Demyelinating disease
  Multiple sclerosis
  AIDS encephalopathy

Miscellaneous
  Subcortical sarcoidosis
  Normal pressure hydrocephalus
  Dementia pugilistica
  Neuro-Behcet's disease

Several vascular syndromes preferentially affect the basal ganglia, thalamus, or adjacent white matter and produce subcortical dementia syndromes. In the lacunar state multiple small deep infarctions arise from occlusion of penetrating branches of the proximal portions of the middle cerebral, posterior cerebral, anterior cerebral, and basilar arteries. The lacunar syndrome is frequently accompanied by subcortical dementia. Thalamic vascular dementia results from bilateral infarction or hemorrhagic injury to the paramedian thalamic nuclei. Binswanger's disease and the clinical syndrome accompanying ischemic injury to the deep hemispheric white matter has not been adequately studied, but preliminary observations suggest that the neuropsychological deficits resemble those of other patients with subcortical dysfunction. The subcortical vascular dementias are described in Chapter 11.

Metabolic conditions typically produce confusional states and result in a mixture of cortical and subcortical disturbances. Two metabolic disorders, Wilson's disease and hypoparathyroidism, have a predominant effect on subcortical structures and produce the clinical syndrome of subcortical dementia. In these two disorders copper and calcium, respectively, are deposited in the basal ganglia (Chapter 14).

The profile of behavioral alterations produced by demyelinating diseases has received relatively little study. Recently, multiple sclerosis (Rao, 1986) and AIDS encephalopathy have been investigated, and both exhibit a subcortical dementia syndrome (Navia et al., 1986; Price et al., 1988). The dementia of multiple sclerosis is described in Chapter 12 and the AIDS dementia complex is presented in Chapter 13. Adult white matter disorders with uncharacterized mental status changes that may have features of subcortical dementia include metachromatic leukodystrophy and adrenoleukodystrophy.

In addition to degenerative, vascular, metabolic, and demyelinating syndromes, subcortical dementia has also been observed in a variety of other conditions including sarcoidosis and other central-nervous-system (CNS) inflammatory disorders (Chapter 14).

Depression shares both motoric and neuropsychologic characteristics of structural disorders with subcortical dementia. Depressed patients exhibit a parkinsonian habitus with psychomotor retardation, stooped posture, masked face, and gait alterations. The dementia syndrome of depression includes memory loss, cognitive dilapidation, and intellectual slowing characteristic of subcortical dementia. The dementia syndrome of depression is explored in Chapter 15.

Normal aging has features suggestive of preferential subcortical dysfunction. The gait, posture, and balance alterations as well as the slowing of cognition and forgetfulness that accompany the aging process indicate that subcortical dysfunction may contribute to some aspects of aging. Subcortical alterations in aging are described in Chapter 16.

Cortical dementias will not be discussed in this volume except as a means of highlighting the contrasting deficits of the subcortical disorders. The principal dementing illness involving cortical dysfunction is DAT. Pick's disease is also primarily a cortical dementia, although its prominent frontal involvement produces several clinical characteristics similar to the frontal-systems disturbances of the subcortical dementias. Vascular, neoplastic, traumatic, infectious, and toxic-metabolic processes may involve both cortical and subcortical structures and produce a mixed clinical syndrome.

CHARACTERISTICS OF CORTICAL AND SUBCORTICAL DEMENTIAS

Two principal patterns of neuropsychological impairment have been identified among the dementia syndromes: a cortical and a subcortical pattern. Cortical dementia syndromes exhibit symptoms indicative of dysfunction of the cerebral cortex including aphasia, amnesia, agnosia, and apraxia. Subcortical dementias manifest a contrasting clinical syndrome characterized by bradyphrenia, defective recall, poor abstraction and strategy formation, and mood abnormalities (Cummings and Benson, 1983, 1984). Table 1-2 contrasts the principal clinical characteristics of cortical and subcortical dementia syndromes.

Memory

Memory dysfunction occurs in both syndromes, but recent studies suggest that the nature of the memory impairment differs in cortical and subcortical dementias. Using DAT as a model of cortical dementia and Huntington's disease and Parkinson's disease as characteristic conditions with subcortical dementia, several distinguishing features in the profile of memory loss in the two syndromes have been described (Table 1-3) (Butters et al., 1983; Dick et al., 1989; Flowers et al., 1984; Moss et al., 1986; Weingartner et al., 1984). In both disorders, spontaneous recall is impaired. In DAT, the recall abnormality reflects a failure to encode the information properly or very rapid decay of memory consolidation, and the patients are not helped by encoding-enrich-

Table 1-2 Contrasting Characteristics of Cortical and Subcortical Dementia Syndromes

Characteristic	Subcortical Dementia	Cortical Dementia
Language	No aphasia (anomia and comprehension deficit when dementia syndrome is severe)	Aphasia early
Memory	Recall impaired; recognition normal or better preserved than recall	Recall and recognition impaired
Visuospatial skills	Impaired	Impaired
Calculation	Preserved until late	Involved early
Frontal systems abilities	Disproportionately affected compared with other neuropsychological abilities	Impaired to a degree consistent with involvement of other abilities
Speed of cognitive processing	Slowed early	Normal until late in disease course
Personality	Apathetic, inert	Unconcerned
Mood	Depressed	Euthymic
Speech	Dysarthric	Normal articulation until late
Posture	Bowed or extended	Upright
Coordination	Impaired	Normal until late
Adventitious movements	Present: chorea, tremor, tics, dystonia	Absent (myoclonus occurs in some cases of DAT)
Motor speed	Slowed	Normal

Table 1-3   Memory Functions in Cortical and Subcortical Dementias

Memory Feature	Cortical Dementia	Subcortical Dementia
Spontaneous recall	Impaired	Impaired
Encoding enrichment	Unhelpful	Helpful
Recognition cueing	Unhelpful	Helpful
Generative effect	Absent	Present
Priming	Absent	Present
Incidental memory	Absent	Present
Remote memory	More severe impairment	Less severe impairment
	Temporal gradient present	Temporal gradient absent
Procedural memory	Intact	Impaired

ment strategies (e.g., embedding the material to be recalled in a story), generative effects (having the patient generate the material to be remembered), or providing category or multiple-choice clues for recall. In addition, patients with DAT do not exhibit priming effects (e.g., do not produce specific responses to partial clues after prior exposure to stimuli containing the clues) and do not exhibit incidental memory for contextual details (e.g., whether the tester was a man or woman, whether the testing was done in the morning or afternoon, etc.). Subcortical disorders produce a deficit in spontaneous recall, but encoding and storage are largely preserved, and recollection is aided by embedding, recognition formats, and priming. In contrast, procedural memory for motor skills is better preserved in DAT than in subcortical dementias. Remote memory in early DAT exhibits a temporal gradient with partial sparing of early-life memories, whereas in subcortical processes remote memory is generally less impaired but exhibits no temporal gradient.

Language

Within the domain of language, aphasia occurs early in the course of cortical dementias, such as DAT, whereas no distinctive aphasia syndromes occur in the subcortical dementias, although patients in the late stages of their illnesses may exhibit difficulties with naming or following auditory commands (Appell et al., 1983; Cummings et al., 1985, 1988). Patients with DAT exhibit progressive language impairment, beginning with anomia and progressing to transcortical sensory aphasia before deteriorating into a terminal language syndrome dominated by echolalia and palilalia (Cummings and Benson, 1983; Cummings et al., 1985). Recent studies comparing patients with DAT with equally demented parkinsonian patients revealed that the DAT patients exhibited more severe anomia and had less information content in spontaneous speech, whereas the Parkinson's disease patients had grammatically simplified utterances with prominent dysarthria (Cummings et al., 1988).

Other Intellectual Functions

Visuospatial skills are impaired in both cortical and subcortical dementias. Preliminary studies suggest that the spatial–organizational deficits exhibited by these two syndromes differ quantitatively and qualitatively. Visuospatial deficits are obvious early in the course of DAT, whereas they are spared or only mildly involved early in the course of most subcortical disorders. In addition, DAT patients have more difficulty with complex constructional tasks, whereas patients with subcortical dementia syndromes such as Huntington's disease are preferentially impaired on tasks involving egocentric space (e.g., the Road Map Test) (Brouwers et al., 1984). Elementary calculation skills are impaired earlier in the course of cortical than subcortical dementias, although development of strategies for the resolution of complex problems may be affected early in the course of either disease.

Tests designed to assess the integrity of frontal systems functions indicated that these are differentially impaired in cortical and subcortical dementias. Mental control tasks are more difficult for patients with subcortical dementias, such as progressive supranuclear palsy, than for patients with DAT even when the patients have comparably severe degrees of dementia (Pillon et al., 1986). Both DAT and Parkinson's disease patients perform poorly on delayed response tests, whereas only the DAT patients have exhibited difficulty with delayed alternation tasks (Freedman and Oscar-Berman, 1986). Slowing of cognitive processing is difficult to quantitate and distinguish from motoric retardation, but bradyphrenia appears to be more prominent in the subcortical dementia syndromes than in DAT (Cummings and Benson, 1986; Rogers et al., 1986).

Personality and Mood

Personality and overall behavioral demeanor are also differentially affected by cortical and subcortical dysfunction. Pillon et al., (1986) demonstrated that patients with the subcortical dementia of progressive supranuclear palsy were more inert, indifferent, and disinterested than patients with DAT. The latter, on the other hand, are more unconcerned and show less insight into their illness. Mood disturbances, particularly depression, are more common in subcortical dementing illnesses such as Parkinson's disease and Huntington's disease than in cortical dementias such as DAT (Caine and Shoulson, 1983; Cummings et al., 1987; Santamaria et al., 1986).

Motor Abilities

In addition to the neurobehavioral differences between cortical and subcortical dementias, there are also marked differences in the degree of motor system dysfunction in the two syndromes. Subcortical dementias manifest prominent motoric abnormalities, including bradykinesia, rigidity, and poor coordination, along with a variety of hyperkinesias much as tremor, chorea, myoclonus, and tics. Dysarthria is often pronounced. Cortical dementing disorders have relatively little effect on motor function, and the patients exhibit normal speech articulation, coordination, tone, posture, and motor speed until late in the clinical course (Cummings and Benson, 1986; Cummings et al., 1988).

CLINICAL RECOGNITION OF SUBCORTICAL DEMENTIA

The clinical recognizability of the subcortical dementia syndrome has been challenged. Mayeux et al. (1983), using a mental status questionnaire, were unable to distinguish between the dementia profiles exhibited by patients with DAT, Parkinson's disease, and Huntington's disease. On this basis, they concluded that the concept of subcortical dementia was misleading and the patterns of neuropsychological impairment manifested in different dementia syndromes were not distinct. Alternative explanations of the results of this study, however, are possible. Dementia severity was more marked in DAT than in Parkinson's disease or Huntington's disease, a finding consistent with the observation that subcortical dysfunction produces less marked intellectual impairment than cortical dysfunction. When the language components of the questionnaire were analyzed separately, the DAT patients were found to have a significant decline as the disease progressed, whereas no linguistic deterioration occurred with the progression of Parkinson's disease or Huntington's disease. Thus, as predicted by the putative profile of subcortical dementia, changes in language function were most characteristic of the cortical dementias and were less marked in the subcortical dementias. Finally, depression was significantly more severe in Parkinson's disease and Huntington's disease than in DAT, conforming to the cortical–subcortical model. Failure to demonstrate other differences among the dementia syndromes may relate to the test methodology. Memory testing, for example, revealed no differences in performance between the cortical and subcortical disorders, but spontaneous recall was the mnemonic function emphasized. Expected differences in recognition memory between the cortical and subcortical disorders could not have been demonstrated using this approach. As noted earlier, recent investigations have demonstrated differences in memory and frontal lobe functions between DAT and subcortical dementias such as Parkinson's disease, Huntington's disease, and progressive supranuclear palsy (Brandt et al., 1988; Cummings et al., 1988; Freedman and Oscar-Berman, 1986; Pillon et al., 1986). These studies indicate that, when the test methodology is sensitive to the abnormalities manifested by the different types of dementias, contrasting profiles of neuropsychological performance are identified.

The neuropsychological differences between cortical and subcortical dementia syndromes are further elaborated in Chapter 6. Unresolved issues in the study of subcortical dementia include identifying appropriate ways of matching groups of patients with the different neuropsychological deficits of subcortical and cortical dementia syndromes for comparison studies and the need to explore differences produced by different subcortical disorders.

SUBCORTICAL INVOLVEMENT IN DEMENTIA OF THE ALZHEIMER TYPE

The discovery of involvement of subcortical structures in DAT challenged the validity of conceptualizing this disease as a cortical dementia and contrasting it with subcortical dementias (Whitehouse, 1986). Senile plaques and neurofibrillary tangles have been identified in the nucleus basalis of Meynert, locus ceruleus, mamillary bodies, striatum, thalamus, cerebellum, hypothalamus, substantia nigra, and raphe nuclei of the brain stem (Bondareff et al., Brun and Gustafson, 1976; Ishii, 1966; McDuff and Sumi, 1985; Rudelli et al., 1984; Tomlinson et al., 1981; Whitehouse et al., 1981, 1982; Yamamoto and Hirano, 1985). In many of these sites, however, not more than 25 percent of the neurons are involved, and symptomatic consequences prior to the terminal phases of the disease are unlikely. Nucleus basalis and locus ceruleus are exceptions and appear to be affected early in the disease course and to a degree commensurate with cortical involvement (Mann et al., 1986). Both these structures project directly to the cerebral cortex. Portions of the locus ceruleus projecting to the cerebral cortex are preferentially atrophic, whereas those portions projecting to basal ganglia, cerebellum, and spinal cord are spared (Marcyniuk et al., 1986). Likewise, nucleus basalis projects diffusely to the cerebral cortex but not to subcortical regions of the hemispheres (Mesulam et al., 1983), and reductions in cholinergic system markers related to nucleus basalis atrophy are limited to the cerebral cortex (Davies, 1978). Studies of glucose metabolism in DAT using positron emission tomography reveal that frontal and parietal metabolism is diminished, whereas the metabolic activity of sub-cortical structures is preserved (Cutler et al., 1985; McGeer et al., 1986; Polinsky et al., 1987). Thus, most of the available evidence indicates the subcortical pathologic alterations in DAT produce cortical dysfunction and are reflected in symptoms indic-ative of cortical disease. The observations emphasize that the cortical–subcortical di-chotomy cannot be regarded as a precise anatomic classification but describes the prin-cipal pattern of functional disruption.

Ontogenic and cytoarchitectonic studies also bear on the relationship of the nucleus basalis to the cerebral cortex and to its importance with regard to the concept of sub-cortical dementia. This nucleus has a "corticoid" structure, and embryologically it is more closely affiliated with the cortex than with striatal structures (Mesulam, 1985). Thus it lacks the characteristics of other subcortical structures and should not be an-alogized with them from a functional perspective.

Finally, the neuropsychological consequences of atrophy of the nucleus basalis and consequent acetylcholine deficiency in DAT have recently been challenged. Scopol-amine, a drug that disrupts central cholinergic function, produces an amnesia but does not reproduce the other aspects of the DAT syndrome such as remote memory loss, aphasia, and visuospatial deficits (Beatty et al., 1986). Spinocerebellar syndromes have been shown to have atrophy of the nucleus basalis of comparable severity to that of DAT with similar low levels of cholinergic function without a corresponding de-mentia syndrome (Kish et al., 1988). Thus, the principal components of the DAT clinical syndrome may be a product of local cortical neuronal loss and plaque and tangle formation rather than subcortical nuclear atrophy and correlative cholinergic deficits.

ANATOMICAL AND BIOCHEMICAL BASIS OF SUBCORTICAL DEMENTIA

The concept of subcortical dementia represents an extension of localization theory from the elementary neurologic to the behavioral domain. Functional specialization within the cerebral cortex has been recognized for over a century and has profitably been explored in the study of aphasias, amnesias, agnosias, and apraxias. The behav-ioral disturbances occurring with focal subcortical lesions have also been increasingly studied (Chapter 5). Investigation of the subcortical syndromes adds another dimension to behavioral research by defining the neurologic role of basal ganglia, thalamus, and brain-stem structures. Division of the dementing disorders into those with cortical or subcortical features is the first step in an increasingly refined understanding of the behavioral contributions of different brain regions.

The principal structure involved in most subcortical dementias is the striatum. This is the predominant site of involvement in Huntington's disease, Wilson's disease, idiopathic basal ganglia calcification, lacunar state, and hypoparathyroidism. The thalamus is also a frequent site of pathologic changes and in a few conditions is the major area where alterations occur, notably in idiopathic thalamic degeneration and thalamic infarction. Other structures commonly involved in the subcortical dementias include the substantia nigra, subthalamic nucleus, ventral tegmental area, locus ceruleus, and deep hemispheric white matter tracts. These structures have robust connections with the limbic system and the cerebral cortex, particularly the frontal lobes. The structure and connections of the striatum are described in Chapter 3.

The lesions of subcortical dementia are located in nuclei that synthesize important neurotransmitters (substantia nigra, locus ceruleus), involve structures that are major transmitter targets (striatum), or affect tracts that serve as ascending transport pathways for transmitters. Dopamine, norepinephrine, serotonin, acetylcholine, and γ-aminobutyric acid are the principal transmitters mediating elements of mood, motivation, motion, and intellectual function disrupted in the subcortical dementias. Recent developments in the subcortical distribution of neurotransmitters and neuromodulators are presented in Chapter 4.

A preliminary model for integrating information regarding cortical–subcortical circuits and neurotransmitters is explored in the final chapter of the book.

FUNDAMENTAL AND INSTRUMENTAL FUNCTIONS

The concept of subcortical dementia has focused attention on the role of subcortical structures in intellectual activity and has contributed to development of neurologically based models of human cognition. Albert (1978) enunciated an important conceptual approach, dividing neuropsychological activities into instrumental and fundamental functions. Instrumental functions include communication, perception, and praxis. Fundamental functions are behaviors such as set shifting and maintenance, attention, concentration, sequencing, and determinants of the rate of information processing. Motivation and mood are closely allied with fundamental functions. Instrumental functions are dependent on the integrity of the cerebral cortex and are disrupted in the cortical dementias. Fundamental functions are mediated by subcortical structures and are the mechanisms disturbed in the subcortical dementias.

Cummings (1986) integrated this approach with the evolutionary model of Yakovlev (1948, 1968), observing that instrumental functions are mediated by phylogenetically recent and ontogenetically late-maturing structures that are organized into cortical regions connected by well-myelinated tracts. Fundamental functions are based on phylogenetically more primitive, ontogenetically precocious nuclear structures connected by shorter projection systems. Instrumental functions are mediated by a cerebral cortical mantle organized into multiple horizontal layers and vertical cellular columns, whereas fundamental functions are subserved primarily by structures with a diffuse or mosaic organization (Yakovlev, 1948, 1968).

The division of the neuropsychological domain into subcortically mediated fundamental functions and cortically mediated instrumental functions also draws attention to one inherent difficulty in studying subcortical dementia: There are excellent tests available for the study of instrumental functions such as memory and language, but the ability to quantify fundamental functions such as speed of cognitive processing, motivation, mood, and set flexibility is limited. Impairment of fundamental functions must often be inferred from the demeanor of the patient and from the pattern of secondary effects on instrumental behavior. The evidence in support of subcortical dementia is often deductive in nature. Nevertheless, there is sufficient converging information derived from a variety of clinical, neuropsychological, pathologic, neuropharmacological, and neuroimaging studies to support the validity of the concept.

IMPORTANCE OF THE CONCEPT OF SUBCORTICAL DEMENTIA

The concept of subcortical dementia has both clinical and theoretical importance. From a clinical perspective, most treatable dementias exhibit the syndrome of subcortical dementia. The mental status alterations of Parkinson's disease can be at least partially improved with levodopa therapy, the dementia of Wilson's disease may be ameliorated or its progression slowed by penicillamine, vascular subcortical dementia syndromes require therapy with antiplatelet aggregation agents, hypoparathyroidism produces a reversible subcortical dementia syndrome, multiple sclerosis and subcortical inflammatory syndromes may require treatment with steroids, the AIDS dementia may be partially reversible with 3'-azido-3'-deoxythymidine (AZT), normal pressure hydrocephalus may improve following ventriculoperitoneal shunting, and the subcortical dementia syndrome of depression responds to antidepressant therapy. Thus, patients presenting features of subcortical dysfunction may be found to have a potentially treatable syndrome. Cortical dementia syndromes (DAT, Pick's disease), in contrast, are irreversible.

Study of the subcortical dementias is advancing understanding of the integrated manner in which brain structures mediate human cognition. The role of the striatum and thalamus in intellectual function, the importance of frontal–subcortical systems in mediating mood and motivation, and the neurochemical underpinnings of thought and emotion are being defined as the subcortical dementias are explored. Neuropsychological studies of subcortical dementias complement information regarding the function, evolution, ontogeny, and structure of the nervous system. The model of cognition based on the distinction of fundamental functions mediated by subcortical structures and instrumental functions mediated by cortical structures is interacting with and enriching other models of cognitive neuropsychology.

REFERENCES

Albert, M.L. Subcortical dementia. In *Alzheimer's Disease: Senile Dementia and Related Disorders*. Katzman R., Terry, R.D., and Bick, K.L. (eds.). Raven Press, New York, 1978, pp. 173–9.

Albert, M.L., Feldman, R.G., and Willis, A.L. The "subcortical dementia" of progressive supranuclear palsy. *J Neurol Neurosurg Psychiatry* 1974; 37:121–30.

American Psychiatric Association. *Diagnostic and statistical manual of mental disorders*. Revised 3rd ed. American Psychiatric Press, Washington, D.C., 1987.

Appell, J., Kertesz, A., and Fisman, M. A study of language functioning in Alzheimer patients. *Brain Lang* 1982; 17:73–91.

Beatty, W.W., Butters, N., and Janowsky, D.S. Patterns of memory failure after scopolamine treatment: implications for cholinergic hypotheses of dementia. *Behav Neural Biol* 1986; 45:196–211.

Boller, F. Mental status of patients with Parkinson disease. *J Clin Exp Neuropsychol* 1980; 2:157–72.

Bondareff, W., Mountjoy, C.Q., and Roth, M. Loss of neurons of origin of the adrenergic projection to cerebral cortex (nucleus locus ceruleus) in senile dementia. *Neurology* 1982; 32:164–8.

Brandt, T., Folstein, S.E., and Folstein, M.F. Differential cognitive impairment in Alzheimer's and Huntington's disease. *Ann Neurol* 1988; 23:555–61.

Brouwers, P., Cox, C., Martin, A., Chase, T., and Fedio, P. Differential perceptual-spatial impairment in Huntington's and Alzheimer's dementias. *Arch Neurol* 1984; 41:1073–6.

Brun, A., and Gustafson, L. Distribution of cerebral degeneration in Alzheimer's disease. *Acta Psychiatr Nervenkr* 1976; 223:15–23.

Butters, N., Albert, M.S., Sax, D.S., Miliotis, P., Nagoda, J., and Sterste, A. The effect of verbal mediators on the pictorial memory of brain-damaged patients. *Neuropsychologia* 1983; 21:307–23.

Caine, E.D., and Shoulson, I. Psychiatric syndromes in Huntington's disease. *Am J Psychiatry* 1983; 140:728–33.

Cummings, J.L. Subcortical dementia. Neuropsychology, neuropsychiatry, and pathophysiology. *Br J Psychiatry* 1986; 149:682–97.

Cummings, J.L. Intellectual impairments in Parkinson's disease: Clinical, pathologic, and biochemical correlates. *J Geriatr Psychiatry Neurol* 1988; 1:24–36.

Cummings, J.L., and Benson, D.F. *Dementia: A Clinical Approach*. Butterworths, Boston, 1983.

Cummings, J.L., and Benson, D.F. Subcortical dementia. Review of an emerging concept. *Arch Neurol* 1984; 41:874–9.

Cummings, J.L., and Benson, D.F. Dementia of the Alzheimer type: An inventory of diagnostic clinical features. *J Am Geriatr Soc* 1986; 34:12–9.

Cummings, J.L., Benson, D.F., Hill, M.A., and Read, S.L. Aphasia in dementia of the Alzheimer type. *Neurology* 1985; 35:394–7.

Cummings, J.L., Darkins, A., Mendez, M., Hill, M.A., and Benson, D.F. Alzheimer's disease and Parkinson's disease: Comparison of speech and language alterations. *Neurology* 1988; 38:680–4.

Cummings, J.L., Miller, B., Hill, M.A., and Neshkes, R. Neuropsychiatric aspects of multi-infarct dementia and dementia of the Alzheimer type. *Arch Neurol* 1987; 44:389–93.

Cutler, N.R., Haxby, J.V., Duara, R., Grady, C.L., Kay, A.D., Kessler, R.M., Sundaram, M., and Rapoport, S.I. Clinical history, brain metabolism, and neuropsychological function in Alzheimer's disease. *Ann Neurol* 1985; 18:298–309.

Davies, P. Studies on the neurochemistry of central cholinergic systems in Alzheimer's disease. In *Alzheimer's Disease: Senile Dementia and Related Disorders*. Katzman, R., Terry, R.D., and Bick, K.L. (eds.). Raven Press, New York, 1978, pp. 453–9.

Dick, M.B., Kean, M.-L., and Sands, D. Memory for internally generated words in Alzheimer-type dementia: Breakdown in encoding and semantic memory. *Brain Cogn* 1989; 9:88–108.

Flowers, K.A., Pearce, Z., and Pearce, J.M.S. Recognition memory in Parkinson's disease. *J Neurol Neurosurg Psychiatry* 1984; 47:1174–81.

Freedman, M., and Oscar-Berman, M. Selective delayed response deficits in Parkinson's and Alzheimer's disease. *Arch Neurol* 1986; 43:886–90.

Ishii, T. Distribution of Alzheimer's neurofibrillary changes in the brainstem and hypothalamus of senile dementia. *Acta Neuropathol (Berl)* 1966; 6:181–7.

Kish, S.J., El-Awar, M., Schut, L., Leach, L., Oscar-Berman, M., and Freedman, M. Cognitive deficits in olivopontocerebellar atrophy: Implications for the cholinergic hypothesis of Alzheimer's dementia. *Ann Neurol* 1988; 24:200–6.

Mann, D.M.A., Yates, P.O., and Marcyniuk, B. A comparison of nerve cell loss in cortical and subcortical structures in Alzheimer's disease. *J Neurol Neurosurg Psychiatry* 1986; 49:310–2.

Marcyniuk, B., Mann, D.M.A., and Yates, P.O. The topography of cell loss from locus coeruleus in Alzheimer's disease. *J Neurol Sci* 1986; 76:335–45.

Mayeux, R., Stern, Y., Rosen, J., and Benson, D.F. Is "subcortical dementia" a recognizable clinical entity? *Ann Neurol* 1983; 14:278–83.

McDuff, T., and Sumi, S.M. Subcortical degeneration in Alzheimer's disease. *Neurology* 1985; 35:123–6.

McGeer, P.L., Kamo, H., Harrop, R., McGeer, E.G., Martin, W.R.W., Pate, B.D., and Li, D.K.B. Comparison of PET, MRI, and CT with pathology in a proven case of Alzheimer's disease. *Neurology* 1986; 36:1569–74.

McHugh, P.R., and Folstein, M.E. Psychiatric syndromes in Huntington's disease. In: *Psychiatric Aspects of Neurologic Disease*. Benson, D.F., and Blumer, D. (eds.). Grune and Stratton, New York, 1975, pp. 267–85.

Mesulam, M.-M. Patterns in behavioral neuroanatomy: Association areas, the limbic system, and hemispheric specialization. In *Principles of Behavioral Neurology*. Mesulam, M.-M., (ed.) F.A. Davis, Philadelphia, 1985, pp. 1–70.

Mesulam, M.-M., Mufson, E.J., Levey, A.F., and Wainer, B.H. Cholinergic innervation of cortex by the basal forebrain: Cyto-chemistry and cortical connections of the septal area, diagonal band nuclei, nucleus basalis (substantia innominata), and hypothalamus in the rhesus monkey. *J Comp Neurol* 1983; 224:170–97.

Moss, M.B., Albert, M.S., Butters, N., and Payne, M. Differential patterns of memory loss among patients with Alzheimer's disease, Huntington's disease and alcoholic Korsakoff's syndrome. *Arch Neurol* 1986; 43:239–46.

Navia, B.A., Jordan, B.D., and Price, R.W. The AIDS dementia complex: I. Clinical features. *Ann Neurol* 1986; 19:517–24.

Pillon, B., Dubois, B., Lhermitte, F., and Agid, Y. Heterogeneity of cognitive impairment in progressive supranuclear palsy, Parkinson's disease, and Alzheimer's disease. *Neurology* 1986; 36:1179–85.

Polinsky, R.J., Noble, H., Di Chiro, G., Nee, L.E., Feldman, R.G., and Brown, R.T. Dominantly inherited Alzheimer's disease: Cerebral glucose metabolism. *J Neurol Neurosurg Psychiatry* 1987;50:752–7.

Price, R.W., Brew, B., Sidtis, J., Rosenblum, M., Scheck, A.C., and Cleary, P. The brain in AIDS: Central nervous system HIV-1 infection and AIDS dementia complex. *Science* 1988; 239:586–92.

Rao, S.M. Neuropsychology of multiple sclerosis: A critical review. *J Clin Exp Neuropsychol* 1986; 8:503–42.

Rogers, D., Lees, A.J., Trimble, M., and Stern, G.M. Concept of bradyphrenia: a neuropsychiatric approach. *Adv Neurol* 1986; 45:447–50.

Rudelli, R.D., Aubler, M.W., and Wisniewski, H.M. Morphology and distribution of Alzheimer neuritic (senile) and amyloid plaques in striatum and diencephalon. *Acta Neuropathol (Berl)* 1984; 64:273–81.

Santamaria, J., Tolosa, E., and Valles, A. Parkinson's disease with depression: A possible subgroup of idiopathic parkinsonism. *Neurology* 1986; 36:1130–3.

Tomlinson, B.E., Irving, D., and Blessed, G. Cell loss in the locus coeruleus in senile dementia of Alzheimer type. *J. Neurol Sci* 1981; 49:419–28.

von Stockert, F.G. Subcorticale demenz. *Arch Psychiatry* 1932; 97:77–100.

Weingartner, H., Burns, S., Diebel, R., and LeWitt, P.A. Cognitive impairment in Parkinson's disease: distinguishing between effort-demanding and automatic cognitive processes. *Psychiatry Res* 1984; 11:223–35.

Whitehouse, P.J. The concept of subcortical and cortical dementia: Another look. *Ann Neurol* 1986; 19:1–6.

Whitehouse, P.J., Price, D.L., Clark, A.W., Coyle, J.T., and DeLong, M.R. Alzheimer disease: Evidence for selective loss of cholinergic neurons in the nucleus basalis. *Ann Neurol* 1981; 10:122–6.

Whitehouse, P.J., Price, D.L., Struble, R.G., Clark, A.W., Coyle, J.T., and DeLong, M.R. Alzheimer's disease and senile dementia: Loss of neurons in basal forebrain. *Science* 1982; 215:1237–9.

Wilson, S.A.K. Progressive lenticular degeneration: A familial nervous disease associated with cirrhosis of the liver. *Brain* 1912; 34:295–507.

Yakovlev, P.I. Motility, behavior and the brain. *J Nerv Ment Dis* 1948; 107:313–35.

Yakovlev, P.I. Telencephalon "impar," "semipar," and "totopar." *Int J Neuro* 1968; 6:245–65.

Yamamoto, T., Hirano, A. Nucleus raphe dorsalis in Alzheimer's disease: Neurofibrillary tangles and loss of large neurons. *Ann Neurol* 1985; 17:573–7.

2

History of Subcortical Dementia

ALAN M. MANDELL AND MARTIN L. ALBERT

An invisible weight seems to be compressing the intellect and slowing perceptions, movements, and ideas, all at the same time.

Ball (1882, p. 26)

Priests, philosophers, and physicians have grappled with the concept of mental infirmity for centuries. In the struggle to understand dementia, the medical literature has suffered from "terminological confusion, as the original terms (e.g., 'dementia,' 'stupidity') acquired additional connotations and new terms were coined to compete with the ancient ones." (Lipowski, 1981). The history of subcortical dementia typifies a focused controversy within the larger question: What is the essence of dementia? One manner of attempting to answer the larger question is to ask another: Is dementia a monolithic phenomenon, or are dementing illnesses distinctive, if overlapping, phenomena?

In this chapter, we wish to address both the larger and the smaller issues. First, we shall address the relatively more specific questions: What is subcortical dementia?, how did it come to be what it is perceived as being?, and why is it controversial? Second, looking through the lens of the subcortical dementia syndrome, we shall attempt to see beyond the plethora of operational definitions (Cummings and Benson, 1983; Hare, 1981; Lipowski, 1981) and ask, what does the history of subcortical dementia tell us about the nature of dementia in general?

REINTRODUCTION OF THE CONCEPT OF SUBCORTICAL DEMENTIA

Legal and literary references to deterioration in mental faculties can be traced back more than 2,500 years, and aspects of the dementia syndrome continued to be recognized by Greek and Roman writers such as Plato, Horace, Celsus, and Cicero. Credit for the first clear medical description of dementia is generally given to Galen (c. A.D. 130–200). Despite abundant literary references (e.g., King Lear), little medical interest in dementia is thereafter recorded until the sixteenth century (Lipowski, 1981). The first adequate clinical descriptions of so-called senile dementia are products of the late eighteenth and early nineteenth centuries, and, by 1911, the essential clinical and pathologic aspects of Alzheimer's disease had been defined (Torack, 1983; Reisberg, 1983).

The association between brain abnormalities and disorders of behavior and intellect had, of course, been previously well documented, beginning principally with Gall, and then primarily by nineteenth century French and German authors (Benson, 1979; Critchley, 1979). Although the concepts of brain-stem dementia and subcortical activation can be traced to the Renaissance, most studies, even those regarding diseases for which we now recognize primary involvement of subcortical structures, had emphasized cortical damage as the major pathologic substrate of mental perturbation (Clarke, 1897; Bruyn, 1968). Bleuler would therefore write in 1916: "Only diffuse disturbances of the cortex cause a real weakening of intelligence, whereas certain affective disturbances can already manifest themselves in (sub)cortical brain lesions, most frequently when it affects the thalamus" (Bleuler, 1924). One can derive from this indirect assertion an implicit recognition that focal subcortical damage may affect at least some aspects of behavior. As will be evident presently, this notion had already been demonstrated in several publications, sometimes quite elegantly.

There is no dearth of historical documentation that subcortical pathology, either exclusively or primarily, can be associated with clinical features of dementia. Thus could Albert, Feldman, and Willis write in 1974: "Descriptions of dementia after subcortical lesions are neither new nor rare." Although the idea of a subcortical dementia was already at least 50 years old (Naville, 1922), and the term itself had been coined just 10 years after Naville had described the syndrome (von Stockert, 1932), it was the controversial and nearly simultaneous articles by Albert et al. (1974) and McHugh and Folstein (1975) that codified the subcortical dementia concept for contemporary analysis and dispute. Their ideas form much of the basis of contemporary "anatomical" classifications of the dementias (Joynt and Shoulson, 1985). A review of their observations and conclusions is therefore in order.

Albert et al. (1974) examined clinically, and in variable detail, five patients with progressive supranuclear palsy (PSP) (Steele et al., 1964). This disease is associated, at least by standard anatomic techniques, with exclusively subcortical pathology. The authors compared their neurobehavioral observations with 42 previously published cases of PSP that provided sufficient descriptions of mental signs and symptoms. Their analysis yielded a composite clinical profile of the dementia syndrome of PSP: forgetfulness, slowness of thought processes, personality alteration (particularly apathy and depression, but also occasional irritability or brief outbursts of rage), and "impaired ability to manipulate acquired knowledge."

They then reviewed individual case reports describing behavioral changes associated with other "degenerative," vascular, neoplastic, and metabolic lesions of subcortical nuclear structures. Some of these behavioral descriptions were very, and occasionally extremely, brief (e.g., Winkelman, 1932). The authors nevertheless felt justified in distilling from the literature a "consistent pattern of dementia characteristic of various neurological syndromes which all have a subcortical pathology." That pattern consisted of the four elements described for their patients with PSP, although "some form of memory defect" was substituted for "forgetfulness." They finally noted that this pattern was remarkably similar to that seen with frontal lobe disease, and that neither their patients, nor any of the other cases, had "higher cortical defects" such as aphasia, apraxia, and agnosia. They emphasized the functional interdependence of cortex and subcortical nuclei, and hypothesized that lesions in subcortical structures and their connections could "deactivate" an otherwise normal cortex. This in turn would result in impaired timing and slowing down of normal intellectual processes.

At approximately the same time, McHugh and Folstein (1975) also discussed the concept of "subcortical dementia." Their study population consisted of eight patients with Huntington's disease (HD), all of whom were residents of a psychiatric hospital. Their eight patients suffered from a dementia syndrome characterized by "a general loss of efficiency in all aspects of thinking including memory functions" ("dilapidation of all cognitive powers"), and a progressive apathy or "loss of initiative." The authors stressed the absence of aphasia, alexia, apraxia, agnosia, and Korsakoff-type amnesia, features they associated more closely with "disorders with prominent cortical pathology." They theorized that degeneration of an ascending cholinergic arousing and altering system could produce both the dementia and the mood disturbances of HD, and they also noted the neuropsychiatric similarities between their patients and those with frontal lobe disease.

Thus, two groups of investigators, working contemporaneously but independently, and studying patients with different diseases, made strikingly similar observations. Each described a dementia syndrome lacking major deficits in "instrumental" cognitive functions, particularly language. Both noted a slowing or "dilapidation" of information processing as well as a prominent mood disturbance, and both hypothesized a disturbance in cortical activation as the underlying mechanism. Both compared their constellation of signs and symptoms to that of the "frontal syndrome." Importantly, each group stressed the interdependency of cortical and subcortical structures in cognitive function. They specifically discarded the notion of dementia as a neuropsychological monolith by asserting the existence of differing patterns of dementia dependent upon separate neurophysiological mechanisms.

At least one intent of these articles was fulfilled; they spurred a debate regarding the validity of two issues. The more literally defined issue could be stated thus: dementia consequent to predominantly or exclusively subcortical pathology is qualitatively different from that secondary to primarily or exclusively cortical disease. This "anatomical subcortical dementia concept" has been both challenged and supported by neuropsychological, imaging, and particularly anatomic–pathologic studies, many of which are discussed in greater detail elsewhere in this volume. The chief criticism of the "anatomical subcortical dementia concept" has been the correct observation that many "subcortical" diseases have cortical pathology (Boller et al., 1980; Leenders et al., 1988; Terry et al., 1978), while "cortical" dementias often show significant subcortical involvement (Whitehouse, 1986).

In a series of articles subsequent to their paper in 1974, Albert and colleagues have attempted to clarify the concept of subcortical dementia. Albert (1978) summarized published accounts of surgical lesions and electrical stimulation of subcortical structures, reviewed clinical observations and neuropsychological studies of patients with known or presumed subcortical lesions, and discussed the use of controversial labels. He noted an overlap between the patterns of intellectual deterioration seen in a normal-aged population and the putative pattern of subcortical dementia, and he discounted the notion that Alzheimer's disease represents an acceleration of normal aging. Signs and symptoms of "subcortical dementia" as components of "cortical dementias" were acknowledged. He noted the difficulty of relating the behavioral defects of Huntington's disease specifically to subcortical dysfunction.

In 1984, Albert reasoned that the clinical concept of subcortical dementia was valid despite strong anatomic, and less strong neuropsychological, evidence against it.

Freedman and Albert (1985) compared the accumulated clinical and neuropsychological data from studies of Parkinson's disease, Huntington's disease, and depressive "pseudodementia," while again reviewing arguments for and against subcortical dementia. Noting the unlikelihood of a pathologically pure cortical dementia and the anatomic indistinctness of "cortical" and "subcortical" terminologies, they proposed elimination of the term *cortical dementia*. The data, nevertheless, supported the existence of *at least* two *clinical patterns* of dementia. The core syndrome of subcortical dementia still consisted of memory loss, impairment of manipulation of acquired knowledge, and, most importantly, an absence of aphasia, apraxia, or agnosia. Slowness of mentation and personality change were frequent, but not invariable, constituents.

Much of the argumentation concerning the existence of subcortical dementia since 1974 has expended energy on the wrong issue. The use of "vague anatomic terms" (Whitehouse, 1986) and their literal interpretation have tended to divert attention from a more fundamental issue: "different neuropsychological patterns of dementia exist and can be identified, and the various clinical patterns may have different pathophysiologic bases" (Albert, 1978). This issue, the classification of dementing illnesses based on sound neurobiological and neuropsychological principles, has only recently been addressed. Here, also, controversies abound.

Cummings (1986, 1988a; Cummings and Benson, 1983, 1984) believes that sufficient evidence exists to support at least a dichotomous taxonomy for the heterogeneous group of dementing disorders. Citing many studies of neuropsychological parameters (e.g., memory, attention, visuospatial skills), neuropsychiatric manifestations, and pathologic, metabolic, and biochemical alterations in various diseases, Cummings concludes that there are qualitative and quantitative differences between "cortical" and "fronto-subcortical" syndromes. "Cortical" dementias involve chiefly instrumental cognitive functions (e.g., language and praxis)—those that are most easily measured. "Subcortical" dementias affect phylogenetically older fundamental functions (e.g., arousal, mood, and motivation) that are more difficult to assess (Cummings, 1986; Albert, 1978).

Whitehouse (1985, 1986) has been less sanguine in his approach to this classification. Surveying history, he seeks not to repeat past mistakes by avoiding "overly simplistic associations between neuroanatomy and psychology." He interprets differently some of the literature cited by Cummings and finds insufficient support at present for "two all-embracing categories of dementia." Referring in particular to the difficulty of matching patient groups according to severity of dementia, he posits that a "subcortical" pattern is reported more often in victims of Parkinson's disease, PSP, and Huntington's disease because their motor disturbances cause them to seek medical attention earlier in their illnesses. Perhaps patients with very early Alzheimer's disease (AD) would exhibit the same pattern if tested. Whitehouse nevertheless stresses the lack of systematic comparative studies in attempts to prove or disprove the two (or more) dementia syndrome concept.

The problem of insufficient data is discussed in detail by Brown and Marsden (1988). The inability to match patients for overall level of dementia is again stressed as a limitation of virtually all previous studies. It is also apparent that, by including severity of behavioral–cognitive deficits as a necessary criterion for a diagnosis of a dementia, Brown and Marsden and many others define dementia differently than do

Cummings and colleagues (Cummings, 1988a; Cummings and Benson, 1983). This bias also hinders comparison.

Brown and Marsden (1988) review many studies of language, memory, visuospatial function, and conceptual ability–behavioral regulation. They conclude that the validity of two broad diagnostic categories has yet to be proved at a formal neuropsychological level. Similarities between Alzheimer's disease and Huntington's disease, and between Alzheimer's disease and Parkinson's disease, seem so far to be just as frequent as those between Huntington's disease and Parkinson's disease. The authors nevertheless highlight articles that document dissociable psychological deficits between diseases with primarily subcortical versus cortical pathology. Indeed, they suggest, as did Albert, that with proper testing each dementing *disease* could be found to have "its own unique pattern of cognitive impairment."

The picture is complicated further by the results of neurochemical investigations into the dementias. Evidence is mounting that intrinsic neurochemical abnormalities (e.g., dopamine deficiency) may cut across traditional diagnostic categories. Phenotypic maladies (e.g., PD and AD) are being subdivided and reclassified on the basis of further neurochemical research (Bachman and Albert, 1984; Whitehouse et al., 1988; Wolfe et al., 1988; Cummings, 1988a, b; Gotham et al., 1988).

In summary, the multiple-pattern concept of dementia, most emblematically portrayed by the cortical–subcortical dichotomy, remains controversial, and, for many behavioral scientists, unsubstantiated. Difficult problems that have plagued most prior studies, and that continue to do so, include a lack of consensus regarding the definition of dementia (Cummings, 1988a; Mayeux, 1982), a lack of experimental designs using patient groups adequately matched for severity of cognitive impairment, and a paucity of studies using instruments sufficiently sensitive to document dissociable neuropsychological deficits among various causes of the dementia syndrome. In the following review of the early studies of subcortical dementia, we hope to demonstrate that this controversy did not arise anew from theoretical formulations of the 1970s.

HISTORICAL REVIEW

The proclivity to split theoretical or ideological constructs is, of course, as old as theory and ideology. In neurology this tendency is evident in such diverse conditions as systems degeneration (Berenberg et al., 1977), aphasia (Benson, 1979; Mandell et al., 1989), and today in various "cortical" dementia syndromes (Neary et al., 1988). It was also apparent in the mid-nineteenth century, as mere acknowledgment of a dementia syndrome evolved gradually into its systematic description.

For example, in the work of Wilhelm Griesinger (1817–1868), the principal organizer of the German "brain psychiatry" movement, we can recognize early attempts to classify divergent clinical aspects of dementia. Griesinger's emphasis on clinical description greatly influenced Kraepelin and other pillars of late nineteenth century psychiatry (Marx, 1972). Perhaps more importantly, he was among the first to label obsolete Esquirol's belief that "pathological anatomy has done nothing towards establishing the material conditions of insanity" (Griesinger, 1867, p. 431). Like many others to follow, he believed that the most constant brain abnormalities in the insane involved the cortex. He nevertheless noted that "many facts also could speak in favor of an essential participation of the ventricular surfaces; but this point is as yet not so well established" (Griesinger, p. 414).

Griesinger devoted almost 100 pages to "states of mental weakness' in his 1861 edition of *Die Pathologie und Therapie der Psychischen Krankheiten*. For him, these states comprised "two great groups—Chronic Mania and Dementia" (Griesinger, 1867, p. 320). "Dementia" consisted of two divisions: démence agitée and démence apathique. Patients with the former retained superficial but considerable "activity of perception" (the patients "still manifest a certain degree of external vivacity and activity in conversation as well as in conduct"), but also had complete indifference, "absence of all actual desires," a Korsakoff-type amnesia, and thoughts that had "degenerated into a disconnected mass of fleeting images and words" (p. 341). Apathetic dementia, on the other hand, represented "the most extreme degrees of mental decay"—a mode of termination of any form of mental weakness, including "senile dementia." Language was "to a great extent forgotten," conduct was "uniform and always the same"; the patients required feeding and lost themselves every moment in their own room (p. 344).

It is not always clear to the modern reader to which type of mental weakness Griesinger referred in his otherwise careful clinical descriptions. What is clear is that his diagnostic term "dementia" encompasses a variety of diseases recognized today by more specific terms (e.g., general paresis, dementia of the Alzheimer type, and schizophrenia). One can nevertheless distill from these descriptions of "dementia" the germination of a syndrome characterized by indifference, preservation of motor activity (until late stages), marked disturbance of judgment and memory, and lack of a significant mood disorder.

In contrast, "chronic mania" (Verrücktheit; La Folie systématisée) was always a "secondary state of insanity" (p. 324) that developed out of melancholia or mania. Many of the characteristics of Griesinger's chronic mania are in fact very similar to those of his "dementia." These patients, however, retained a "chronic state of modified melancholia or maniacal excitement" for many years, until very late did not exhibit incoherence, and exhibited "a dullness and weakness of all physical reaction." They were "forgetful" of great ideas, while weakness of thought was "sometimes moderate and sometimes increased" (p. 327). Their chronic morbid delusions "falsified" all their thoughts (p. 329). Although he did not provide a coherent distinction akin to the current subcortical–cortical dichotomy, Griesinger nevertheless explicitly recognized broad clinical differences in the expression of dementia among large groups of patients. His descriptions of the intellectual and personality changes of chronic mania foreshadowed by a century the much more exact characterizations of subcortical dementia.

By the turn of the century, sociodemographic factors—including improved general health and hygiene, better medical treatment, and increased longevity—allowed more systematic and prolonged study of behavior in normal and psychiatrically impaired persons. It became increasingly apparent that the elderly were particularly prone to dissolution of mentation characterized by memory loss, language disorder, personality change, and diminished judgment, and these perturbations were in great part related to the cortical brain pathology being described at the same time by Blocq and Marinesco, Alzheimer, Fischer, and others (Stam, 1985). Discussion of dementia syndromes became more common. Schott (1904), for example, noted "a special type of dementia . . . in which there gradually developed a weakness of memory and skill, with loss of initiative and insight and with deterioration in habits"; Tuke (1892): ". . . a state of dullness . . . [that] may take place with a certain mental enfeeblement"; and Maudsley (1895): a moral blunting and "some degree of impairment of intellectual memory" (all cited and/or quoted by Hare, 1981).

Still other contemporary writers recognized clinical and pathologic differences in their demented patients and attempted to systematize their observations into coherent syndromes. "Terminologic confusion" was, however, particularly rife at this time. Kahlbaum, Wernicke, Kraepelin, and Bleuler were among those who either equated or distinguished between diagnoses such as presbyophrenia, senile psychosis, senile dementia, and Alzheimer's disease (Bleuler, 1924, p. 294; Stam, 1985). Their classifications were anything but elucidating. During these years, the mental changes of Huntington's disease were based upon still-uncertain pathology, the dementia of "tetanoid chorea" (Wilson, 1912) went almost unnoticed, the cognitive decline of PSP had received hardly a sentence (Posey, 1904), the existence of a dementia syndrome in Parkinson's disease was already a matter of debate (Ball, 1881; Parant, 1883), and Kraepelin had "split" dementia praecox from manic-depressive insanity (Hare, 1981).

In 1912, S.A.K. Wilson became the first to distinguish clearly, albeit with circumspection, a dementia pattern different from those associated with the common "senility," general paresis, or dementia praecox. Three of his 212 pages summarize the mental symptoms of progressive lenticular degeneration. These were frequent, but "perhaps not an integral part of the clinical picture" (p. 447). Wilson remarked upon the variability in either the presence or the type of mental disturbance in individual cases. He nevertheless emphasized that the "dementia" (quotes by Wilson), when present, never included apraxia or agnosia. Rather, it consisted of a "narrowing of the mental horizon," which Wilson linked to the early stages of Huntington's disease. He also noted that "within the limits of this constricted mental field his powers of perception and recognition are good" (p. 448). Wilson also noted an affective disturbance, partly characterized by pathological laughter. The patients were facile, docile, childish, and seemed "unable to deliberate or pass judgment on what is presented." Wilson in later years interestingly hesitated to attribute the mental changes of some parkinsonians to subcortical pathology. He favored "psychological" explanations, including an "unwillingness to exert" oneself (Rogers, 1986; Rogers et al., 1986).

At the time of Wilson's seminal paper, Eugen Bleuler also described a symptom constellation including slowness of thinking, memory disorder, and behavioral disturbances consequent to demonstrable (or presumed) brain pathology. He referred to this in his 1916 textbook as the "Psycho-organisches Syndrom." In the rather tortured prose of the English translation (Bleuler, 1924), the description of the psycho-organic syndrome is more akin to what modern terminology designates as acute confusional state or delirium. Bleuler apparently modified his formulation in the ensuing years, as, by the posthumous 1949 edition, he had described the psycho-organic syndrome as a dilapidation of intellect and an affective disturbance very similar to that of the syndrome of subcortical dementia. He specifically related the psycho-organic syndrome to the dementia of Huntington's disease (p. 155), and to parkinsonism and bradyphrenia (p. 195; following discussion).

The characteristics of the psycho-organic syndrome that most closely link it to subcortical dementia were perhaps best articulated by Bleuler's son, Manfred, who lamented the use of several equivalent labels while adding yet another: the "chronic amnestic syndrome." He believed that "the amnestic syndrome generally is the expression of a very diffuse brain damage and has not much connexion with any particular localization." However, its neuropsychological characteristics were invariable and independent of the underlying causes, which included senile and arteriosclerotic dementia, alcoholism, the simple form of general paresis, and cerebral tumor (M. Bleuler, 1951). The symptoms and signs were memory and personality impairment, narrowing of ideational margins, impoverished concept formation, perseveration, fatigability, and general loss of interest. Not included in Bleuler's psycho-organic syndrome were signs such as aphasia, apraxia, and agnosia, which are "more of a neurological than a psychological nature."

As a confusing but interesting side issue, Manfred Bleuler vaguely distinguished from the psycho-organic syndrome a "frontal psychosyndrome" (less memory impairment, more personality change), which, despite its name, had for him little anatomic localizing value. He then proceeded to emphasize its similarities with those of a (brain) "stem" psychosyndrome: "both lead to changes of emotions, of mood, of impulses and instinct, and any psychic symptom of the one can also be found in the other." "Cortical" signs were again not mentioned (Bleuler, 1951).

The Bleulers, therefore, described under the rubric *psycho-organic syndrome* a cluster of behavioral signs and symptoms similar to those subsumed under the contemporary label of subcortical dementia. For them, this syndrome was generally caused by diffuse brain malfunction of any etiology, including senile dementia. When caused by a "local" brain lesion, frontal or brain-stem sites seemed more likely. Apraxia, agnosia, and aphasia were not present.

In the midst of the encephalitis pandemic, Naville (1922) described a psychiatric syndrome that "is completely new," and that "does not fit any of the established categories." He did not speculate upon its pathophysiology but noted a "constant relationship between motor and intellectual slowness" (p. 425). It consisted of reduction in voluntary attention, spontaneous interest, initiative, and capacity for work and effort, along with fatigability and a slight, subjective diminution in memory (p. 373). There was also a loss of "psychic tone" and a chronic lethargy that could appear late in the illness "even when not preceded by the classic somnolent lethargy" of the acute stage. An akinetic mute state could be seen in severe cases. Most authors insist, said Naville, that "the intellect is spared despite a deficit in the domain of initiative and a capacity for intellectual work" (p. 375); furthermore, "despite their appearance, these patients never had a true apraxia" (p. 374).

Naville felt that this syndrome of psychomotor retardation had not attracted enough scientific attention, and that, unlike Bleuler, it was "pathognomonic—found in no other organic, psychiatric or functional illness, except perhaps in a few cases of classical Parkinsonism." We emphasize here that Naville proposed little clinico-anatomic correlation; the pathologic substrate of encephalitis lethargica was still to be realized. Rather, he claimed credit for giving this specific cluster of behavioral signs and symptoms coherence (p. 428) but was unsure about what to call it. He did not like *brady-psyche,* because this prejudged the syndrome's etiologic nature. He rejected *chronic lethargy,* as it had already been used to describe other states, and he disapproved of *dysergia* (a term used by Hippocrates), *dysergophrenia,* and *adynamophrenia.* Naville considered these too vague. He finally settled upon *la bradyphrenie,* a purely descriptive term. Rogers (1986) recounts at length the subsequent history and various meta-morphoses of bradyphrenia, emphasizing its relationships to Parkinson's disease; however, further clarification is required at this point.

Like other labels, *bradyphrenia* has suffered from terminological confusion. We demonstrate, as did Rogers (1986), that, 50 years before Albert and McHugh and Folstein rediscovered the syndrome of subcortical dementia, Naville more or less described the same syndrome. He called it *bradyphrenia*. This use of the word is not congruent with its current, more limited, meaning. Scatton et al. (1984) define bradyphrenia as "slowness of thought processes" and relate it to frontal lobe disease and cortical dopaminergic deficiency. *Dementia,* which includes loss of memory, is for them a product of cortical cholinergic deficiency and can be seen in parkinsonians who *also* have significant Alzheimer pathology. Scatton et al. are in effect saying that parkinsonian patients, at least those early in the illness, suffer cognitive abnormalities unlike those associated with Alzheimer's disease, but that such abnormalities do not of themselves constitute a dementia. If indeed the behavioral disturbances of Parkinson's disease and other diseases with primarily subcortical pathology differ only quantitatively from those of Alzheimer's disease, then this terminological inconsistency is of little import. But if, as Albert et al. (1974) and McHugh and Folstein (1975) have asserted, and Brown and Marsden (1988) have concurred, there are differing dementing illnesses with differing neuropsychological patterns, then the term *bradyphrenia* should be employed according to Naville's original description, or "another, more satisfactory label should be agreed upon" (Albert, 1978).

Naville was not, of course, the only worker to study the phenomenon of epidemic encephalitis. Stern described its pathology in 1928, von Economo gave it landmark status in 1929, and several of Naville's contemporaries supported his concept of bradyphrenia (Cloake, 1925; von Stockert, 1932).

In the course of publishing about 150 articles and books on a variety of neurologic and psychological subjects, Franz Günter von Stockert coined the term "Subcorticale Demenz" in 1932. The term appears in the title, but nowhere else in his paper. It referred to a post-encephalitic thought disturbance (Denkstörung) in a patient who had, like some of Naville's patients, none of the motor signs of parkinsonism. Von Stockert depicted a memory disorder, slowness, a personality change, and a disturbance of affect, all of which he related to a severe "impairment of the mental attitude" (Einstellungsstörung). He associated this syndrome with the bradyphrenia of Naville (1922) and attributed it to the recently described pathologic disturbances of the substantia nigra. The cognitive disorder was described as a "total fixation of attention . . . independent of stimuli" (p. 97).

In virtually concurrent publications, Stertz strengthened the emerging concept of subcortical dementia by linking a special dementia syndrome with the incomplete inactivation of an otherwise undisturbed cerebral cortical apparatus. This inactivation produced a "lowering (Senkung) of the general psychic level of energy which acts on all psychic performances"; this in turn yielded a Korsakoff-like amnesia, a "flat euphoria," with apathy and lack of initiative that could "even reach a kind of stupor" (Stertz, 1931, p. 632). Stertz shortly thereafter explicitly related this "psychic transformation" (psychische Veränderung) to subcortical structures. His findings allowed him to "oppose a cortical dementia (Hirnmanteldemenz) from a brain-stem dementia (Hirnstammdemenz)" (Stertz, 1933, p. 441). This subcortical dementia could result from a variety of specific afflictions, including tumors, hydrocephalus, abscess, syphilis, trauma, encephalitis, and multiple sclerosis. These associations have been highlighted by many recent studies (Cummings and Benson, 1983; Graff-Radford et al., 1985; Rao, 1986; Navia et al., 1986; Katz et al., 1987), which are summarized elsewhere in this volume.

The decades from the early 1930s to the mid-1970s provide a deep reservoir of articles that relate dementia to subcortical pathology, and these have been reviewed elsewhere (Albert et al., 1974; Cummings, 1986; Freedman and Albert, 1985). There is relatively little published material in these years that distills consistent patterns of cognitive loss into coherent syndromes. There were, nevertheless, important contributions. Hassler coined the term *psychic akinesia* in 1953 to describe parkinsonian psychological deficits; these were similar to those of Naville's bradyphrenia, and were related to cell loss in the substantia innominata (Rogers, 1986). Faust (1960) described a subcortical dementialike syndrome as a frequent outcome of head trauma, and he specifically cited Stertz in distinguishing *Rindendemenz* (cortical dementia) from *Stammhirndemenz* (brain-stem dementia). Contantinidis et al. (1970) analyzed the "pseudodementia" of PSP and noted reduced interest and speech, slowness, marked perturbation of "practical efficiency," and increase in response latencies. There was no aphasia or apraxia. In concluding that their patient was "certainly not demented," they linked his neuropsychological abnormalities to "motor impairment and difficulties with visuo-perceptual activity which . . . slow and fragment the process of thought." More recently, a similar dichotomous concept, "dementia of the frontal type" (distinct from "posterior cortical dementia") has also been proposed (Neary et al., 1988).

COMMENT

We have attempted to develop two major threads in this chapter. The first concerns the contemporary problem of subcortical dementia. Especially since the mid-1970s there has been increasing clinical awareness that diverse brain disorders may be associated with a cluster of behavioral–cognitive changes that differs from that of Alzheimer's disease. Historical analysis shows that this specific behavioral–cognitive syndrome was well defined as early as 1922 and has been recognized repeatedly in the succeeding half-century. Various labels have been attached to this syndrome and its variants: dysergia, bradyphrenia (Naville, 1922), psycho-organic syndrome, chronic amnestic syndrome (E. Bleuler, 1924, 1949; M. Bleuler, 1951), psychic akinesia (Hassler, 1953, as cited by Rogers, 1986), subcortical dementia (von Stockert, 1932; Albert et al., 1974; McHugh and Folstein, 1975), brain-stem dementia (Stertz, 1931, 1933; M. Bleuler, 1951), fronto-subcortical dementia (Freedman and Albert, 1985).

Considerable time, effort, and printer's ink have been expended on the question: Does the syndrome exist? That question has yet to be conclusively answered, for reasons previously summarized. Nevertheless, recently developed online neuropsychological techniques are indeed beginning to document reproducible differential deficits among patients suffering from different dementing illnesses (Brandt et al., 1988; Brown and Marsden, 1988; Dubois et al., 1988; Milberg and Albert, 1989), while systematic neuropathologic studies are uncovering the anatomic bases of individual aspects of the dementia syndrome (Zubenko and Moossy, 1988).

The second thread concerns the relationship between the subcortical dementia controversy and our understanding of dementia in general. The essence of dementia has yet to be defined. There is no consensus regarding which behavioral or cognitive parameters, if any, are necessarily abnormal in each and every "demented" person. A historical review of the subcortical dementia concept demonstrates that, for well over a century, there has been at least an implicit wisdom that dissolution of mentation is not phenomenologically identical in all individuals. The dichotomy exemplified by the "subcortical–cortical" distinction serves as an initial step—a coarse triage—in elucidating mechanisms underlying the (likely) distinctive neurochemical–neuropsychological profiles of each dementing illness.

To paraphrase James Parkinson, experimentation into the dementias is replacing conjecture. The past and present originators of the subcortical dementia concept would, we believe, have repined "at no censure which the precipitate publication of mere conjectural suggestions may occur; but shall think (themselves) fully rewarded by having excited the attention of those, who may point out the most appropriate means of relieving a tedious and most distressing malady" (Parkinson, 1817).

ACKNOWLEDGMENTS

Preparation of this paper was supported by the NIH Center Grant #NS06209, the Medical Research Service of the Veterans Administration, and the Seidel Fund for Research in Dementia. We are indebted to Dr. Theodor Landis, who graciously sought out and translated several key German articles on subcortical dementia. We also thank Professor Arthur Benton, who provided many useful suggestions.

REFERENCES

Albert, M.L. Subcortical dementia. In *Alzheimer's Disease: Senile Dementia and Related Disorders.* Katzman, R., Terry, R.D., and Bick, K.L., (eds.). Raven Press, New York, 1978.

Albert, M.L. *The controversy of subcortical dementia. Neurology and Neurosurgery Update Series, Vol. 5.* Continuing Professional Education Center, Inc., Princeton, 1984.

Albert, M.L., Feldman, R.G., and Willis, A.L. The "subcortical dementia" of progressive supranuclear palsy. *J Neurol Neurosurg Psychiatry* 1974; 37:121–30.

Bachman, D.L., and Albert, M.L. The dopaminergic syndromes of dementia. In *Brain Pathology, Vol. 1.* Pilleri, G., and Tagliavini, F., (eds.). Brain Anatomy Institute, Bern, Switzerland, 1984, pp. 91–119.

Ball, B. De l'insanité dans la paralysie agitante. *L'Encéphale* 1882; 2:22–32.

Benson, D.F. *Aphasia Alexia and Agraphia.* Churchill Livingstone, Inc., New York, 1979.

Berenberg, R.A., Pellock, J.M., Dimauro, S., et al. Lumping or splitting? "Ophthalmoplegia-plus" or Kearns-Sayre syndrome? *Ann Neurol* 1977; 1:37–54.

Bleuler, E. *Textbook of Psychiatry,* Brill, A.A. (trans.). MacMillan Co., New York, 1924.

Bleuler, E. *Lehrbuch der Psychiatrie, Eighth Edition.* Springer, Berlin, 1949.

Bleuler, M. Psychiatry of cerebral diseases. *Br Med J* 1951; 2:1233–8.

Boller, F., Tomohiko, M., Rocssmann, U., and Gambetti, P. Parkinson disease, dementia, and Alzheimer disease: Clinicopathological correlations. *Ann Neurol* 1980; 329–35.

Brandt, J., Folstein, S.E., and Folstein, M.F. Differential cognitive impairment in Alzheimer's disease and Huntington's disease. *Ann Neurol* 1988; 23:555–61.

Brown, R.E., and Marsden, C.D. "Subcortical dementia": The neuropsychological evidence. *Neuroscience* 1988; 25:363–87.

Bruyn, G.W. Huntington's chorea: A historical, clinical and laboratory synopsis. In *Handbook of Clinical Neurology, Vol. 6*. Vinken, P.J., and Bruyn, G.W. (eds.). North Holland Publishing Co., Amsterdam, 1968, pp. 298–378.

Clarke, J.M. On Huntington's Chorea. *Brain* 1897; 20:22–34.

Cloake, P.C. Discussion on the mental sequelae of encephalitis lethargica. *Proc R Soc Med* 1925; 18:26–31, 37–8.

Constantinidis, J., Tissot, R., and de Ajuriaguerra, J. Dystonie oculo-facio-cervicale ou paralysie progressive supranucléaire de Steele-Richardson-Olszewski. *Rev Neurol (Paris)* 1970; 122:249–62.

Critchley, M. God and the brain: Medicine's debt to phrenology. In *The Divine Banquet of the Brain*. Raven Press, New York, 1979.

Cummings, J.L. Subcortical dementia. Neuropsychology, neuropsychiatry, and pathophysiology. *Br J Psychiatry* 1986; 149:682–97.

Cummings, J.L. Intellectual impairment in Parkinson's disease: clinical, pathologic and biochemical correlates. *J Geriatr Psychiatry* 1988a; 1:24–36.

Cummings, J.L. The dementias of Parkinson's disease: Prevalence, characteristics, neurobiology, and comparison with dementia of the Alzheimer type. *Eur Neurol* 1988b; 28(suppl. 1):15–23.

Cummings, J.L., and Benson, D.F. *Dementia. A Clinical Approach*. Butterworths, Boston, 1983.

Cummings, J.L., and Benson, D.F. Subcortical dementia. Review of an emerging concept. *Arch Neurol* 1984; 41:874–9.

Dubois, B., Pillon, B., Legault, F., Agid, Y., and Lhermitte, F. Slowing of cognitive processing in progressive supranuclear palsy. *Arch Neurol* 1988; 45:1194–9.

Faust, C. Die psychischen Störungen nach Hirntraumen. In *Psychiatrie der Gegenwart. Forschung und Praxis. Band 2: Klinische Psychiatrie*. Gruhle, H.W., Jung, R., and Mayer-Gross, W. (eds.). Springer, Berlin, 1960.

Freedman, M., and Albert, M.L. Subcortical dementia. In *Handbook of Clinical Neurology, Vol. 46: Neurobehavioral Disorders*. Viken, P.J., Bruyn, G.W., Klawans, H., and Fredericks, J.A.M., (eds.). Elsevier Science Publishers, Amsterdam, 1985:311–6.

Gotham, A.M., Brown, R.G., and Marsden, C.D. "Frontal" cognitive function in patients with Parkinson's disease "on" and "off" levodopa. *Brain* 1988; 111:299–321.

Graff-Radford, N.R., Damasio, H., Yamada, T., Eslinger, P.J., and Damasio, A.R. Nonhaemorrhagic thalamic infarction. *Brain* 1985; 108:485–516.

Griesinger, W. *Mental Pathology and Therapeutics* (1867). Robertson, C.L. and Rutherford, J. (trans.). Hafner Publishing Co., New York, 1965.

Hare, E. The two manias: A study of the evolution of the modern concept of mania. *Br J Psychiatry* 1981; 138:89–99.

Joynt, R.J., and Shoulson, I. Dementia. In *Clinical Neuropsychology, Second edition*. Heilman, K.M., and Valenstein, E. (eds.). Oxford University Press, New York, 1985, pp. 453–80.

Katz, D.I., Alexander, M.P., and Mandell, A.M. Dementia following strokes in the mesencephalon and diencephalon. *Arch Neurol* 1987; 44:1127–33.

Leenders, K.L., Frackowiak, R.S.J., and Lees, A.J. Steele-Richardson-Olszewski syndrome. Brain energy metabolism, blood flow and fluorodopa uptake measured by positron emission tomography. *Brain* 1988; 111:615–30.

Lipowski, Z.J. Organic mental disorders: Their history and classification with special reference to DSM-III. In *Senile Dementia* Miller, N.E., Cohen, E.D. (eds.). *Aging, Vol. 15.* Raven Press, New York, 1981, pp. 37–45.

Mandell, A.M., Alexander, M.P., and Carpenter, S. Creutzfeldt-Jakob disease presenting as isolated aphasia. *Neurology* 1989; 39:55–8.

Marx, O.M. Wilhelm Griesinger and the history of psychiatry: A reassessment. *Bull Hist Med* 1972; 46:519–44.

Mayeux, R. Depression and dementia in Parkinson's disease. In *Movement Disorders.* Marsden, C.D., and Fahn, S. (eds.). Butterworth, London, 1982.

McHugh, P.R., and Folstein, M.F. Psychiatric syndromes of Huntington's chorea: A clinical and pharmacologic study. In *Psychiatric Aspects of Neurologic Disease,* Chapter 13. Benson, D.F., and Blumer, D. (eds.). Grune & Stratton, New York, 1975.

Milberg, W.P., and Albert, M.S. Cognitive differences between patients with PSP and Alzheimer's disease. *J Clin Exp Neuropsychol* 1989; in press.

Navia, B.A., Jordan, B.D., and Price, R.W. The AIDS dementia complex: I. Clinical features. *Ann Neurol* 1986; 19:517–24.

Naville, F. Etudes sur les complications et les séquelles mentales de l'encéphalite épidémique. La bradyphrénie. *L'Encéphale* 1922; 17:369–75, 423–36.

Neary, D., Snowden, J.S., Northern, B., and Goulding, P. Dementia of the frontal type. *J Neurol Neurosurg Psychiatry* 1988; 51:353–61.

Parant. La paralysie agitante. Examinée comme cause de folie. *Ann Med Psychol (Paris)* 1883; 10:45–62.

Parkinson, J. An essay on the shaking palsy (1817). *Medical Classics* 1938; 2:964–97.

Posey, W.C. Paralysis of the upward movements of the eyes. *Ann Ophthamol* 1904; 13:523–9.

Rao, S.M. Neuropsychology of multiple sclerosis: A critical review. *J Clin Exp Neuropsychol* 1986; 8:503–42.

Reisberg, B. The clinical syndrome. In *The Martin Steinberg Memorial Symposium on Alzheimer's Disease and Related Disorders,* The Hebrew Home for the Aged, Riverdale, New York, 1983, pp. 7–17.

Rogers, D. Bradyphrenia in parkinsonism: A historical review. *Psychol Med* 1986; 16:257–65.

Rogers, D., Lees, A.J., Trimble, M., and Stern, G.M. Concept of bradyphrenia: A neuropsychiatric approach. In *Advances in Neurology, Vol. 45.* Yahr, M.D., and Bergmann, K.J. (eds.). Raven Press, New York, 1986, pp. 447–50.

Scatton, B., Javoy-Agid, F., and Agid, Y. Reply from the authors. *Neurology* 1984; 34:265–6.

Stam, F.C. Senile dementia and senile involution of the brain. In *Handbook of Clinical Neurology, Vol. 46.* Vinken, P.J., Bruyn, G.W., Klawans, H., Frederiks, J.A.M. (eds.). Elsevier Science Publishers, Amsterdam, 1985, pp. 283–8.

Steele, J.C., Richardson, J.C., and Olszewski, J. Progressive supranuclear palsy. *Arch Neurol* 1964; 10:333–59.

Stertz, G. Über den Anteil des Zwischenhirns an der Symptomgestaltung organischer Erkrankungen des Zentralnervensystems: ein diagnostisch brauchbares Zwischenhirnsyndrom. *Dtsch Z Nervenheilk* 1931; 117:630–65.

Stertz, G. Probleme des Zwischenhirns. *Arch für Psychiat* 1933; 98:441–4.

Terry, R.D., Victor, M., et al. Discussion of subcortical dementia. In *Alzheimer's Disease: Senile Dementia and Related Disorders* Katzman, R., Terry, R.D., and Bick, K.L. (eds.). *Aging, Vol. 7.* Raven Press, New York, 1978:194–7.

Torack, R.M. The early history of senile dementia. In *Alzheimer's Disease. The Standard Reference.* Reisberg, B. (ed.). The Free Press, New York, 1983.

von Stockert, F.G. Subcorticale Demenz. *Arch Psychiatry* 1932; 97:77–100.

Whitehouse, P.J. Theodor Meynert: Foreshadowing modern concepts of neuropsychiatric pathophysiology. *Neurology* 1985; 35:389–91.
Whitehouse, P.J. The concept of subcortical and cortical dementia: Another look. *Ann Neurol*
1986; 19:1–6.
Whitehouse, P.J., Martino, A.M., Marcus, K.A., et al. Reductions in acetylcholine and nicotine
binding in several degenerative diseases. *Arch Neurol* 1988; 45:722–4.
Wilson, S.A.K. Progressive lenticular degeneration: A familial nervous disease associated with
cirrhosis of the liver. *Brain* 1912; 34:296–508.
Winkelman, N.W. Progressive pallidal degeneration. *Arch Neurol Psychiatry* 1932; 27:1–21.
Wolfe, N., Katz, D.I., Albert, M.L. et al. Neuropyschological profile linked to low dopamine
in Alzheimer's disease, major depression, and Parkinson's disease. Presented at the Annual Meeting of the Society for Neurosciences, 1988.
Zubenko, G.S., and Moossy, J. Major depression in primary dementia. Clinical and neuropathologic correlates. *Arch Neurol* 1988; 45:1182–6.

3

Subcortical Anatomy: The Circuitry of the Striatum

VALERIE B. DOMESICK

The striatum, globus pallidus, and substantia nigra undergo degeneration in subcortical dementia (Cummings and Benson, 1983). Since these structures and their connections may comprise the underlying neural substrate of subcortically mediated intellectual functions, our work on the afferent and efferent connections of these structures is relevant to understanding the pathophysiology of subcortical dementia. In this chapter we will examine the circuitry of the striatum and related anatomical structures.

The striatum is large, receiving a wide variety of afferents, including input from most areas of cortex. Until recently, the striatum was conceptualized as the wide mouth of a funnel where a large number of inputs, by means of convergence, were channeled to the globus pallidus, which served to provide output pathways from the striatum. During the past few years the results of several studies have suggested that cortical impulses from different cortical areas do not converge in the striatum but are inter-digitated to follow separate parallel circuits through the striatum and globus pallidum to the thalamus and back to the cortex. Moreover, there is an analogous parallel circuit through the ventromedial striatum and nucleus accumbens that projects to the ventral pallidum, and by way of the mediodorsal nucleus of the thalamus to the frontal cortex (Alexander et al., 1986). Until these pathways were described, the thalamic circuits of the striatum were thought to subserve primarily motor functions. Identification of these parallel circuits uniting frontal cortex and striatum with thalamus provides a basis for hypothesizing the mediation of cognitive functions by these structures. Goldman-Rakic (1987) has emphasized that it may be more helpful to understand the functions of a given area of cortex in terms of its distributed cortical networks rather than as a specialized area at the end of a chain of hierarchical connections. The frontal-striatal circuit through the medial dorsal nucleus is of major interest in understanding demen-tias, since the frontal cortex has a well-documented role in cognition and higher mental function.

In the following sections the intrinsic organization of the striatum, the portion of the striatum with predominant limbic system connections, the afferent and efferent connections of the striatum, and the projection systems through the globus pallidus and substantia nigra are described. The concept of discrete parallel circuits mediating cognitive, limbic-emotional, and motor functions will be emphasized throughout.

THE STRIATUM

The term *striatum* refers to the caudate nucleus and putamen, which in all primate and many nonprimate mammals, are separated by the plate-like internal capsule. Bands or bridges of gray matter perforating the capsule create the appearance of striations. The caudate nucleus and ventromedial putamen are continuous with each other around the ventromedial margin of the internal capsule. Anteriorly, this ventral region is contiguous with the nucleus accumbens, which is directly continuous ventrally with the small-celled core of the olfactory tubercle by way of cell bridges perforating the interposed fiber layer of olfactory radiations situated above the olfactory tubercle (Heimer, 1978; Nauta and Haymaker, 1969; Newman and Winans, 1980). The putamen has the same cytological features as the caudate nucleus but is physically continuous with the globus pallidus. The lens-shaped structure formed by the putamen and the globus pallidus is referred to as the lentiform nucleus. Together, the striatum (caudate and putamen) and globus pallidus comprise the corpus striatum. All of our studies involve rats where the striatum is not subdivided by the internal capsule into a caudate and putamen, but appears as a continuous sheet referred to as the caudatoputamen. The caudatoputamen and the nucleus accumbens are continuous and exhibit the same basic cytoarchitecture in various preparations by stains for fibers, Nissl, or acetylcholinesterase (Heimer, 1978). At present there are no structural or connectional criteria that delimit the various subdivisions of the striatum from each other. The similar connections and pattern of neurogenesis shared by the nucleus accumbens and caudatoputamen support the notion that all three regions are subdivisions of a single striatal complex (Swanson and Cowan, 1975).

LIMBIC STRIATUM

One can subdivide the striatal complex into two parts determined by their afferent connections: (1) a *dorsolateral sector,* receiving its major cortical input from the motor cortex, and (2) a *ventromedial sector* delineated by the projections from a variety of limbic structures in the forebrain, including the hippocampal formation (Kelley and Domesick, 1982), the basolateral nucleus of the amygdala (Kelley et al., 1982), the cingulate cortex (Domesick, 1969; Beckstead, 1979), the prefrontal cortex (Leonard, 1969), and the midbrain, particularly the ventral tegmental area and dorsal raphe (Beckstead et al., 1979). The ventromedial sector is also characterized by higher somatostatin levels (Beal et al., 1983) and is labeled by LAMP (an antibody for limbic-associated membrane protein developed from hippocampal membrane protein) (Leavitt, 1984). Thus, the striatum has prominent limbic system connections that indicate a role in the processing of emotionally-relevant information.

   The limbic striatum corresponds to the ventral striatum and nucleus accumbens. The term *ventral striatum* is used here to refer to the entire ventral territory of the striatum exclusive of the nucleus accumbens and olfactory tubercle; it includes the ventrolateral and ventromedial caudatoputamen. In a recent study, outlines of the striatum from serial coronal sections through its anteroposterior extent were used to reconstruct the three regions of the striatum—the dorsolateral, ventromedial, and nucleus accumbens—and showed that the limbic striatum comprises about 33 percent of the striatum (Domesick, 1988).

AFFERENT CONNECTIONS OF THE STRIATUM

The striatum receives afferents from diverse areas of the telencephalon, diencephalon, and mesencephalon. Most telencephalic afferents to the nucleus accumbens originate from the hippocampus and amygdala, structures within the circuitry of the limbic system. Virtually all sensory, motor, limbic, and associational areas of neocortex (Webster, 1961; Carmen et al., 1963), as well as several subcortical limbic structures, project upon the caudate and putamen (Domesick, 1988). The convergence of projections from association and limbic cortex as well as from primary motor and sensory areas suggest a crucial role for the striatum in the integration of many types of information. In addition to descending telencephalic projections, the striatum receives ascending fibers from the substantia nigra and raphe nuclei.

Telencephalic Afferents

Neocortex

All regions of the cerebral cortex project to the caudatoputamen in a topographically organized pattern that largely preserves the topology of the cortical mantle. Yeterain and Van Hoesen (1978) suggested that cortical areas that enjoy reciprocal cortical connections exhibit converging projections in the striatum. By means of doubling techniques—injecting two labeled markers (tritiated amino acids and horseradish peroxidase {HRP}) in a single hemisphere—in the monkey, it has been shown that projections terminating in the same general location interdigitate rather than overlap or converge (Selemon and Goldman-Rakic, 1985). Distinct zones of the caudate nucleus receive projections from the dorsolateral prefrontal, orbital prefrontal, and cingulate cortex (Alexander et al., 1986). The putamen receives projections from the motor cortex (Kunzle, 1975). Afferents from the limbic regions of the cortex are also prominent in the striatum: for example, a dorsomedial region of the caudatoputamen receives a projection from the medial prefrontal and cingulate cortex (Domesick, 1969; Beckstead, 1979).

Amygdala

In an attempt to outline the borders of the nucleus accumbens in terms of its afferent input, autoradiographic and HRP studies of the amygdala were initiated (Kelley et al., 1982). The projections from the amygdala, however, were shown to spread far beyond the accumbens region and involve most areas of the striatum with a predominance of projections to the ventral striatal areas. A similar range of amygdala projections to the ventromedial caudate and putamen has also been demonstrated in the primate and cat. This wide distribution extends beyond the traditional borders of the nucleus accumbens into caudatoputamen indicating that the concept of the limbic striatum must be expanded to include ventral territories of the caudatoputamen, a well as the nucleus accumbens.

Fornix

The nucleus accumbens receives afferents from the hippocampal formation by way of the precommissural fornix (Nauta, 1956; Swanson and Cowan, 1977). The fornix projection is confined to the most medial part of the nucleus accumbens, abutting against the septum, with limited distribution to more lateral and dorsal areas (Kelley and Domesick, 1982).

Diencephalic Afferents to the Striatum

The nucleus accumbens, caudatoputamen, and olfactory tubercle receive thalamic projections (Groenwegen et al., 1980; Hemphill et al., 1981). The caudatoputamen is projected upon by intralaminar nuclei: the parafascicular nucleus, nucleus centralis lateralis, and nucleus paracentralis. The nucleus accumbens, by contrast, is projected upon by more medially situated nonspecific thalamic cell groups, including the nuclei parataenialis, paraventricularis, and reniens, as well as the most medial part of the parafascicular nucleus that lies medial to fasciculus retroflexus. Both the septum and the amygdala project to the parataenial nucleus, which thus provides a second, indirect route for hippocampal, septal, and amygdala inputs to the nucleus accumbens (Kelley and Domesick, 1982).

Substantia nigra

It is now well established that the cells of the pars compacta of the substantia nigra and ventral tegmental area of Tsai (1925) are dopaminergic neurons. They have been categorized by Dahlstrom and Fuxe (1964) into dopamine cell groups A8, A9, and A10 and have been shown to project to the striatum (Anden et al., 1966). The continuity of these midbrain cell groups is easily demonstrated by placing small HRP injections in various parts of the striatum. A cell group overlying the medial lemniscus corresponds to the cell group labeled retrorubral nucleus and serves as a "bridge" between cell groups A8, A9, and A10. It is continuous with A9 laterally around the lateral margin of the lemniscus, and with A10 medially; it continues caudally over a short distance so as to appear as an independent nucleus in the ventrolateral tegmentum at a level behind the caudal pole of the substantia nigra proper. The mesencephalic cell groups containing dopamine-synthesizing cells are included in the term *nigral complex*.

Tracing studies have shown a consistent medial-to-lateral topography of the projection from the pars compacta of the substantia nigra to the caudatoputamen (Fallon and Moore, 1978; Beckstead et al., 1979). Beckstead et al. (1979) demonstrated the near absence of an anteroposterior topography in the nigro-striatal connection; each locus of the nigral dopamine complex projects to tissue extending through the anteroposterior length of the striatum. Each of the variously placed tracer injections of the ventral tegmental area was found to label fibers distributed not only to the nucleus accumbens and olfactory tubercle but to the entire length of the ventral striatal region. Moreover, the A10 projection, in gradually diminishing volume, extends dorsally from the ventral region to involve the ventromedial and ventrolateral sectors of the caudatoputamen. It overlays the nigrostriatal projection from the medial half of the pars compacta. The extent of overlap or interdigitation of these has not been determined. Thus, the nigrostriatal projection from nuclear groups A8 and A10, although distributed in greatest volume to the ventral striatum, overlaps the nigrostriatal projection from the pars compacta throughout most of the larger part of the striatum. These findings are largely in agreement with the schema first suggested by Anden et al. (1966) and Ungerstedt (1971) that the mesencephalic dopamine system consists of two parts: (1) a nigrostriatal system from the pars compacta to the caudatoputamen, and (2) a mesolimbic system consisting of the projection from A10 to the nucleus accumbens, olfactory tubercle, central amygdaloid nucleus, and septum. Although A9 appears to project only to the caudatoputamen, call group A10 apparently projects not only to structures implicated in the circuitry of the limbic system (including the nucleus accumbens) but also to a large area of the caudatoputamen included in limbic striatum.

Raphe nuclei

Both the nucleus accumbens and the caudatoputamen are projected upon by the dorsal raphe nucleus (Miller et al., 1975). The extent to which this projection is serotonergic has not been fully documented, but it appears to account for the serotonin found in all parts of the striatum.

EFFERENT CONNECTIONS OF THE STRIATUM

The projections from the striatum are basically to two major targets, the pallidum and the nigral complex. The limbic-versus-nonlimbic dichotomy in the innervation of the striatum is reflected in their projection to the pallidum (Domesick et al., 1986). The striatopallidal projection from the "nonlimbic" sector projects to the dorsal pallidum and entopeduncular nucleus; the limbic, ventromedial striatal region projects to the entire ventral pallidum. The nucleus accumbens has additional projections to a variety of subcortical structures associated with the limbic system, including the ventral tegmental area. Throughout the efferent projection systems striatal output is arranged in parallel circuits constructed of discrete systems capable of mediating differential functions (Alexander et al., 1986).

Globus Pallidus

The caudatoputamen projects massively to the main (supracommissural) part of the external segment of the globus pallidus and the internal segment (entopeduncular nucleus of nonprimates) of the globus pallidus. Like the spokes of a wheel, the projections originate from the dorsal-to-ventral caudatoputamen and maintain their dorsal-to-ventral arrangement as they converge onto the globus pallidus in a radial fashion.

Ventral Pallidum

Originally viewed as a component of the preoptic region or substantia innominata, its pallidal nature was not recognized until reports indicated that the ventral pallidum receives a dense striatofugal projection from the nucleus accumbens, the ventral stiatum, and the subthalamic nucleus (Heimer and Wilson, 1975). The ventral pallidum, like the overlying dorsal pallidum, has a high iron content (Hill and Switzer, 1984) and strong enkephalin-like and glutamic-acid-decarboxylase-like immunoreactivity (Switzer et al., 1982; Haber and Elde, 1981; Haber and Nauta, 1983). The ventral pallidum can be distinguished from the dorsal pallidum by its dense substance P-positive fiber plexus (Switzer et al., 1982; Haber and Elde, 1981; Haber and Nauta, 1983), and its efferent projections (Haber et al., 1985).

Striatofugal fibers pass caudomedially through the external segment of the globus pallidus in an orderly radial pattern. The nucleus accumbens, as the most anteroventral striatal region, projects only to the ventral pallidum. The latter appears grossly to be a component of the substantia innominata but was identified on cytological grounds as part of the external pallidum (Heimer and Wilson, 1975). The ventral pallidum lies below the anterior commissure, bounded by the bed nucleus of the stria terminalis medially and by a small subcommissural pocket of the striatum laterally. Fibers from the caudatoputamen continue through the internal capsule to the entopeduncular nucleus. In contrast, the fibers from the nucleus accumbens take a course through the medial forebrain bundle that largely bypasses the entopeduncular nucleus.

Substantia Nigra

The topography of the striatonigral projection is remarkable in that fibers preserve their dorsal-to-ventral order in the globus pallidus and invert the dorsoventral coordinate of the striatum in the substantia nigra (Nauta and Domesick, 1979). The pars compacta lies as a dorsal cap over the larger ventral nigral component, the pars reticulata. From observations based on small isotope injections throughout the striatum, we concluded that the most dorsal striatal regions project to the most ventral zones of the pars reticulata, whereas middle-depth strata project to middle zones of the pars reticulata, and the most ventral zone of the striatum including the nucleus accumbens project to the most dorsal zone of the pars reticulata and to the dorsally adjacent pars compacta.

If nigral cells were completely governed by feedback from the striatum, it would be necessary for all points in the striatum receiving a nigral projection to reciprocate with a return "feedback" loop. The topography of the striatonigral projection and the arrangement of dopaminergic and nondopaminergic cells in the substantia nigra suggest, however, that the striatal connections are not limited to feedback systems. The majority of the dopaminergic cells lie in the dorsal nigra (pars compacta) (Phillipson, 1979; Palkovits and Jacobowitz, 1974), creating a dorsal-to-ventral gradient of the density of dopamine cells. The topography of the connections suggest that "open" or "nonloop" connections exist in which nigrostriatal contacts have no reciprocating striatonigral feedback or in which striatonigral projections lack corresponding nigrostriatal input. Two other types of connection that do not participate in the nigro-striato-nigral return loop exist in this system. First, the extensive projection to the caudatoputamen from cell groups A8 and A10 is not reciprocated by the caudatoputamen. These neurons are, instead, influenced by the nucleus accumbens, as well as by limbic afferents from the septo-preoptico-hypothalamic continuum (Swanson, 1976). Second, the nucleus accumbens projects most massively to the pars compacta of the substantia nigra from which it receives only a very sparse return projection. Since the nucleus accumbens receives its telencephalic afferents for the most part from the hippocampus and amygdala, this "open loop" may be another avenue by which the limbic system affects the nigrostriatal system. Nondopaminergic cells in the pars reticulata affected by the striatonigral fibers might include interneurons contacting dopaminergic neurons of the pars compacta, and hence intercalated in a nigro-striatal-nigral feedback loop. It must be emphasized, however, that this suggested indirect mode of closure of the loop at the nigral level is almost certain to be paralleled by direct closure: light microscopic observations persuasively indicate the existence of striatonigral fibers terminating directly on pars compacta dendrites protruding into the pars reticulata. Thus, open loop, direct closed loop, and indirect closed loop circuitry unite the nigra and the striatum.

Limbic System

Whereas the topography of the striatopallidal and striatonigral projection expresses the continuity of the dorsal with the ventral striatum, including the nucleus accumbens, long descending fibers from the nucleus accumbens and adjoining parts of the ventral striatum can be distinguished from the overlying striatum. They follow the trajectory of the medial forebrain bundle, which is the main route of descent for fibers from the septum, preoptic area, substantia innominata, and hypothalamus (Nauta et al., 1978; Conrad and Pfaff, 1976a,b; Swanson and Cowan, 1979; Nauta and Domesick, 1982). The descending accumbens efferents pass through and appear to partially terminate in the preoptic area, the hypothalamus, and the thalamus. At the level of the substantia nigra, most of the remaining fibers are distributed to cell groups A8 and A10 as well as to pars compacta and the most dorsal strata of the pars reticulata of the substantia nigra; longer fibers extend beyond the limits of the nigral complex to the mesencephalic tegmentum, central gray substance, and medial raphe nuclei (Steinbusch, 1981). Cell groups A8 and A10 lie directly in the path of the descending fibers from both the nucleus accumbens and the hypothalamus; the striatofugal fibers arising in the more dorsally located caudatoputamen do not directly involve either cell groups A8 or A10 or any nonnigral part of the mesencephalon.

PROJECTIONS THROUGH THE PALLIDUM

The dualism of the nonlimbic and limbic and sectors of the striatum reflects itself in the existence of two partly segregated striatofugal conduction lines projecting through the globus pallidus and ventral pallidum, respectively. The parallel organization of cortico-striatal circuits remains evident as the efferents through the pallidum and substantia nigra to serially arranged telencephalic and diencephalic structures are delineated.

Subthalamic Nucleus

The dorsolateral sector of the anterior striatum, receiving only sparse afferents of limbic origin and heavily innervated by the sensorimotor cortex, projects to an anterodorsolateral region of the main, supra-, and retrocommissural mass of the globus pallidus; this pallidal region (dorsal pallidum) in turn gives rise to a projection that forms part of the classical pallidofugal pathway descending to the subthalamic nucleus and substantia nigra. By contrast, the heavily limbic-innervated anteroventromedial striatal region projects largely to the infracommissural, ventral pallidum, from which efferents pass to the subthalamic nucleus.

Thalamus and Cortex

There is a remarkable parallel between the "limbic" and "nonlimbic" trans-striatal conduction lines through the thalamus and back to the cortex. The familiar "extrapyramidal motor circuit," motor cortex–striatum–pallidum–thalamic VA-VL complex–premotor cortex–motor cortex appears to have limbic counterparts in the sequences: limbic system–striatum–ventral pallidum–amygdala, and: limbic system–striatum–ventral pallidum–thalamic mediodorsal nucleus–frontal and anterior limbic cortex. It is considered likely on the basis of long-known anatomical connections that the function of the striatum expresses itself in part through a major circuit affecting the mechanisms of the motor cortex. More recent anatomical data make it appear no less likely that the striatum through an analogous, though less massive circuit, can affect the mechanisms of the prefrontal cortex, and thus, a class of functions more likely to be cognitive than skeletomuscular. Alexander et al. (1986) indicate that projections from the dorsolateral prefrontal, orbital prefrontal, frontal eye fields, supplementary motor, and anterior cingulate cortex terminate in topographically segregated areas within the caudate and putamen, and this segregation is maintained in the conduction lines through the pallidal-thalamo-cortical loop, creating parallel circuits mediating cognitive, motor, eye movement, and emotional functions.

Limbic System

Projections through the ventral pallidum involve not only the subthalamic nucleus and thalamus but also various limbic system associated structures including the amygdala, medial frontal and cingulate cortex, lateral habenular nucleus, mediodorsal thalamic nucleus, hypothalamus, ventral tegmental area, and caudal and dorsal regions of the midbrain tegmentum. These are the structures receiving direct projections from the nucleus accumbens. Thus, projections from the nucleus accumbens and the ventral pallidum join limbic as well as extrapyramidal circuits.

PROJECTIONS THROUGH THE SUBSTANTIA NIGRA

Much more certain is the anatomical basis of feed-forward systems in the striatonigral projection, since the striatum projects massively to the ventral nigra (pars reticulata) where it very likely contacts the prevalent nondopaminergic cell type that projects in turn to the thalamus, superior colliculus, or brainstem reticular formation. In addition to the feedback lines from the nigra to the striatum, striatal feed-forward projections reach the ventromedial nucleus of the thalamus, the deeper layers of the superior colliculus, and the pedunculopontine nucleus of the midbrain reticular formation via the nigral pars reticulata. There is conclusive electron microscopic evidence that striatonigral fibers contact pars reticulata neurons projecting to either the thalamus or superior colliculus (Somogyi et al., 1981). The projection of the ventromedial nucleus to a large expanse of the outer layer of the neocortex (layer one) suggests that the striato-nigral feed-forward mechanism may also exert an important influence on cortical function.

Less unequivocal is the evidence that a similar striatal feed-forward involves the nigra's pars compacta. Beckstead et al. (1979) have suggested the existence of pars compacta projections to the midbrain, specifically to the parabrachial nuclei, the central gray substance, and the dorsal raphe nucleus. Whether these compacta projections are dopaminergic in nature requires further study.

CONCLUSION

Intellectual dysfunction in dementia of the Alzheimer type can be ascribed to the neuronal pathology and biochemical deficiencies of the cerebral cortex. The disturbances of language, memory, praxis, and perceptual recognition evident in this disease correspond to the deficits observed with localized cerebral cortical injuries in patients with stroke or other focal cortical lesions. Diseases affecting subcortical structures, however, also affect intellectual function and produce abnormalities of memory, motivation, speed of information processing, executive ability, and mood. These cognitive disorders cannot be attributed to direct cortical involvement and may result from indirect effects of subcortical dysfunction on cortical activity, disruption of local information processing at the subcortical level, or both. The antomical connections discussed previously provide insight into the cortical-subcortical circuits that may mediate the deficits of subcortical dementia syndromes.

Animal models have been sought to elucidate the anatomical underpinnings of behavioral disturbances associated with subcortical lesions. Investigators have found that lesions of the frontal lobe cortex and the striatum produce deficits analogous to those observed in subcortical dementias. Jacobson (1936) originally discovered that frontal lobe lesions disrupt a monkey's ability to solve correctly delayed response tasks involving the monkey's ability to predict the site of a patterned stimulus after an intervening distraction. Similar deficits have been demonstrated following frontal lobe damage in a variety of species (Kolb, 1984; Rosvold and Szwarcbart, 1964; Rosvold et al., 1961). Striatal lesions also disrupt delayed response capabilities (Divac, 1977; Divac et al., 1967; Rosvold et al., 1961). The striatal lesions disrupt both the fiber tracts descending from the frontal cortex as well as the tissue of the striatum involved in processing information received from the frontal lobe. These observations indicate that interruption of either the frontal origination or striatal destination of frontal-subcortical connections produces equivalent deficits in at least some aspects of behavior. Furthermore, it has been shown that monkeys can perform the delayed response task in spite of the presence of frontal lobe lesions if the frontal lesions are made in stages or are performed in infancy, suggesting that in specific circumstances the striatum may partially or completely assume the mediation of these functions (Butters et al., 1973; Goldman and Galkin, 1978; Kolb and Nonneman, 1978). Thus, animal models support the hypothesis derived from anatomical observations in humans that the frontal lobe and the striatum are part of a complex frontal-subcortical circuit and share important behavioral functions.

Current evidence does not definitively indicate whether it is the disruption of local processing or the de-afferentation of the striatum that is primarily responsible for the ensuing behavioral alterations. As suggested by Alexander et al. (1986), essential processing contributions may be made by all of the structures of the functional circuit comprised of the frontal cortex, striatum, pallidum, and thalamus. Interruption of any of these structures or their connections will result in similar behavioral deficit syndromes.

Biochemical as well as structural changes may contribute to the behavioral syndromes observed with subcortical dysfunction. Involvement of dopaminergic projections from the substantia nigra to the striatum may disrupt the frontal-subcortical circuit with resulting behavioral changes. Manipulation of dopamine levels in the cortex, striatum, and ventral tegmental area have been shown to effect performance on delayed response tasks (Brozoski et al., 1979; Simon et al., 1980). There is also ample evidence that dopamine levels in the ventral striatum and nucleus accumbens play a major role in regulating general activity levels (Iversen, 1975). Involvement of these dopaminergic systems may contribute to the subcortical dementia of parkinsonian syndromes where dopamine depletion is the primary biochemical abnormality.

Structural and biochemical circuitry involving the striatum, frontal cortex, and limbic system provide an anatomical basis for understanding the cognitive consequences of subcortical dysfunction and the similarities between subcortical dementia and frontal lobe syndromes. In addition, the limbic input to the striatum provides an interpretive framework for neuropsychiatric disturbances that commonly accompany subcortical dementia.

REFERENCES

Alexander, G.E., DeLong, M.R., Strick, P.L. Parallel organization of functionally segregated circuits linking basal ganglia and cortex. *Ann Rev Neurosci* 1986; 9:357–81.

Anden, N.E., Dahlsatrom, A., Fuxe, A., Larsson, K., Olson, L., Ungerstedt, U. Ascending monoamine neurons to the telencephalon and diencephalon. *Acta Physiol Scand* 1966; 67:313–26.

Beal, M.F., Domesick, V.B., Martin, J.B. Regional somatostatin distributions in the rat striatum. *Brain Res* 1983; 278:103–8.

Beckstead, R.M., Domesick, V.B., Nauta, W.J.H. Efferent connections of the substantia nigra and ventral tegmental area in the rat. *Brain Res* 1979; 175:191–217.

Beckstead, R.M. An autoradiographic examination of cortico-cortical and subcortical projections of the mediodorsal-projection (prefrontal) cortex in the rat. *J Comp Neurol* 1979; 184:43–62.

Brozoski, T.J., Brown, R.M., Rosvold, H.E., Goldman, P.S. Cognitive deficit caused by regional depletion of dopamine in prefrontal cortex of rhesus monkey. *Science* 1979; 205:929–31.

Butters, N., Butter, C., Rosen, J., Stein, D. Behavioral effects of sequential and one-stage ablations of orbital prefrontal cortex in the monkey. *Exp Neurol* 1973; 39:204–14.

Carmen, J.B., Cowan, W.M., Powell, T.P.S. The organization of cortico-striate connections in the rabbit. *Brain* 1963; 86:525–62.

Conrad, L.C.A., Pfaff, D.W. Efferents from medial basal forebrain and hypothalamus in the rat. I. An autoradiographic study of the anterior hypothalamus. *J Comp Neurol* 1976a; 169:221–62.

Conrad, L.C.A., Pfaff, D.W. Efferents from medial basal forebrain and hypothalamus in the rat. I. An autoradiographic study of the medial preoptic area. *J Comp Neurol* 1976b; 169:185–220.

Cummings, J.L., Benson, D.F. *Dementia: A clinical approach.* Butterworths, Boston, 1983.

Dahlstrom, A., Fuxe, K. Evidence for the existence of monoamine-containing neurons in the central nervous system. I. Demonstration of monoamines in the cell bodies of brainstem neurons. *Acta Physiol Scand* 1964; 62 (Suppl 232):1–55.

Divac, I., Rosvold, H.E., Szwarcbart, M.K. Behavioral effects of selective ablation of the caudate nucleus. *J Comp Physiol Psychol* 1967; 63:184–90.

Divac, I. Does the neostriatum operate as a functional entity? In *Psychobiology of the striatum.* Cools, A.R., Lohman, A.H.M., van der Bercken, J.H.L. (eds.). Elsevier, Amsterdam, 1977, pp. 21–30.

Domesick, V.B. Projections from the cingulate cortex in the rat. *Brain Res* 1969; 12:296–320.

Domesick, V.B. Neuroanatomical organization of dopamine neurons in the ventral tegmental area. In *The mesocortical dopamine system.* Kalivas, P.W., Nemeroff, C.B. (eds.). Ann New York Acad Sci, New York, 1988, pp. 10–26.

Domesick, V.B., Paskevich, P., Matthysse, S.W. *Neurosci Abst* 1986.

Fallon, J.H., Moore, R.Y. Catecholamine innervation of the basal forebrain. IV. Topography of the dopamine projection to the basal forebrain and neostriatum. *J Comp Neurol* 1978; 180:545–80.

Goldman, P.S.D., Galkin, T.W. Prenatal removal of frontal association cortex in the rhesus monkey: anatomical and functional consequences in postnatal life. *Brain Res* 1978; 152:451–85.

Goldman-Rakic, P.S. Circuitry of the frontal association cortex and its relevance to dementia. *Arch Gerontol Geriatr* 1987; 6:299–309.

Groenewegen, H.J., Becker, N.E.H.M., Lohman, A.H.M. Subcortical afferents to the nucleus accumbens septi in the cat, studied with retrograde axonal transport of horseradish peroxidase and bisbenzimid. *Neuroscience* 1980; 5:1903–16.

Haber, S., Elde, R. Correlation between met-enkephalin and substance P immunoreactivity in the primate globus pallidus. *Neuroscience* 1981; 6:1291–7.

Haber, S.N., Groenewegen, H.J., Grove, E.A., Nauta, W.J.H. Efferent connections of the ventral pallidum: Evidence of a dual striato pallidofugal pathway. *J Comp Neurol* 1985; 235:322–35.

Haber, S.N., Nauta, W.J.H. Ramifications of the globus pallidus in the rat as indicated by patterns of immunohistochemistry. *Neuroscience* 1983; 9:245–60.

Heimer, L. The olfactory cortex and the ventral striatum. In *Limbic mechanisms.* Livingston, K.E., Hornykiewicz, O. (eds.). New York, Plenum Press, 1978, pp. 95–187.

Heimer, L., Wilson, R.D. The subcortical projections of the allocortex. Similarities in the neural associations of the hippocampus, the piriform cortex, and the neocortex. In *Golgi centennial symposium: Perspectives in neurology.* Santini, M., (ed.). New York, Raven Press, 1975, pp. 177–93.

Hemphill, M., Holm, G., Crutcher, M., DeLong, M.R., Hedreen, J. Afferent connections of the nucleus accumbens in the monkey. In *Neurobiology of the nucleus accumbens.* Chronister, R., DeFrance, J. (eds.). Brunswich, Maine, Haer Inst. Press, 1981, pp. 75–81.

Hill, J.M., Switzer, R.C. The regional distribution and cellular localization of iron in the rat brain. *Neuroscience* 1984; 11:595–603.

Iversen, L.L. Dopamine receptors in the brain. *Science* 1975; 188:1084–1089.

Jacobsen, C.F. Studies of cerebral function in primates: I. The functions of the frontal association areas in monkeys. *Comp Psychol Monogr* 1936; 13:3–60.

Kelly, A.E., Domesick, V.B. The distribution of the projection from the hippocampal formation to the nucleus accumbens in the rat: An anterograde- and retrograde-horseradish peroxidase study. *Neuroscience* 1982; 7:2321–35.

Kelly, A.E., Domesick, V.B., Nauta, W.J. The amygdalostriatal projection in the rat—an anatomical study of anterograde and retrograde tracing methods. *Neuroscience* 1982; 7:615–30.

Kolb, B. Functions of the frontal cortex of the rat: a comparative view. *Brain Res Rev* 1984; 8:65–98.

Kolb, B., Nonneman, A.J. Sparing of function in rats with early prefrontal cortex lesions. *Brain Res* 1978; 151:135–48.

Kunzle, H. Bilateral projections from precentral motor cortex to the putamen and other parts of the basal ganglia. An autoradiographic study in *Macaca fascicularis*. *Brain Res* 1975; 88:195–209.

Leavitt, P. A monoclonal antibody to limbic system neurons. *Science* 1984; 223:299–301.

Leonard, C.M. The prefrontal cortex of the rat. I. Cortical projection of the mediodorsal nucleus. II. Efferent connections. *Brain Res* 1969; 12:3211–343.

Miller, J.J., Richardson, T.L., Fibiger, H.C., McLennon, H. Anatomical and electrophysiological identification of a projection from the mesencephalic raphe to the caudate putamen in the rat. *Brain Res* 1975; 97:133–8.

Nauta, W.J.H. An experimental study of the fornix system in the rat. *J Comp Neurol* 1956; 104:247–71.

Nauta, W.J.H., Domesick, V.B. The anatomy of the extrapyramidal system. In *Dopaminergic ergot derivatives and motor function.* Fuxe, K., Calne, D.B. (eds.). Oxford, Pergamon Press, 1979.

Nauta, W.J.H., Domesick, V.B. In *Neural substrates of behavior.* Beckman, A., (ed.). New York, Spectrum Publications, 1982, pp. 175–206.

Nauta, W.J.H., Haymaker, W. Hypothalamic nuclei and fiber connections. In *The hypothalamus.* Haymaker, W., Anderson, E., Nauta, W.J.H. (eds.). Springfield, Illinois, CC Thomas Publisher, 1969, pp. 136–209.

Nauta, W.J.H., Smith, G.P., Faull, R.L.M., Domesick, V.B. Efferent connections and nigral afferents of the nucleus accumbens septi in the rat. *Neuroscience* 1978; 3:385–401.

Newman, R., Winans, S.S. An experimental study of the ventral striatum of the golden hamster. I. Neuronal connections of the nucleus accumbens. *J Comp Neurol* 1980; 191:167–92.

Palkovits, M., Jacobowitz, D.M. Topographic atlas of catecholamine and acetylcholinesterase-containing neurons in the rat brain. II. Hindbrain (mesencephalon, rhombencephalon). *J Comp Neurol* 1974; 157:29–42.

Phillipson, O.T. The cytoarchitecture of the interfascicular nucleus and ventral tegmental area of Tsai in the rat. *J Comp Neurol* 1979; 187:85–98.

Ricardo, J. Efferent connections of the rubrothalamic region in the rat. I. The subthalamic nucleus of Luys. *Brain Res* 1980; 202:257–71.

Rosvold, H.E., Szwarcbart, M.K., Mirsky, A.F., Mishkin, M. The effect of frontal-lobe damage on delayed response performance in chimpanzees. *J Comp Physiol Psychol* 1961; 54:368–74.

Rosvold, H.E., Szwarcbart, M.K. Neural structures involved in delayed-response performance. In *The frontal granular cortex and behavior.* Warren, J.M., Akert, K. (eds.). McGraw-Hill, New York, 1964, pp. 1–15.

Selemom, W., Goldman-Rakic, P.S. Longitudinal topography and interdigitation of cortico-striatal projections in the rhesus monkey. *J Neuroscience* 1985; 5:776–84.

Simon, H., Scatton, B., Le Moal, M. Dopaminergic A10 neurons are involved in cognitive functions. *Nature* 1980; 286:150–1.

Somogyi, P., Bolam, J.P., Smith, A.D. Monosynaptic cortical input and local axon collaterals to identified striatonigral neurons. A light and electron microscopic study using the Golgi-peroxidase transport degeneration procedure. *J Comp Neurol* 1981; 195:567–84.

Steinbusch, H.W.M. Distribution of serotonin-immunoreactivity in the central nervous system of the rat—cell bodies and terminals. *Neuroscience* 1981; 6:557–618.

Swanson, L.W. An autoradiographic study of the efferent connections of the preoptic region in the rat. *J Comp Neurol* 1976; 167:227–56.

Swanson, L.W., Cowan, W.M. A note on the connections and development of the nucleus accumbens. *Brain Res* 1975; 92:324–30.

Swanson, L.W., Cowan, W.M. An autoradiographic study of the organization of the efferent connections of the hippocampal formation in the rat. *J Comp Neurol* 1977; 172:49–84.

Swanson, L.W., Cowan, W.M. The connections of the septal region in the rat. *J Comp Neurol* 1979; 186:621–56.

Switzer, R.C., Hill, C.J., Heimer, L. The globus pallidus and its rostroventral extension into the olfactory tubercle of the rat: A cyto- and chemoarchitectural study. *Neuroscience* 1982; 7:1891–1904.

Tsai, C. The optic tracts and centers of the opossum, *Didelphys virginiana*. *J Comp Neurol* 1925; 39:173–216.

Ungerstedt, U. Stereotaxic mapping of the monoamine pathways in the rat brain. *Acta Physiol Scand* 1971; 197 (Suppl 367):1–48.

Webster, K.E. Cortico-striate interrelations in the albino rat. *J Anat* 1961; 95:532–45.

Yeterian, E.H., Van Hoesen, G.W. Corticostriate projections in the rhesus monkey: the organization of certain cortico-caudate connections. *Brain Res* 1978; 139:43–63.

4

Subcortical Chemical Neuroanatomy

ROBERT Y. MOORE

Over the past 20 years there have been striking advances in methodology that have elevated neuroanatomical tract tracing from an arcane and difficult endeavor to a precise and powerful tool of modern neurobiology. Many modern anatomical methods are generally useful, but others are selective, and these have been particularly powerful in the identification of neural circuits on the basis of the chemicals produced by neurons for the process of synaptic transmission. The basis of this chemical neuroanatomy is a long series of observations that established chemical neurotransmission as a fundamental principle of nervous system organization and function. Within this context a major discovery that stimulated the development of subcortical chemical neuroanatomy was the identification of dopamine as a transmitter in the nigrostriatal system and the demonstration of a relatively selective loss of nigrostriatal dopamine neurons in Parkinson's disease (cf. Hornykiewicz, 1966, for a review). At present, this remains a model for a subcortical disease process in which the pathology is predominantly associated with the loss of a single chemically identified neuronal system.

The first substances demonstrated to be chemical neurotransmitters were acetylcholine (ACH) and norepinephrine (NE). Subsequently, a relatively small number of additional small-molecule transmitters, either amino acids or amines derived from amino acids, has been identified (Table 4-1). These substances vary from being present in a relatively high proportion of central neurons to being found in very limited populations. In addition, there are several other amino acids, particularly aspartate and taurine, for which there is some evidence, none of it definitive, for participation in the process of synaptic transmission. Typically, small-molecule transmitters produce either inhibitory or excitatory postsynaptic potentials. The postsynaptic effects depend upon the receptors, second message systems, and ion channels activated. In the presynaptic neuron, small-molecule transmitters have a typical intraneuronal distribution with highest concentration in axon terminals and a low, or relatively low, concentration in preterminal axons and the cell body. The distribution of small-molecule transmitters was often determined initially by chemical assay, but most have been identified more recently either by use of an antiserum generated against the substance itself or an antiserum against an enzyme necessary for its synthesis. And, although substantial progress has been made, the anatomical localization of amino acid transmitters has been more difficult than that of the amines. For example, glutamate clearly is present in metabolic pools other than for release as a neurotransmitter and is present both in neurons and in glia. Gamma-aminobutyric acid (GABA) may also be present in glia.

Table 4-1   Small-Molecule Neurotransmitters

Transmitter	Estimated Percentage of CNS Neurons[a]
GABA[b]	35
Glutamate	35
Acetylcholine	10
Serotonin	5
Dopamine	2
Norepinephrine	1
Glycine	< 1
Histamine	< 1

[a]The estimates are obtained from several sources and are based on currently available information on the rodent nervous system. They should be taken as only very rough approximations; no definitive quantitative data are available.
[b]GABA, gamma-aminobutyric acid.

Another limitation is the availability of sensitive and specific antisera against amino acids. Nevertheless, it is clear that the major small-molecule transmitters have been identified, and substantial progress has been made in determining their localization and function.

Another area of striking recent advance has been in the identification and characterization of peptides as neuroactive substances. These substances, ranging in size from 3 to more than 40 amino acids, appear to have a variety of postsynaptic effects that differ in their time course of action from brief, transmitterlike activity to longer-term modification of the action of small-molecule transmitters and, finally, to quite prolonged "trophic" functions. The number of peptides identified in the mammalian nervous system has grown very rapidly and now includes more than 100 substances. The rapidity with which knowledge is being generated about both small-molecule transmitters and peptides is exemplified by the five volumes already published in the *Handbook of Chemical Neuroanatomy* series. As might be expected from the distribution of small-molecule transmitters, they are frequently colocalized with peptides, including many instances in which more than one peptide is produced with a small-molecule transmitter in the same neuron (cf. Hokfelt et al., 1986, for a review). Examples of small-molecule transmitter and peptide colocalization are shown in Table 4-2.

Indeed, the phenomenon of colocalization is so common, and new peptides are discovered so rapidly, that it seems likely to be a general principle of nervous system organization. That is, it appears reasonable to conclude that most neurons will eventually be shown to contain a small-molecule transmitter and one or more peptides, indicating that the chemical communication between neurons is likely to be shown to be a very complex process.

In addition to differences in localization and colocalization, there are significant differences in the neurobiology of small-molecule transmitters and peptides. Small-molecule transmitters are either synthesized in axon terminals, or taken up into terminals, and stored. They are released on stimulation, interact with pre- or postsynaptic receptors, and are then either taken up by the terminals releasing them by specific reuptake mechanisms or catabolyzed by degradative enzymes. Peptides, in contrast, must be produced in the cell body, packaged in vesicles, and transported to the axon terminal prior to release. Peptides also interact with receptors but are not taken up by

Table 4-2   Colocalization of Neuroactive Substances

Small-Molecule Neurotransmitters	Peptides[a]
GABA	SS, NPY, ENK, SP
Glutamate	SP
Serotonin	SP, TRH, GAL
Dopamine	CCK, NT
Norepinephrine	NPY, GAL, ENK
Acetylcholine	VIP, GAL, CGRP
Epinephrine	NPY, GAL, ENK

[a]Peptides that have been shown to be colocalized with the small-molecule transmitter noted. CCK, cholecystokinin; CGRP, calcitonin gene-related peptide; ENK, enkephalin; GAL, galanin; NT, neurotensin; NPY, neuropeptide Y; SP, substance P; SS, somatostatin; VIP, vasoactive intestinal polypeptide.

the axons releasing them and must be inactivated and degraded by postsynaptic processes. Thus small-molecule transmitters are a recyclable neuronal resource, whereas peptides must be synthesized, transported, and stored in sufficient amounts to meet reasonable functional requirements. Although peptides generally appear to have the same intraneuronal distribution as small-molecule transmitters, there are exceptions (Moore and Gustafson, 1989). In addition, peptides are produced from large precursor molecules that may contain more than one peptide or multiple copies of a single peptide. The regulation of peptide production and processing is a relatively new area of investigation in which substantial advances are being made. Similarly, although peptide receptors have been demonstrated, the analysis of their localization, characterization, and mechanism of action is not nearly so far advanced as for small-molecule transmitter receptors.

This brief introduction forms a background for the review that follows. It should be evident that the chemical neuroanatomy of subcortical structures is likely to be very complex, and to continue to grow more so in the immediate future. If one simply takes our current knowledge of neural circuitry, which is considerable, and adds to it the complications of a chemical coding for each circuit, the magnitude of the problem is evident. From this perspective it is certainly clear that one could not review all of the known localization of neuroactive substances in subcortical structures. Rather, I shall select two sets of pathways to exemplify the increments in understanding obtained from the analysis of chemical neuroanatomy. To illustrate some of the anatomical connections potentially involved in cognitive processes, I shall describe the organization of the nonthalamic subcortical projections to the cerebral cortex that have been characterized by their content of classical neurotransmitters. To illustrate further the utility of chemical neuroanatomy, I shall also describe the complex organization of the striatum and its interconnections with rostral midbrain.

NONTHALAMIC SUBCORTICAL–CORTICAL PROJECTIONS

The cerebral cortex and dorsal thalamus are a functional unit. Until relatively recently, it was believed that the majority of subcortical projections to the cortex arose from the dorsal thalamus. One of the interesting achievements of chemical neuroanatomy has been the demonstration of pontine, mesencephalic, hypothalamic, and basal forebrain projections to the cerebral cortex. Strikingly, these projections have been identified and characterized by their neurotransmitter content, whereas the transmitters produced by thalamic projection neurons remain to be identified. The general organization of each of these systems will be described.

Locus Coeruleus–Norepinephrine

The locus coeruleus is a compact nucleus of the isthmic tegmentum. In virtually all mammals it is composed of NE-producing neurons located in the central gray and the adjacent reticular formation (Moore and Card, 1984). In humans, neurons of the locus coeruleus contain neuromelanin, and the nucleus is one of the pigmented brain-stem nuclei. Although much of it is located within the reticular formation and central gray in humans, there is a large component that extends along the surface of the superior medullary velum (Braak, 1975). The NE content of locus coeruleus neurons was first noted by Dahlstrom and Fuxe (1964), and the organization and projections of the locus have been studied intensively (cf. Moore and Card, 1984, for a review). The locus coeruleus projects predominantly to suprasegmental structures (Figure 4-1). Axons arising from locus coeruleus neurons take one of three pathways. The first, largely from neurons located ventrally in the locus, descends into the brain stem and the spinal cord. The second ascends via the superior cerebellar peduncle to provide a widespread innervation to cerebellar cortex. The third, and major, pathway ascends in the midbrain as the dorsal catecholamine bundle. Projections are given off to brain-stem sensory nuclei (Levitt and Moore, 1979), with the major pathway continuing in the medial forebrain bundle. A major site of projection is the dorsal thalamus (Lindvall et al., 1974). Virtually all thalamic nuclei are innervated, with the density of the terminal plexus varying from sparse (ventrobasal complex, lateral complex) to dense (anterior

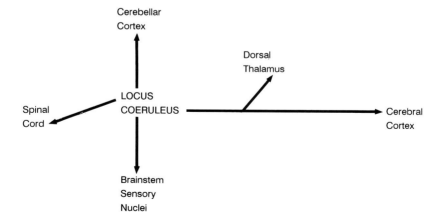

NOREPINEPHRINE

Figure 4-1   Diagram depicting the organization of locus coeruleus NE projections.

nuclei). Most studies have been carried out on the rat, but there are data indicating that the patterns of innervation are similar in primates, including humans. One significant difference is that the moderately dense innervation of the dorsal lateral geniculate nucleus (Kromer and Moore, 1980) does not appear to be present in primates (R.Y. Moore, unpublished).

NE-containing axons ascending in the medial forebrain bundle take three primary pathways to the cortex: a ventral pathway along the ventral amygdaloid bundle to the temporal lobe, a rostral and lateral pathway along the external capsule, and a medial pathway along the cingulum. The pattern of terminal plexuses varies according to the region innervated. The greatest variation is among allocortical areas, amygdala, olfactory cortex, and hippocampus. In rodents the pattern of neocortical innervation is fairly uniform (Levitt and Moore, 1978), whereas in primates there are major differences among areas (Lewis et al., 1987). The typical pattern is a fairly dense plexus in the molecular layer and loose plexuses throughout the remainder of the cortex.

There have been a number of studies of the topography of locus coeruleus projections. These demonstrate a limited topography, particularly with respect to the projections to the spinal cord (Loughlin et al., 1986), but it appears most likely that individual locus neurons have widespread projections. Recent studies (Ashton-Jones et al., 1986) indicate that afferent projections to the locus coeruleus are very restricted and limited to brain-stem nuclei that themselves receive input from widespread regions. Thus the locus coeruleus NE system can be viewed as one that has input from diverse areas and projects to widespread, suprasegmental components of the neuraxis.

Locus coeruleus neurons also contain peptides. In the rat approximately one half of the neurons contain neuropeptide Y (NPY; Everitt et al., 1984; Moore and Gustafson, 1989), and nearly all contain galanin (Holets et al., 1988; Moore and Gustafson, 1989). It is of interest that the perikaryal content of galanin, for example, appears quite high but that little, if any, galanin can be demonstrated in axons in terminal fields in the cerebral and cerebellar cortices or dorsal thalamus (Moore and Gustafson, 1989).

Midbrain Raphe Nuclei—Serotonin

Neurons that produce 5-hydroxytryptamine (5-HT, serotonin) are located in the raphe nuclei, a series of midline nuclei extending from the midbrain to the caudal medulla. At the present time, it appears that the largest and most rostral of these nuclei, the dorsal raphe nucleus and the central superior nucleus, project predominantly to forebrain structures (Figure 4-2). Like all of the raphe nuclei, these contain a combination of 5-HT–producing and non–5-HT–producing neurons, but it appears that the non–5-HT neurons have largely short, local projections (Moore et al., 1978). The ascending pathways used by 5-HT neuron axons to reach terminal sites are very similar to those used by locus coeruleus NE neuron axons. The major ascending pathway is the medial forebrain bundle with branches into the areas shown in Figure 4-2. The 5-HT innervation of the diencephalon and telencephalon is much more widespread than the locus coeruleus NE innervation. In particular, there are relatively dense projections to the hypothalamus, striatum, and basal forebrain, in addition to the widespread projections to the thalamus and cerebral cortex. In the cortex, the 5-HT innervation is generally dense but with some variation from area to area (Berger et al., 1988). The general pattern of 5-HT innervation in brain has been reviewed by Steinbusch (1981).

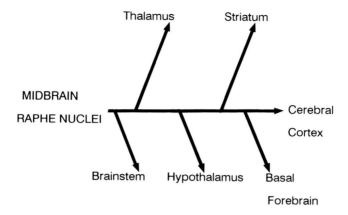

SEROTONIN

Figure 4-2 Diagram depicting the organization of midbrain raphe 5-HT projections.

The ultrastructural organization of 5-HT neuron innervation of the forebrain has been studied extensively by Descarries and his colleagues (Descarries et al., 1975; Soghomonian et al., 1989). In contrast to innervation from other sources, 5-HT terminals are reported to participate in relatively few synaptic complexes in either the neocortex or striatum. This would suggest that the effects of serotonin release might be distributed more widely than an immediate postsynaptic element. 5-HT neurons have also been described to contain peptides, substance P, and thyrotropin releasing hormone (Johanssen et al., 1981), which presumably are released and participate in the postsynaptic actions of 5-HT neurons in the areas innervated.

Substantia Nigra—Ventral Tegmental Area—Dopamine

The existence of a dopaminergic projection from the substantia nigra, pars compacta (SNc), to the neostriatum was demonstrated by Swedish workers using the fluorescence histochemical method (cf. Moore and Bloom, 1978; Bjorklund and Lindvall, 1984, for a review). The SNc is composed primarily of a population of dopamine (DA) neurons that is continuous medially with DA neurons in the ventral tegmental area (VTA) and caudally with DA neurons in the midbrain reticular formation (the A9, A10, and A8 groups, respectively, of Dahlstrom and Fuxe, 1964). These groups and their projections have subsequently been designated the mesotelencephalic DA systems (Moore and Bloom, 1978; Bjorklund and Lindvall, 1984). They project in a highly topographically organized pattern to most of the telencephalon (cf. Fallon and Moore, 1978; Fallon and Loughlin, 1987, for reviews). The mesotelencephalic system has three components that differ with respect to cells of origin and regions innervated: the mesocortical, mesolimbic, and nigrostriatal DA systems (Figure 4-3). The mesocortical system arises principally from VTA neurons, and it is now apparent that virtually all cortical areas receive some DA innervation that varies markedly in density and

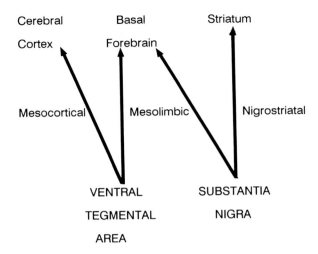

DOPAMINE

Figure 4-3   Diagram depicting the organization of mesotelencephalic DA projections.

laminar organization between areas (Fallon and Loughlin, 1987; Lewis et al., 1987; Berger et al., 1988). For example, there is very dense DA innervation in the monkey in the precentral gyrus and the inferior parietal labule, whereas the innervation of the postcentral gyrus is sparse and the visual area very sparse (Lewis et al., 1987). Similar differences occur in rat neocortex (Berger et al., 1988).

The mesolimbic DA system arises from VTA and SNc neurons. The areas innervated include the nucleus accumbens, septal nuclei, olfactory tubercle, amygdala, entorhinal cortex, piriform cortex, cingulate cortex, and hippocampal formation. The pattern of innervation is quite different among areas. In the nucleus accumbens and olfactory tubercle, there is a dense distribution of terminals similar to the neostriatal nuclei. Within the septal nuclei and amygdala there is a variable innervation that is regionally specific, as is the laminar pattern within the cortical areas (Bjorklund and Lindvall, 1984; Fallon and Loughlin, 1987). Very few DA fibers are present in the hippocampal formation.

The most extensively analyzed DA system is the nigrostriatal projection (Figure 4-4). DA neurons of the SNc project in a highly topographically organized manner on the neostriatum. The DA innervation of caudate nucleus and putamen is very dense and represents about 20 percent of the total terminal field. During development, DA neurons initially project to restricted areas, "patches," of neostriatum (Olson et al., 1972). These zones, also termed striosomes, are acetylcholinesterase rich in development and form a fundamental component of the functional organization of the neostriatum (cf. Penney and Young, 1986, for a review). In the adult brain, the nigrostriatal innervation is very homogeneous, with terminals predominantly on dendrites of striatal neurons. Although the majority of the nigrostriatal projection is to the neo-

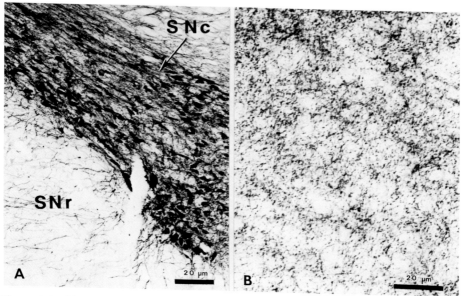

Figure 4-4 Photomicrograph illustrating the DA neurons of the SNc (A) in the rat and (B) their terminal plexus in the caudate nucleus of the monkey demonstrated by tyrosine hydroxylase immunohistochemistry. Densely packed neurons are present in the SNc with fine dendrites extending into SNr (A). The very fine, punctate terminals form a dense plexus in the neostriatum (B).

striatum, there is a relatively small projection to the globus pallidus. As with other catecholamine neurons, peptides have been demonstrated in DA neurons of the SNc and VTA. Cholecystokinin has been found in a subpopulation of SNc-VTA DA neurons, predominantly medially (Hokfelt et al., 1980), and subsequently shown to coexist with neurotensin (Fallon and Loughlin, 1987).

Nucleus Basalis—Diagonal Band Complex—Acetylcholine

ACH was identified early as a neurotransmitter produced by motor neurons, but the elucidation of central cholinergic pathways was not accomplished until the past few years and was possible because of the availability of antisera to the ACH-synthesizing enzyme, choline acetyltransferase. In retrospect, the work of Shute and Lewis (1967) using acetylcholinesterase histochemistry as a marker for cholinergic pathways provided a remarkably close approximation of the pathways demonstrated by choline acetyltransferase immunohistochemistry (Mesulam et al., 1983a,b, 1984). There are two primary sets of cholinergic neurons that provide a subcortical and cortical innervation (Figure 4-5).

The laterodorsal tegmental nucleus (LTN) and pedunculopontine nucleus (PPN) are brain-stem nuclei among a complex group of pontine and mesencephalic reticular nuclei projecting to the diencephalon and telencephalon (Rye et al., 1987). The LTN and PPN contain ACH neurons that project to the hypothalamus, ventral thalamus, and dorsal thalamus (Rye et al., 1987). There is a major projection to the thalamus, in-

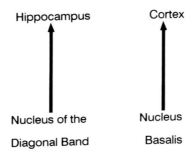

ACETYLCHOLINE

Figure 4-5   Diagram depicting the organization of the nucleus of the diagonal band–nucleus basalis ACH projections to cortical structures.

cluding the midline-intralaminar nuclei and the reticular nucleus, with virtually all major groups receiving afferents (Levey et al., 1987; Hallanger et al., 1987). Input to the LTN and PPN is from ascending lemniscal sensory pathways and reticular formation so that the cholinergic projections to the thalamus relay a wide variety of information and should have a major influence on thalamic and, hence, cortical function.

The principal forebrain cholinergic group is the nucleus basalis (NB)–nucleus of the diagonal band (NDB) complex (Mesulam et al., 1983a,b, 1986; Mesulam and Geula, 1988). Afferents to the NB-NDB complex arise from a widespread set of brainstem (reticular formation, midbrain raphe, locus coeruleus, and substantia nigra), basal forebrain (amygdala, piriform, and entorhinal cortex), thalamic (midline nuclei), hypothalamic (preoptic area), and neocortical (temporal, insular, and orbitofrontal) structures (Mesulam and Mufson, 1984; Russchen et al., 1985). The NB-NDB cholinergic neurons project widely on the cortex (Mesulam et al., 1983a,b, 1986).

The involvement of these neurons in Alzheimer's disease is well known. It is worth noting that a subdivision of the NDB cholinergic neurons, the medial septal group, provides the cholinergic projection to the hippocampal formation. The pattern of projection to the hippocampus is quite specific and differs significantly from that to the cortex.

ORGANIZATION OF STRIATAL CONNECTIONS

The striatal complex has been studied extensively, and recent work has greatly advanced our knowledge of its chemical neuroanatomy (Figure 4-6). The neostriatum consists largely of medium-sized to small neurons that produce GABA and one or more peptides, primarily substance P, enkephalin, and dynorphin (cf. Penney and Young, 1986, for a review). These neurons have spiny dendrites and are the projection neurons. In addition to these, there are two groups of striatal interneurons, large aspiny

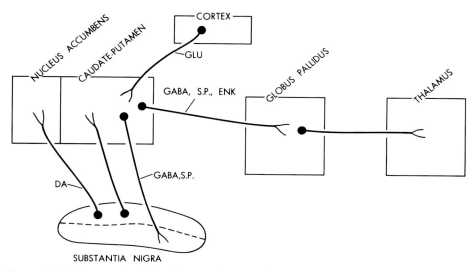

Figure 4-6 Diagram depicting the organization of connections of the striatal complex.

neurons that are cholinergic and small aspiny neurons that contain somatostatin and neuropeptide Y (Figure 4-7B).

The organization of striatal projections is shown in Figure 4-6. A major input to the neostriatum, in addition to those already described, arises in cerebral cortex and appears to be glutamatergic (Otterson and Storm-Mathisen, 1984). Corticostriatal connections arise from nearly all neocortical areas. The neostriatum has two primary areas of projection, globus pallidus and substantia nigra, pars reticularis. Both areas show a typical pattern of afferents characterized by dense, linear axodendritic terminal arrays on proximal dendrites (Fig. 4-7A). Since the globus pallidus and substantia nigra, pars reticularis, both project to the ventral thalamic nuclei, they form two components of an interconnected set of structures that influences not only the activity of the motor cortex but the frontal lobe as well (cf. Young and Penney, 1988, for a review). All pallidal neurons appear to use GABA as a transmitter.

As noted previously, the neostriatum has an additional component of organization revealed by chemical neuroanatomy. This is a mosaiclike organization of striosomes within a matrix (Graybiel and Ragsdale, 1978; Graybiel et al., 1981). These develop as dopamine islands in the fetus that are acetylcholinesterase-dense, and striosome neurons appear with different birth dates from those in the matrix (Graybiel and Hickey, 1982). There are now substantial data to indicate that the connections of striosome and matrix neurons are different. The neurons of striosomes appear to receive DA input primarily from the dorsal SNc and project back to SNc and not to pars reticularis (Gerfen, 1985; Gerfen et al., 1985, 1987). Cortical input to striosomes appears to be predominantly from the frontal cortex rather than from other areas, whereas matrix neurons receive input from motor, sensory, and association cortices and from intralaminar thalamic nuclei (Donoghue and Herkenham, 1986; Ragsdale and Graybiel, 1981; Goldman-Rakic, 1982). Neurons in striosomes contain GABA and either dynorphin or neurotensin (Penney and Young, 1986). Neurons in the matrix

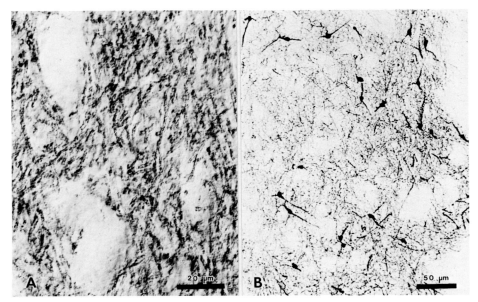

Figure 4-7 Photomicrographs illustrating patterns of organization of immunohistochemically identified neurons. (A) GABA-containing terminals of neostriatal neurons projecting to globus pallidus in the monkey brain. (B) Neuropeptide Y–containing neurons and axons in the rat neostriatum.

contain GABA and either enkephalin or substance P and project to the substantia nigra, pars reticulata, or to globus pallidus (Figure 4-8). Neuropeptide Y–somatostatin neurons are apparently restricted to the matrix. The extent to which there are interconnections between striosome and matrix neurons is unclear. These observations indicate that there is great complexity in the organization of the striatum and its connections.

SUMMARY

The functions of the nervous system can be viewed in two contexts, physiological regulation and maintenance of the internal milieu and behavioral adaptation to the environment. The complex behaviors of humans, and other mammals, require a precise integration of these functions, and the mediation of the most complex behaviors requires the integration of subcortical and cortical activities. The intent of this review has been to provide examples of how chemical neuroanatomy has extended our understanding of the functional organization of subcortical–cortical interactions. In this I have emphasized two sets of information that exemplify the utility of a chemical subcortical neuroanatomy. These are the organization of nonthalamic subcortical projections to the cortex and the organization of the basal ganglia.

Prior to the development of methods to study chemical neuroanatomy, it was believed that all subcortical projections to the cortex arose from the dorsal thalamus. It is now evident that there are at least four major systems with widespread influences on cerebral cortical function. These differ somewhat in organization. For example, the

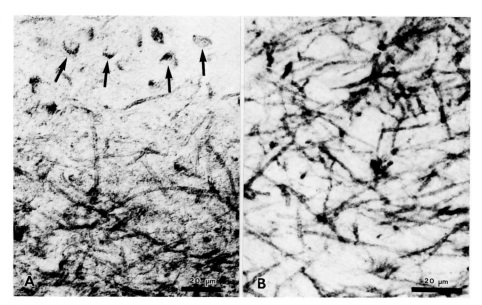

Figure 4-8 Photomicrographs illustrating patterns of termination of the axons of neostriatal neurons. (A) Human substantia nigra with melanin-containing neurons of SNc (arrows) and a plexus of substance P–containing terminals in SNr. These are in linear arrays along large proximal dendrites. (B) Human globus pallidus with a similar pattern of enkephalin-containing terminals.

locus coeruleus NE system and the raphe 5-HT system have quite widespread, diffuse projections on the cortex, whereas the midbrain DA and, particularly, the basal forebrain ACH systems are more precisely organized.

The beginning of chemical neuroanatomy was the discovery of the nigrostriatal system. It is now apparent that the striatal complex has an extremely intricate organization that would not have been discovered without methods to analyze chemical organization. This is exemplified by the complex interaction of striatal striosomes and matrix with afferent and efferent connections. Thus it is clear that chemical neuroanatomy provides new insights into the organization of the nervous system, and it has one further advantage: It provides a rational basis for the development of therapies in diseases in which specific, chemically identified systems are involved.

REFERENCES

Ashton-Jones, G., Ennis, M., Pieribone, V.A., Nickel, W.T., and Shipley, M.T. The brain nucleus coeruleus: Restricted afferent control of a broad efferent network. *Science* 1986; 234:734–7.

Berger, B., Trottier, S., Verney, C., Gasparj, P., and Alvarez, C. Reginal and lamnor distribution of the dopamine and serotonin innervation in the macaque cerebral cortex. A radioautographic study. *J Comp Neurol* 1988; 273:99–119.

Bjorklund, A., and Lindvall, O. Dopamine-containing systems in the CNS. In *Handbook of*

Chemical Neuroanatomy, Vol. 2. Bjorklund, A., and Hokfelt, T. (eds.). Elsevier, Amsterdam, 1984, pp. 55–122.

Braak, H. On the pars cerebellaris loci coerulei within the cerebellum of man. *Cell Tissue Res* 1975; 160:279–83.

Dahlstrom, A., and Fuxe, K. Evidence for the existence of monoamine-containing neurons in the central nervous system. *Acta Physiol Scand* 1964; 62 (Suppl. 232):1–55.

Descarries, L., Beaudet, A., and Watkins, K.C. Serotonin nerve terminals in adult rat neocortex. *Brain Res* 1975; 100:567–88.

Donoghue, J.P. and Herkenham, M.R. Neostriatal projections from individual cortical fields conform to histochemically distinct striatal compartments in the rat. *Brain Res* 1986; 365:397–403.

Everitt, B.J., Hokfelt, T., Teremius, L., Tatemoto, K., Mutt, V., and Goldstein, M. Differential coexistence of neuropeptide-like immunoreactivity with catecholamines in the central nervous system of the rat. *Neuroscience* 1984; 11:443–62.

Fallon, J.H., and Loughlin, S.E. Monoamine innervation of the cerebral cortex and a theory of the role of monoamines in cerebral cortex and basal ganglia. In *Cerebral Cortex, Vol. 6.* Jones, E.G., and Peters, A. (eds.). Plenum, New York, 1987, pp. 41–127.

Fallon, J.H., and Moore, R.Y. Catecholamine innervation of the basal forebrain. IV. Topography of dopamine cell projections to the basal forebrain and neostriatum. *J Comp Neurol* 1978; 180:545–80.

Gerfen, C.R. The neostriatal mosaic. I. Compartmental organization of projections from the striatum to the substantia nigra in the rat. *J Comp Neurol* 1985; 236:454–76.

Gerfen, C.R., Bainbridge, K.G., and Miller, J.J. The neostriatal mosaic: Compartmental distribution calcium binding protein and parvalbumin in the basal ganglia of rat and monkey. *Proc Natl Acad Sci USA* 1985; 82:8780–4.

Gerfen, C.R., Herkenham, M.R., and Thibault, J. The neostriatal matrix. II. Path- and matrix-directed mesostriatal dopaminergic and non-dopaminergic systems. *J Neurosci* 1987; 7:3915–34.

Goldman-Rakic, P.S. Cytoarchitectonic heterogeneity of the primate neostriatum. Subdivision into island and matrix cellular compartments. *J Comp Neurol* 1982; 205:398–413.

Graybiel, A.M., and Hickey, T.L. Chemospecificity of ontogenetic units in the striatum. Demonstration combining (³H) thymidine neuronography and histochemical staining. *Proc Natl Acad Sci USA* 1982; 79:198–202.

Graybiel, A.M., Pickel, V.M., Joh, T.H., Reis, D.J., and Ragsdale, C.W., Jr. Direct demonstration of the correspondence between the dopamine islands, and acetylcholinesterase patches in the developing neostriatum. *Proc Natl Acad Sci USA* 1981; 78:5871–5.

Graybiel, A.M., and Ragsdale, C.W. Histochemically distinct compartments in striatum of monkey and cat demonstrated by acetylthiocholinesterase staining. *Proc Natl Acad Sci USA* 1978; 75:5723–6.

Hallanger, A.E., Levey, A.I., Lee, H.J., Rye, D.B., and Wainer, B.H. The origins of cholinergic and other subcortical afferents to the thalamus in the rat. *J Comp Neurol* 1987; 262:105–24.

Hokfelt, T., Holets, V.R., Staines, W., Meister, B., Melander, T., and Schalling, M. Coexistence of neuronal messengers: An overview. *Prog Brain Res* 1986; 68:33–70.

Hokfelt, T., Skorboll, L.R., Rehfeld, J.F., Goldstein, M., Markey, K., and Dann, O. A subpopulation of mescencephalic dopamine neurons projecting to limbic areas contains a cholecystokinin-like peptide. *Neuroscience* 1980; 5:2093–124.

Holets, V., Hokfelt, T., Rokaeus, A., Terenius, L., and Goldstein, M. Locus coeruleus neurons in the rat containing neuropeptide Y, tyrosine hydroxylase or galanin and their projections to the spinal cord, cerebral cortex or hypothalamus. *Neuroscience* 1988; 24:893–906.

Hornykiewicz, O. Dopamine (3-hydroxytryptamine) and brain function. *Pharmacol Rev* 1966; 18:925–64.

Johanssen, O., Hokfelt, T., Pernov, B., Jeffcoate, S.L., White, W., Steinbusch, H., Verhofstad, A., Emson, P.C., and Spindel, E. Immunohistochemical support for three putative transmitters in one neuron: Coexistence of 5-hydroxytryptamine, substance P, and thyrotropin releasing hormone-like immunoreactivity in medullary neurons projecting to spinal cord. *Neuroscience* 1981; 6:1857–81.

Kromer, L.F., and Moore, R.Y. A study of the organization of the locus coeruleus projections to the lateral geniculate nucleus in the albino rat. *Neuroscience* 1980; 5:255–71.

Levey, A.I., Hallanger, A.E., and Wainer, B.H. Choline acetyltransferase immunoreactivity in the rat thalamus. *J Comp Neurol* 1987; 257:317–32.

Levitt, P.R., and Moore, R.Y. Noradrenaline neuron innervation of the neocortex in the rat. *Brain Res* 1978; 139:219–31.

Levitt, P.R., and Moore, R.Y. Origin and organization of brainstem catecholamine innervation in the rat. *J Comp Neurol* 1979; 186:505–28.

Lewis, D.A., Campbell, M.J., Foote, S.L., Goldstein, M., and Morrison, J.H. The distribution of tyrosine hydroxylase-immunoreactive fiber in primate neocortex is widespread but regionally specific. *J Neurosci* 1987; 7:279–90.

Lindvall, O., Bjorklund, A., Nobin, A., and Stenevi, U. The adrenergic innervation of the rat thalamus as revealed by the glyoxylic acid fluorescence method. *J Comp Neurol* 1974; 154:317–48.

Loughlin, S.E., Foote, S.L., and Grzanna, R. Efferent projections of the nucleus locus coeruleus. Morphologic subpopulations have different targets. *Neuroscience* 1986; 18:307–20.

Mesulam, M.M., and Geula, C. Nucleus basalis (Ch4) and cortical cholinergic innervation in the human brain: observations based on the distribution of acetylcholinesterase and choline acetyltransferase. *J Comp Neurol* 1988; 275:216–40.

Mesulam, M.M., and Mufson, E.J. Neural inputs into the nucleus basalis of the substantia innominata (Ch4) in the rhesus monkey. *Brain* 1984; 107:253–74.

Mesulam, M.M., Mufson, E.J., Levey, A.I., and Waimer, B.H. Cholinergic innervation of the cortex by the basal forebrain. Cytochemistry and cortical connections of the septal diagonal band, nucleus basalis (substantia innominata) and hypothalamus in the rhesus monkey. *J Comp Neurol* 1983a; 214:170–97.

Mesulam, M.M., and Mufson, E.J., and Wainer, B.H. Three-dimensional representation and cortical projection topography of the nucleus basalis (Ch4) in the macaque. *Brain Res* 1986; 367:301–4.

Mesulam, M.M., Mufson, E.J., Wainer, B.H., and Levey, A.I. Central cholinergic pathways in the rat: An overview based on an alternative nomenclature (Ch1–Ch6). *Neuroscience* 1983b; 10:1185–201.

Moore, R.Y. Catecholamine neuron systems in brain. *Ann Neurol* 1982; 12:321–7.

Moore, R.Y., and Bloom, F.E. Central catecholamine neuron systems: Anatomy and physiology of the dopamine systems. *Annu Rev Neurosci* 1978:1 129–69.

Moore, R.Y., and Card, J.P. Noradrenaline-containing neuron systems. In *Handbook of Chemical Neuroanatomy, Vol. 2.* Bjorklund, A., and Hokfelt, T. (eds.). Elsevier, Amsterdam, 1984, pp. 123–56.

Moore, R.Y., and Gustafson, E.L. The distribution of dopamine-β-hydroxylase, neuropeptide Y and galanin in locus coeruleus neurons. *J Chem Neuroanat* 1989; 2:95–106.

Moore, R.Y., Halaris, A.E., and Jones, B.E. Serotonin neurons of the midbrain raphe: Ascending projections. *J Comp Neurol* 1978; 180:417–38.

Olson, L., Seiger, A., and Fuxe, K. Heterogeneity of striatal and limbic dopamine innervation: Highly fluorescent islands in developing and adult rats. *Brain Res* 1972; 44:283–8.

Otterson, O.P., and Storm-Mathisen, J. Neurons containing or accumulating amino acids. In *Handbook of Chemical Neuroanatomy, Vol. 3.* Bjorklund, A., Hokfelt, T., and Kuhar, M.J., (eds.). Elsevier, Amsterdam, 1984, pp. 141–246.

Penney, J.B., Jr., and Young, A.B. Striatal inhomogeneities and basal ganglia function. *Movement Disorders* 1986; 1:3–15.

Ragsdale, C.W., and Graybiel, A.M. The frontostriatal projection in cat and monkey and its relationship to inhomogeneities established by acetylcholinesterase histochemistry. *Brain Res* 1981; 208:259–66.

Russchen, F.T., Amaral, D.G., and Price, J.L. The afferent connections of the substantia innominata in the monkey *Macaca fascicularis. J Comp Neurol* 1985; 242:1–27.

Rye, D.B., Saper, C.B., Lee, H.J., and Wainer, B.H. Pedunculopontine tegmental nucleus of the rat: Cytoarchitecture, cytochemistry, and some extrapyramidal connections of the mesopontine tegmentum. *J Comp Neurol* 1987; 259:483–528.

Shute, C.C.D., and Lewis, P.R. The ascending cholinergic reticular system: neocortical, olfactory and subcortical projections. *Brain* 1967; 90:497–520.

Soghomonian, J.-J., Descarries, L., and Watkins, K.C. Serotonin innervation in the adult rat neostriatum. II. Ultrastructural features. *Brain Res* 1989; 481:67–86.

Steinbusch, H.W.M. Distribution of serotonin immunoreactivity in the central nervous system of the rat: cell bodies and terminals. *Neuroscience* 1981; 6:557–618.

Young, A.B., and Penney, J.B., Jr. Biochemical and functional organization of the basal ganglia. In *Parkinson's Disease and Movement Disorders.* Jenkovic, J., and Tolosa, E. (eds.). Urban and Schwartzenberg, Baltimore, 1988, pp. 1–11.

5

Neurobehavioral Effects of Focal Subcortical Lesions

CHRISTOPHER M. FILLEY AND JAMES P. KELLY

Dementia is typically due to widespread or diffuse damage to cerebral areas, and the term *subcortical dementia* refers to a group of diseases that primarily affect subcortical regions. In contrast, more restricted neurobehavioral syndromes, such as aphasia and amnesia, are often due to focal cerebral pathology, and an enormous body of literature has evolved describing syndromes associated with discrete cortical damage. Focal subcortical lesions, however, have not been extensively studied, although many lines of evidence suggest that specific neurobehavioral syndromes may be associated with damage to certain subcortical structures. This chapter will summarize existing knowledge of the neurobehavioral effects of focal subcortical lesions and explore points of contention that remain unresolved.

The syndrome that has attracted the most interest is subcortical aphasia, descriptions of which have appeared in increasing numbers over the past decade. The study of amnesia related to focal subcortical disease has also advanced, and limited information on visuospatial deficits, cognitive impairments, and emotional disorders is available. The major neuroanatomic areas under scrutiny have been the thalamus, basal ganglia, and subcortical white matter, regions seen with increasing clarity using high-resolution imaging techniques such as computerized tomography (CT), magnetic resonance imaging (MRI), and positron emission tomography (PET).

APHASIA

Although the role of subcortical structures in the production of aphasia has long been suspected (Marie, 1906), only recently has systematic clinical investigation of this possibility begun in earnest. Aphasias have, of course, been regarded classically as linguistic syndromes related to left-hemisphere cortical injury. In his influential paper on disconnection syndromes, however, Geschwind postulated that conduction aphasia was due to a lesion in the arcuate fasciculus, a white matter tract projecting from temporoparietal association cortex to premotor frontal cortex (Geschwind, 1965). Since then, interest in the participation of subcortical structures in language function has steadily grown.

Aphasia in the context of focal subcortical disease has most often been noted after

deep left-hemisphere intracerebral hemorrhage (Hier et al., 1977; Alexander and
LoVerme, 1980), but more recent studies have focused on aphasias following ischemic
infarction (Naeser et al., 1982; Damasio et al., 1982; Graff-Radford et al., 1984).
Studies of patients undergoing stereotactic surgery (Riklan and Levita, 1969) and thalamic stimulation (Ojemann et al., 1968) have contributed information, as have reports
on patients with subcortical neoplasms (Cheek and Taveras, 1966). The following
review will emphasize the vascular etiologies and concentrate on aphasias that have
been ascribed to lesions in the thalamus, basal ganglia, and subcortical white matter.

Thalamus

The first clear description of the clinical syndrome related to thalamic hemorrhage was
that of Mohr et al. (1975). A profile of somnolence and fluctuating alertness was
described, accompanied by fluent, paraphasic speech, anomia, relatively good auditory comprehension, and preserved repetition (Mohr et al., 1975). Reynolds et al.
(1979) and Alexander and LoVerme (1980) observed a similar syndrome, with inattention, dysarthric but fluent speech, anomia, relatively preserved auditory comprehension, and intact repetition. The similarity of this syndrome to classical transcortical
aphasia has often been noted (Alexander and LoVerme, 1980; Cappa and Vignolo,
1979), although the variable preservation of fluency and auditory comprehension ren-
ders difficult a further classification into transcortical motor, transcortical sensory, or
mixed transcortical aphasia. Additional features in these cases have included perseveration (Mohr et al., 1975), neologisms (Reynolds et al., 1979), dysgraphia (Cappa
and Vignolo, 1979), right hemineglect (Alexander and LoVerme, 1980), echolalia
(Mohr et al., 1975), and memory impairment (Alexander and LoVerme, 1980). Although these cases were all associated with left thalamic lesions, one case of right
thalamic hemorrhage with aphasia has been reported (Kirshner and Kistler, 1982); in
this patient, a converted sinistral, the aphasia was similar to those cited earlier. Recovery has often been observed to be complete or nearly so within weeks to months.
   Ischemic lesions of the left thalamus have also been studied clinically, and again
the preservation of repetition is the striking feature (McFarling et al., 1982; Graff-
Radford et al., 1984; Gorelick et al., 1984; Tuszynski and Petito, 1988). Syndromes
identifiable as transcortical sensory aphasia (Graff-Radford et al., 1984; Gorelick et
al., 1984), transcortical motor aphasia (McFarling et al., 1982), and mixed transcortical aphasia (McFarling et al., 1982; Tuszynski and Petito, 1988) have been described.
The case of Tuszynski and Petito (1988) was examined post mortem, and pathology
was confined to the left thalamus; dorsomedial (DM), lateral posterior, and ventral
lateral nuclei appeared to be involved.
   Stereotactic thalamotomies performed for movement disorders commonly cause
postoperative dysarthria and hypophonia (Riklan and Levita, 1969). These deficits
only occur with left-sided lesions. Anomia has also been observed in up to 42 percent
of such patients, but other language functions are not significantly compromised, and
the word-finding difficulties generally improve (Selby, 1967). Studies of left thalamic
stimulation have supported the concept of language function mediated by the thalamus;
stimulation of the pulvinar, which is connected to temporoparietal language cortex,
has resulted in anomia (Ojemann et al., 1968).

Patients with thalamic tumors have been described as aphasic (Cheek and Taveras, 1966), in association with other deficits such as inattention, hypophonia, perseveration, and memory disturbance. In these cases, however, the effects of a mass lesion on surrounding tissue may often be significant.

Basal Ganglia

In general, speech disturbances such as dysarthria, hypophonia, and palilalia are known to occur with disease of the basal ganglia (Darley et al., 1975), but language disorders have been less clearly related. Most of the information pertains to lesions of the striatum, particularly the putamen, and many cases appear to demonstrate damage to adjacent white matter as well.

An early report described aphasia ("total aphasia" or "echolalia") in five of seven noncomatose patients with left putaminal hypertensive hemorrhage (Hier et al., 1977). A more detailed study (Alexander and LoVerme, 1980) concluded that six patients with similar lesions had transcortical aphasia that was not decisively different from the aphasia noted in nine patients from the same study who had thalamic hemorrhage.

Several reports on ischemic lesions of the basal ganglia have become available. Brunner et al. (1982) noted a pattern of transcortical motor aphasia in patients with left basal ganglia infarctions. Naeser et al. (1982) carefully described nine patients with left internal capsule/putaminal lesions (eight infarcts and one hemorrhage). Three profiles emerged:

1. Capsular/putaminal with anterior–superior white matter extension.
2. Capsular/putaminal with posterior white matter extension.
3. Capsular/putaminal with both anterior–superior and posterior extension (Naeser et al., 1982).

Whereas the last group had global aphasia, the first two had syndromes that were difficult to classify; overall, the first group had better comprehension than fluency, and the second group had the reverse (Naeser et al., 1982). It is notable that repetition was impaired in all nine patients (Naeser et al., 1982). Another report (Damasio et al., 1982) reached similar conclusions after considering 11 patients with nonhemorrhagic lesions in the basal ganglia and internal capsule; classification of syndromes into traditional aphasia types was not possible, and aphasia features themselves, such as impaired repetition, were quite variable. A notable feature was frequent dysarthria, and the authors made a general comment that the syndromes resembled those described in thalamic and putaminal hemorrhage (Damasio et al., 1982). One reason why these patients had a more elusive syndrome was the small size of the lesions compared with the patients in the study by Naeser et al. (1982).

An investigation of 12 cases of subcortical aphasia (six infarcts and six hemorrhages) tentatively supported Naeser and colleagues (Cappa et al., 1983). These investigators distinguished between anterior subcortical lesions, involving the putamen and anterior limb of the internal capsule, which are sometimes associated with atypical nonfluent aphasias, and posterior subcortical lesions, involving the putamen and posterior limb of the internal capsule, which are sometimes associated with atypical fluent aphasias (Cappa et al., 1983).

White Matter

Lesions of the subcortical white matter have been neglected in discussions of aphasia until recently, despite the emphasis placed upon white matter tracts by Geschwind (1965). The rarity (Almos-Lau et al., 1977) or inapparent nature (Filley et al., 1989) of aphasic disturbance in multiple sclerosis may account for some of this bias. Alexander et al. (1987), after a presentation of 19 cases of subcortical infarcts or hemorrhages and a review of 61 published cases, concluded that lesions in white matter were critical for all components of aphasia. These authors then provided an elegant model for the understanding of language function related to white matter tracts: Fluency is dependent on superior periventricular and internal capsule white matter, speech initiation on white matter pathways from the supplementary motor area to Broca's area, repetition on external and extreme capsules and/or the arcuate fasciculus, and auditory comprehension on the temporal isthmus and auditory association pathways in the corpus callosum (Alexander et al., 1987).

Despite the recent growth of interest in subcortical aphasia, the data are still too few to permit firm conclusions about the type(s), or even the presence, of aphasia associated with subcortical lesions. Criticism of the concept comes from several viewpoints.

The clinical variability of syndromes is striking, even though a transcortical type of aphasia with normal repetition has often been found. It is perhaps not surprising that subcortical syndromes often do not fit classical "cortical" categories, but this ambiguity pervades the available clinical information. One consistent feature, however, is that predominantly left subcortical lesions are associated with aphasia.

Pathologic verification of clinically detected lesions has been notably lacking, substantiating the criticism that the exact areas damaged are not well delineated, despite the improvements in localization offered by CT, MRI, and PET. The case of Tuszynski and Petito (1988) may signal a welcome change in this trend.

Perhaps the most significant doubts relate to the possible influence of other pathology associated with the primary lesion. Geschwind (1967) expressed reservations about the existence of thalamic aphasia, pointing out that pressure and edema from the acute lesion could explain language dysfunction. Alexander and LoVerme (1980) also raised this possibility and queried in addition whether transient ischemic effects could occur in left-hemisphere cortical areas. A PET study of three patients with a subcortical lesion and aphasia disclosed that all had cortical metabolic changes in addition to subcortical hypometabolism (Metter et al., 1983). Even more impressive was a regional cerebral blood flow study of 18 patients with left subcortical lesions; 8 had aphasia that was accompanied by low-flow areas in the overlying cortex, while 10 had no aphasia and normal overlying cortical flow (Skyhoj Olsen et al., 1986). The authors contended that the aphasia was not due to subcortical disease, but to hypoperfusion in a related cortical area (the "ischemic penumbra") critical to language function. The good recovery of many subcortical aphasics is another point in favor of transient cortical dysfunction.

Aphasia associated with subcortical lesions is a controversial syndrome. Many authorities accept the existence of this entity, but debate centers on what type(s) of aphasia exist(s) and what the relative contribution of subcortical and cortical regionsis. Lesions of the left subcortical area appear to be associated with aphasia much more

Table 5-1 Common Features of Subcortical Aphasia

Fluent paraphasic speech
Mild or absent comprehension deficit
Intact repetition
Anomia
Inattention/neglect
Dysarthria
Perseveration
Memory impairment

than those on the right, but often only mild anomia or speech deficits may be present, or the patient may even be normal in terms of speech and language function. If a single profile of subcortical aphasias can be tentatively proposed, it is that of a transcortical aphasia (Table 5-1), although many other aphasias have been described.

AMNESIA

Amnesia is a disturbance of memory characterized by impaired learning of new verbal or nonverbal material (anterograde amnesia), usually with less prominently impaired retrieval of long-term memories (retrograde amnesia). Excellent reviews of the subject have been written by Butters and Miliotis (1985) and Signoret (1985). The debate over the neuroanatomic basis of memory revolves around temporal lobe and limbic system structures. The structure most commonly accepted as the locus of the new memory formation is the hippocampus, deep within the medial temporal lobe. It is generally accepted that bilateral lesions of the medial temporal lobes can cause severe amnesic states. The work of Scoville and Milner (1957) and Penfield and Milner (1958) established the hippocampal memory hypothesis through careful studies of patients undergoing temporal lobectomy for control of seizures. Lesions confined to more anterior temporal regions involving only the uncus and amygdala did not produce amnesia. Resections involving the hippocampus produced an amnesic disorder, with the posterior extent of the lesion determining the severity of the memory deficit; that is, the more posterior the lesion, the more impaired were the patient's memory functions. However, both cortical and subcortical temporal lobe structures were resected in these procedures, and a critique of the hippocampal memory hypothesis has been provided by Horel (1978).

There have been several reports of focal subcortical lesions associated with disorders of memory. Most studies of amnesia related to diencephalic lesions concentrate on the mamillary bodies or their connections (Kahn and Crosby, 1972). The nystagmus, ophthalmoplegia, ataxia, and transient confusional state of Wernicke's encephalopathy, along with the more persistent amnesic syndrome associated with apathy, confabulation, and loss of insight of Korsakoff's syndrome, is a well-recognized neurologic condition. The cause of the Wernicke-Korsakoff syndrome is a nutritional disorder of thiamine deficiency, most commonly seen in alcoholics. Lesions are seen in the mamillary bodies, anterior columns of the fornix, portions of the hypothalamus, and portions of the thalamus including the DM nucleus, dorsolateral (DL) nucleus,

(DL) nucleus, and medial pulvinar. Victor et al. (1971) theorized that involvement of the DM nucleus was central to the development of amnesia, as those patients with mamillary body lesions but intact DM nuclei had no memory disturbance. Other investigators found contradictory evidence in patients with Korsakoff's amnesia. Mair et al. (1979) followed two alcoholic patients with Korsakoff's psychosis for 3 or more years, employing detailed measures of memory and intelligence. Both patients had relative sparing of short-term memory and other cognitive functions while long-term memory was significantly impaired. Post mortem pathologic examination revealed gliosis and atrophy in the medial nuclei of the mamillary bodies as well as gliosis between the DM nucleus and the wall of the third ventricle. The DM nucleus itself was spared, raising the question of whether the DM nucleus must be involved directly or if its disconnection from limbic structures is sufficient to cause Korsakoff's amnesic state.

McEntee et al. (1976) reported the case of a patient exhibiting severe amnesia associated with a metastatic tumor involving bilateral medial and posterior thalamic nuclei. In this case the mamillary bodies, mamillothalamic tracts, anterior thalami, and Ammon's horn configuration were normal bilaterally. These findings supported the hypothesis of Victor et al. (1971) that lesions of the DM nucleus can cause amnesic syndromes without mamillary body involvement. Subsequent reports have documented unilateral lesions of the DM nucleus associated with specific memory impairment. Squire and Moore (1979) reported the case of a young man who suffered a stab wound with a miniature fencing foil that entered the cranial cavity by piercing the ethmoid bone through the right nostril. The focal lesion identified in a CT scan was in the left DM nucleus of the thalamus, sparing the fornix and mamillary bodies. His memory deficit involved anterograde amnesia for verbal material. Speedie and Heilman (1982) described a patient with left thalamic infarction associated with similar anterograde amnesia for verbal information. Other authors have criticized these studies because of the uncertainty of lesion location, which was typically determined by CT scan only. Mori et al. (1986) reported disturbances of verbal memory processing in a 41-year-old right-handed man. Using recently developed CT stereotactic techniques and MRI with three-directional sectioning, they localized their patient's infarct to the left ventrolateral nucleus, centromedian–parafascicular nuclei complex, internal medullary lamina, and mamillothalamic tract. Speedie and Heilman (1983) later described a patient exhibiting anterograde amnesia for visuospatial information after infarction of the right DM nucleus. Three patients reported by Choi et al. (1983) were found to have a prominent memory disturbance following hemorrhagic destruction of the medial thalamus as noted on CT scans.

Ziegler et al. (1977) reported a less convincing case of memory deficit in a patient with glioblastoma multiforme involving both thalami and the medial aspects of both temporal lobes. While the authors suggested that their patient's retrograde amnesia and inability to recognize some familiar faces were due to right thalamic tumor, pathologic examination found the mass to be infiltrating many diencephalic and limbic structures. Moonis et al. (1988) proposed the notion that transient global amnesia, as seen in a case of left thalamic hemorrhage, can be due to pressure effects and/or secondary ischemia rather than direct tissue damage, but this phenomenon had not been reported previously.

Kooistra and Heilman (1988) have recently reported a case of severe persistent verbal memory deficit resulting from an infarct in the posterior limb of the left internal capsule. The authors speculated that this lesion caused memory disturbance by effectively disconnecting the DM nucleus from amygdaloid and prefrontal areas. Lesions of the internal capsule had not previously been reported to cause amnesia. This report raises the possibility that memory disturbance associated with other diseases of white matter, such as multi-infarct dementia and multiple sclerosis, might be the result of similar pathway disconnection.

NEGLECT

The preponderance of evidence suggests that the right hemisphere is dominant for visuospatial integration and directed attention (Mesulam, 1985; Heilman et al., 1985; Denny-Brown and Chambers, 1958). Recently, the role of the right hemisphere in vigilance and arousal has been documented (Heilman et al., 1978). It is widely accepted that lesions of the right hemisphere produce a neglect syndrome much more commonly than do similar lesions of the left hemisphere (Mesulam, 1985; Heilman et al., 1985). In brief, the neglect syndrome is the failure to respond to stimuli presented to the side opposite the brain lesion in the absence of motor or sensory deficits. Features of the syndrome include hemi-inattention, extinction to double simultaneous stimulation, hemispatial agnosia, hemiakinesia, and anosognosia.

Historically, this syndrome had been described in association with lesions of the right parietal lobe, both in humans and in experimental animals (Eidelberg and Schwartz, 1971). This phenomenon has since been noted following lesions of the nondominant frontal lobe (Heilman and Valenstein, 1972). More recent literature has focused on the role of subcortical structures in mechanisms of attention.

Watson et al. (1974) created discrete unilateral mesencephalic reticular formation lesions in monkeys and produced profound contralateral tactile, visual, and auditory neglect. The alerting function of the reticular formation was therefore linked to attentional mechanisms of higher structures. These data lent support to the theory that neglect could be produced by unilateral lesions in a corticolimbic–reticular activating loop. Watson et al. (1973) had previously demonstrated that neglect could be produced by cingulectomy, suggesting that the syndrome could result from corticolimbic–reticular activating disconnection. In a review of 24 patients who had suffered putaminal hemorrhage, 12 of the 16 noncomatose patients presented with some form of neurobehavioral dysfunction (Hier et al. 1977). There was a variety of nondominant hemisphere syndromes in patients with right putaminal hemorrhage, including unilateral neglect, apractognosia, and anosognosia.

Watson and Heilman (1979) described three patients with right thalamic hemorrhage resulting in contralateral neglect as well as with anosognosia, visuospatial disorders, and emotional flattening. The same group later reported neglect in a patient who had suffered ischemic infarction of the right medial thalamus (Watson et al., 1981). They proposed that the mesencephalic reticular activating system produces tonic arousal by inhibiting the nucleus reticularis thalami, and that selective attention is mediated by cortical input to the same thalamic nucleus. Soon thereafter, Healton et al. (1982) reported the first autopsy-confirmed example of neglect resulting from hemorrhagic infarction of the striatum and adjacent deep white matter. They proposed a modification of the Watson and Heilman theory, suggesting that the striatum may mediate intention (motor activation) after selective attention and arousal. Thus, symptoms of neglect may appear as a pathophysiological consequence of damage to the striatum.

COGNITIVE IMPAIRMENTS

A careful study of residual neuropsychological deficits detected after small unilateral thalamic lesions was conducted by Wallesch et al. (1983). This group applied a thorough battery of neuropsychological tests to 13 right-handed patients who had CT evidence of small, well-demarcated unilateral thalamic lesions caused by either ischemia or hemorrhage. Included in their design were comparisons of test performance with age-matched normal controls and age-matched patients with white matter lesions of larger size than those of the thalamic lesion subjects. Some of their results are unexpected in view of other reports mentioned in this chapter.

First, the performance of patients with left thalamic lesions was worse than that of patients with right thalamic lesions on all test measurements, even though the average lesion size for the two groups was nearly identical. The authors also made the point that their findings offered no supportive evidence of the lateralization of verbal functions to the left and visuoconstructive or visuospatial functions to the right. These results are in direct contradiction with those of authors cited previously (Speedie and Heilman, 1982; Speedie and Heilman, 1983; Mori et al., 1986; Squire and Moore, 1979).

Furthermore, small thalamic lesions were found to produce general impairment of cognitive function, while similar but less pronounced deficits were noted with significantly larger white matter lesions. Those who theorize an entirely cortical representation of cognition would have anticipated the reverse association (i.e., cortico-cortical disconnection due to a white matter lesion would be expected to produce greater cognitive deficits than a smaller thalamic lesion).

Finally, there appeared to be some evidence for dissociation of cognitive functions between rostral and caudal lesion location within the thalamus. Rostral thalamic lesions were associated with disturbance of memory and learning, while caudal lesions produced deficits of abstract conceptualization and categorization. These findings support the work of Victor et al. (1971), who contended that lesions of the DM nucleus are associated with memory disturbance.

MOOD DISORDERS

An analysis of mood disorders following stroke has been advanced by Starkstein et al. (1987). Well over 200 patients with thromboembolic cerebral infarction or intracerebral hemorrhage were assessed for evidence of mood changes after CT scans were obtained to distinguish cortical from subcortical lesion location. The results indicated that subcortical lesions in the left hemisphere were associated with similar frequency and severity of depression as cortical lesions. Right hemisphere lesions did not correlate with depression but were associated with a higher incidence of undue cheerfulness. Measures of cognitive function employed in this study demonstrated no significant difference between right–left or cortical–subcortical groups.

A subsequent study by the same group found that patients with unilateral left-sided basal ganglia infarcts or hemorrhages had significantly higher frequency and severity of depression than those with right-sided basal ganglia or thalamic (left- or right-sided) lesions (Starkstein et al., 1988). Damage to ascending biogenic amine pathways or to frontocaudate projections may be responsible for this finding (Starkstein et al., 1988).

CONCLUSION

Focal subcortical lesions offer a unique opportunity to observe a variety of syndromes in behavioral neurology. Table 5-2 displays the subcortical structures that have been implicated in several of these syndromes. Although experience is limited, these structures may represent deep portions of cerebral circuits devoted to specific neurobehavioral capacities. This hypothesis finds anatomical support, for example, in the known connections between pulvinar and posterior language cortex, or the connections between the DM nucleus of the thalamus and the hippocampus. Thus there may be specific subcortical contributions to individual neurobehavioral functions; Mesulam (1985) has described these "channel-dependent" functions as based upon cortical–subcortical interactions. This theory does not, of course, deny the existence of more general, nonspecific subcortical activities such as arousal, attention, and motivation, which Mesulam has termed "state-dependent" functions. On the basis of the available data, it would seem most reasonable to consider that the subcortex may participate in both general cortical activation and in specific neurobehavioral functions.

The considerable variability of focal subcortical syndromes, coupled with uncertain lesion localization and questions about remote effects on cortical structures, con-

Table 5-2 Subcortical Structures Implicated in Selected Neurobehavioral Syndromes

Syndrome	Structure(s)
Aphasia[a]	Thalamus
	Striatum
	White matter
Amnesia	DM thalamic nucleus
	Mamillary bodies
Neglect[b]	Mesencephalic reticular formation
	Cingulate gyrus
	Striatum
	Thalamus
Cognitive Impairment	Caudal thalamus
Mood Disorder	Anterior subcortical regions

[a]Typically with left hemisphere lesions.
[b]More notably with right hemisphere lesions.

tinue to becloud this intriguing topic. Nevertheless, clinical evidence has strongly suggested a crucial role for subcortical structures in the process of intellect and behavior. It may no longer be appropriate to use the term *higher cortical function* in discussing the cerebral basis of language, memory, and other abilities. Further research, using sophisticated neuroimaging technology, careful clinical evaluation, long-term follow-up, and pathologic verification whenever possible, should permit further exploration of the neurobehavioral significance of subcortical regions.

REFERENCES

Alexander, M.P., and LoVerme, S.R. Aphasia after left hemispheric intracerebral hemorrhage. *Neurology* 1980; 30:1193–202.

Alexander, M.P., Naeser, M.A., and Palumbo, C.L. Correlations of subcortical CT lesion sites and aphasia profiles. *Brain* 1987; 110:961–91.

Almos-Lau, N., Ginsberg, M.D., and Geller, J.B. Aphasia in multiple sclerosis. *Neurology* 1977; 27:623–6.

Brunner, R.J., Kornhuber, H.H., Seemuller, E., et al. Basal ganglia participation in language pathology. *Brain Lang* 1982; 16:281–99.

Butters, N., and Miliotis, P. Amnesic disorders. In *Clinical Neuropsychology.* Heilman, K.M., and Valenstein, E. (eds.). Oxford, New York, 1985, pp. 403–52.

Cappa, S.F., Cavallotti, G., Guidotti, M., et al. Subcortical aphasia: two clinical CT-scan correlation studies. *Cortex* 1983; 19:227–41.

Cappa, S.F., and Vignolo, L.A. "Transcortical" features of aphasia following left thalamic hemorrhage. *Cortex* 1979; 15:121–30.

Cheek, W.R., and Taveras, J.M. Thalamic tumors. *J Neurosurg* 1966; 24:505–13.

Choi, D., Sudarsky, L., Schachter, S., et al. Medial thalamic hemorrhage with amnesia. *Arch Neurol* 1983; 40:611–3.

Damasio, A.R., Damasio, H., Rizzo, M., et al. Aphasia with nonhemorrhagic lesions in the basal ganglia and internal capsule. *Arch Neurol* 1982; 39:15–20.

Darley, F.L., Aronson, A.E., and Brown, J.R. *Motor Speech Disorders.* W.B. Saunders, Philadelphia, 1975.

Denny-Brown, D., and Chambers, R.A. *The Parietal Lobe and Behavior. Research Publications: Association for Research in Neurones and Mental Disease.* Vol. 36. 1958, pp. 35–117.

Eidelberg, E., and Schwartz, A.J. Experimental analysis of the extinction phenomenon in monkeys. *Brain* 1971; 94:91–108.

Filley, C.M., Heaton, R.K., Nelson, L.M., et al. A comparison of dementia in Alzheimer's Disease and multiple sclerosis. *Arch Neurol* 1989; 46:157–61.

Geschwind, N. Disconnexion syndromes in animals and man. *Brain* 1965; 88:237–94, 585–644.

Geschwind, N. Discussion of cerebral connectionism and brain function. In *Brain Mechanisms Underlying Speech and Language.* Millikay, C.H., and Darley, F.L. (eds.). Grune and Stratton, New York, 1967, pp. 71–2.

Gorelick, P.B., Hier, D.B., Benevento, L., et al. Aphasia after left thalamic infarction. *Arch Neurol* 1984; 41:1296–8.

Graff-Radford, N.R., Eslinger, P.J., Damasio, A.R., and Yamada, T. Nonhemorrhagic infarction of the thalamus: behavioral, anatomic, and physiologic correlates. *Neurology* 1984; 34:14–23.

Healton, E.B., Navarro, C., Bressman, S., and Brust, J.C.M. Subcortical neglect. *Neurology* 1982; 31:776–8.

Heilman, K.M., Schwartz, H.D., and Watson, R.T. Hypoarousal in patients with neglect syndrome and emotional indifference. *Neurology* 1978; 28:229–32.

Heilman, K.M., and Valenstein, E. Frontal lobe neglect in man. *Neurology* 1972; 22:660–4.

Heilman, K.M., Watson, R.T., and Valenstein, E. Neglect and related disorders. In *Clinical Neuropsychology.* Heilman, K.M., and Valenstein, E. (eds.). Oxford, New York, 1985, pp. 243–93.

Hier, D.B., Davis, K.R., Richardson, E.P., and Mohr, J.P. Hypertensive putaminal hemorrhage. *Ann Neurol* 1977; 1:152–9.

Horel, J.A. The neuroanatomy of amnesia: A critique of the hippocampal memory hypothesis. *Brain* 1978; 101:403–45.

Kahn, E., and Crosby, E.C. Korsakoff's syndrome associated with surgical lesions involving the mammillary bodies. *Neurology* 1972; 22:117–25.

Kirshner, H.S., and Kistler, K.H. Aphasia after right thalamic hemorrhage. *Arch Neurol* 1982; 39:667–9.

Kooistra, C.A., and Heilman, K.M. Memory loss from a subcortical white matter infarct. *J Neurol Neurosurg Psychiatry* 1988; 51:866–9.

Mair, W.G.P., Warrington, E.K., and Weiskrantz, L. Memory disorder in Korsakoff's psychosis: a neuropathological and neuropsychological investigation of two cases. *Brain* 1979; 102:749–83.

Marie, P. Revision de la question de l'aphasie. *Semaine Med* 1906; 26:241–7, 493–500, 565–71.

McEntee, W.J., Biber, M.P., Perl, D.P., and Benson, D.F. Diencephalic amnesia: A reappraisal. *J Neurol Neurosurg Psychiatry* 1976; 39:436–41.

McFarling, D., Rothi, L.J., and Heilman, K.M. Transcortical aphasia from ischaemic infarcts of the thalamus: a report of two caes. *J Neurol Neurosurg Psychiatry* 1982; 45:107–12.

Mesulam, M.-M. *Principles of Behavioral Neurology.* F.A. Davis, Philadelphia, 1985, pp. 1–70, 125–68.

Metter, E.J., Riege, W.H., Hanson, W.R., et al. Comparison of metabolic rates, language, and memory in subcortical aphasias. *Brain Lang* 1983; 19:33–47.

Mohr, J.P., Watters, W.C., and Duncan, G.W. Thalamic hemorrhage and aphasia. *Brain Lang* 1975; 2:3–17.

Moonis, M., Jain, S., Prasad, K., et al. Left thalamic hypertensive haemorrhage presenting as transient global amnesia. *Acta Neurol Scand* 1988; 77:331–4.

Mori, E., Yamadori, A., and Mitani, Y. Left thalamic infarction and disturbance of verbal memory: A clinicoanatomical study with a new method of computed tomographic stereotaxic lesion localization. *Ann Neurol* 1986; 20:671–6.

Naeser, M.A., Alexander, M.A., Helm-Estabrooks, N., et al. Aphasia with predominantly subcortical lesion sites: description of three capular/putaminal aphasia syndromes. *Arch Neurol* 1982; 29:2–14.

Ojemann, G.A., Fedio, P., and VanBuren, J.M. Anomia from pulvinar and subcortical white matter stimulation. *Brain* 1968; 91:99–116.

Penfield, W., and Milner, B. Memory deficit produced by bilateral lesions in the hippocampal zone. *Arch Neurol Psychiatry* 1958; 79:475–97.

Reynolds, A.F., Turner, P.T., Harris, A.B., et al. Left thalamic hemorrhage with dysphasia: A report of five cases. *Brain Lang* 1979; 7:62–73.

Riklan, M., and Levita, E. *Subcortical Correlates of Human Behavior: A Psychological Study of Basal Ganglia and Thalamic Surgery.* Williams and Wilkins, Baltimore, 1969.

Scoville, W.B., and Milner, B. Loss of recent memory after bilateral hippocampal lesions. *J Neurol Neurosurg Psychiatry* 1957; 20:11–21.

Selby, G. Stereotactic surgery for the relief of Parkinson's disease. Part 2. An analysis of the results in a series of 303 patients (413 operations). *J Neurol Sci* 1967; 5:343–75.

Signoret, J.L. Memory and amnesias. In *Principles of Behavioral Neurology.* Mesulam, M.-M. (ed.). F.A. Davis, Philadelphia, 1985, pp. 169–92.

Skyhoj Olsen, T., Bruhn, P., and Oberg, G.E. Cortical hypoperfusion as a possible cause of "subcortical aphasia." *Brain* 1986; 109:393–410.

Speedie, L.S., and Heilman, K.M. Amnestic disturbance following infarction of the dorsomedial nucleus of the thalamus. Read before the International Neuropsychological Society, Pittsburgh, Pennsylvania, Feb. 5, 1982.

Speedie, L.J., and Heilman, K.M. Anterograde memory deficits for visuospatial material after infarction of right thalamus. *Arch Neurol* 1983; 40:183–6.

Squire, L.R., and Moore, R.Y. Dorsal thalamic lesion in a noted case of human memory dysfunction. *Ann Neurol* 1979; 6:503–6.

Starkstein, S.E., Robinson, R.G., Berthier, M.L., et al. Differential mood changes following basal ganglia vs thalamic lesions. *Arch Neurol* 1988; 45:725–30.

Strakstein, S.E., Robinson, R.G., and Price, T.R. Comparison of cortical and subcortical lesions in the production of poststroke mood disorders. *Brain* 1987; 110:1045–59.

Tuszynski, M.H., and Petito, C.K. Ischemic thalamic aphasia with pathologic confirmation. *Neurology* 1988; 38:800–2.

Victor, M., Adams, R.D., and Collins, G.H. *The Wernicke-Korsakoff Syndrome.* F.A. Davis, Philadelphia, 1971.

Wallesch, C.W., Kornhuber, H.H., Kunz, T., and Brunner, R.J. Neuropsychological deficits associated with small unilateral thalamic lesions. *Brain* 1983; 106:141–52.

Watson, R.T., and Heilman, K.M. Thalamic neglect. *Neurology* 1979; 29:690–4.

Watson, R.T., Heilman, K.M., Cauthen, J.C., and King, F.A. Neglect after cingulectomy. *Neurology* 1973; 23:1003–7.

Watson, R.T., Heilman, K.M., Miller, B.D., and King, F.A. Neglect after mesencephalic reticular formation lesions. *Neurology* 1974; 24:294–8.

Watson, R.T., Valenstein, E., and Heilman, K.M. Thalamic neglect: Possible role of the medial thalamus and nucleus reticularis in behavior. *Arch Neurol* 1981; 38:501–6.

Ziegler, D.K., Kaufman, A., and Marshall, H.E. Abrupt memory loss associated with thalamic tumor. *Arch Neurol* 1977; 34:545–8.

6

Neuropsychological Assessment of Subcortical Dementia

STEVEN J. HUBER AND EDWIN C. SHUTTLEWORTH

The dementia syndrome is characterized by an acquired, persistent, and usually progressive impairment of intellect. Both the clinical features and underlying pathophysiology, however, may vary systematically among different diseases. In this chapter neuropsychological features characteristic of cortical and subcortical dementias are outlined, and assessment techniques appropriate for detecting and exploring subcortical dementias are emphasized.

Cortical dementias occur in disorders having pathologic changes predominantly in neocortical association areas with relative sparing of subcortical structures other than the hippocampus, and dementia of the Alzheimer type (DAT) is the most common example. Subcortical dementias have pathologic changes located primarily in deep structures such as the basal ganglia, thalamus, and brain stem, with relative sparing of the cerebral cortex. Subcortical dementia syndromes have most notably been associated with progressive supranuclear palsy (PSP) (Albert et al., 1974), Huntington's disease (HD) (McHugh and Folstein, 1975), Parkinson's disease (PD) (Albert, 1978; Marsden, 1978; Benson, 1983; Cummings and Benson, 1984), multiple sclerosis (MS) (Rao, 1986; Huber et al., 1987), multi-infarct dementia (MID) (Cummings and Benson, 1983), depressive dementia (Folstein and McHugh, 1978; Caine, 1981), and the acquired immune deficiency syndrome (AIDS) dementia complex (Navia et al., 1986).

Subcortical dementias differ clinically from cortical dementias both quantitatively and qualitatively. Quantitatively, cortical dementias tend to have more severe impairment of memory, cognition, and visuospatial function. Subcortical disorders, on the other hand, tend to manifest greater impairment in procedural memory, speed of information processing, and concept formation, and disturbances of mood, including apathy and depression. Qualitatively, subcortical disorders lack the symptoms of aphasia, agnosia, and apraxia typical of patients with cortical dysfunction.

CLINICAL FEATURES AND ASSESSMENT METHODS

Memory

Impairment of memory in dementia is nearly universal and is usually the initial symptom. Immediate memory, the ability to retain information when given constant attention, is typically preserved in demented patients with normal attentiveness. The digit-span task (Wechsler, 1945) is a common method used to assess immediate memory function. In the digits-forward procedure, subjects are presented with increasingly longer strings of numbers, and the task is to repeat them in their original order. Normal performance is on the order of 7 ± 2 items (Miller, 1956). Performance on the digit-span task is not significantly impaired in patients with DAT (Rosen, 1983; Storandt et al., 1984; Huber et al., 1986a; Pillon et al., 1986), PD (Huber et al., 1986a,b; Pillon et al., 1986), HD (Caine et al., 1977; Butters et al., 1978), and MS (Rao et al., 1984; Huber et al., 1987). Pillon et al. (1986), however, did find impairment in the digit-span task for patients with PSP.

Recent memory, the ability to retrieve newly acquired information, is almost always impaired. Auditory verbal recent memory is most often assessed by the paired-associates procedure (Wechsler, 1945). In this test word pairs that are related (easy) and unrelated (hard) are read to the subject, and the task is to recall the second item when provided with the first. Because the easy items are semantically related (e.g., north-south), it is questionable whether this portion of the task is of much value. A better measure of recent memory might be the distractor procedure developed by Peterson and Peterson (1959). Three consonants are presented to the subject, followed immediately by a distractor task. This involves counting backwards from 100 by 3s for anywhere from 3 to 18 seconds, the intent being to prevent rehearsal of the to-be-remembered items.

Impairment of recent memory is present in patients with DAT (Rosen, 1983; Storandt et al., 1984; Huber et al., 1986a), PD (Pirozzolo et al., 1982; Huber et al., 1986b), HD (Caine et al., 1977; Josiassen et al., 1983; Huber and Paulson, 1987), and MS (Rao et al., 1984; Huber et al., 1987; Beatty et al., 1988). Two studies found impairment of recent memory to be more severe in patients with DAT compared with PD (Gainotti et al., 1980; Huber et al., 1986a), but Pillon et al. (1986) did not.

Impairment of recent memory in patients with PD and HD is associated with both encoding and retrieval difficulties (Caine et al., 1977; Tweedy et al., 1982; Huber and Paulson, 1987), as ascertained by a failure to exhibit release from proactive interference during recall. In patients with HD, the emergence of these memory-processing impairments is also associated with progressive slowing of information processing (Huber and Paulson, 1987).

Remote memory, the ability to recall information learned prior to the onset of disease, can be assessed by a standardized procedure developed by Albert and associates (1979). This procedure examines knowledge of famous people and news events from the 1920s to the 1970s. Remote memory is impaired in patients with DAT (Moscovitch et al., 1981; Albert et al., 1981a), PD (Huber et al., 1986b), HD (Albert et al., 1981b), and MS (Beatty et al., 1988). One report (Moscovitch et al., 1981) found a temporal gradient of remote memory in DAT. Very remote memories were spared relative to more recent information, a finding similar to that seen in amnestic patients (Korsakoff's syndrome). Another report, however, found equal impairment of remote memory across decades for patients with DAT (Albert et al., 1981a). All reports on patients with PD, HD, and MS found that impairment of remote memory is equally severe for all decades.

Inability to remember both recently learned and remote information is well documented in patients with dementia. However, the types of memory function that are preserved in these patients are not well understood. In patients with amnesia (Korsakoff's syndrome), memory for general information in the form of procedural or skill learning seems well preserved, but memory for the contents of a learning episode (declarative information) is often forgotten (Cohen and Squire, 1980; Squire, 1982). In a task that involved reading of mirror-image words, amnestic patients improved with practice at a rate comparable to controls; memory for the test stimuli, however, was significantly impaired. In contrast, Martone et al. (1984) found patients with HD to have impairment of generalized skill acquisition relative to controls and amnestic patients, but the patients with HD did benefit from the repetition of material during skill learning and could recognize this information subsequent to the learning sessions at a higher rate than amnestic patients. The question of whether other subcortical dementias also show impaired skill learning, and whether the pattern of procedural/declarative memory offers differential value among dementia syndromes is unknown but deserves research attention.

Bradyphrenia

Slowed information processing or mental inertia is a cardinal feature of subcortical dementia and may occur to a lesser extent in patients with DAT. The term *bradyphrenia* is used to describe the mental correlate of slowed movement (bradykinesia) often seen in patients with subcortical syndromes.

Slowed information processing in patients with PD has been demonstrated with measures of memory scanning rate (Wilson et al., 1980) and reaction-time tasks (Evarts et al., 1981). Patients with HD have significant slowing on choice-reaction time tasks that increases with progression of the disease (Huber and Paulson, 1987). Performance on the Symbol-Digit Modalities Test, which measures the speed of processing information, was the most common impairment seen in a recent study of patients with MS (Beatty et al., 1988).

Mid- and long-latency auditory evoked potentials can also be employed to measure the speed of cognitive processing. Goodin and Aminoff (1986) found differences among patients with DAT, PD, and HD. The N2 and P3 components had prolonged latencies for all groups. N1 and P2 latencies were normal in patients with DAT, but N1 latencies were prolonged in patients with HD and PD, and P2 was prolonged only in patients with HD.

Cognition

Cognition refers to the ability to manipulate previously acquired information. Impairment of cognition can be measured by tasks such as the calculation subtest of the Mini-Mental State Examination (MMSE) (Folstein et al., 1975), but this task also depends on attentiveness and may be affected by anxiety and other noncognitive factors (Smith, 1967). Judgment of similarities and differences, as listed, for example, in Cummings and Benson (1983, p.30) or Strub and Black (1977, p.112), can also be used to assess abstract reasoning. Both of these tasks are impaired in patients with DAT (Storandt et al., 1984), and impairment of calculation is more severe in patients with DAT compared with patients with PD (Huber et al., 1986a).

Patients with the subcortical syndrome show consistent impairment on tasks of "executive" function that involve concept formation and the ability to shift mental sets. Lees and Smith (1983) found impairment on the Wisconsin Card Sorting Task, which examines the ability to acquire and shift conceptual sets, even in patients with PD who were early in their clinical course and who had no evidence of generalized intellectual impairment. A similar task, the Odd Man Out test, which requires shifting of two rules on a given trial, is also performed poorly by patients with PD (Flowers and Robertson, 1985). Patients with PSP, HD, and depressive dementia also have difficulty with abstract reasoning and the ability to shift conceptual sets (Rafal and Grimm, 1981; Caine, 1981; Josiassen et al., 1983; Maher et al., 1985). By way of comparison, Pillon et al. (1986) found that patients with PD or PSP performed significantly worse than patients with DAT on the Wisconsin Card Sorting Task when the three patient groups were matched for severity of dementia. Thus "executive" function appears to be more severely affected in patients with subcortical dementia.

Just the opposite pattern was seen when cognitive processes required to detect picture absurdities (Wells and Ruesch, 1972) were examined. Patients with a cortical dementia (DAT) had significantly greater impairment on this task compared with patients with subcortical dementias (MID and depressive dementia) when the three groups were matched for dementia severity (Shuttleworth and Huber, 1988a).

Verbal fluency (word-list generation) requires the patient to name as many words as possible that begin with a common letter (controlled word association test) or words from a specific semantic category (category naming test) (Rosen, 1980). Patients with PD and HD have impaired verbal fluency (Matison et al., 1982; Taylor et al., 1986), which is evident early in the course of the disease (Butters et al., 1978; Lees and Smith, 1983). Patients with MS and DAT also exhibit impaired verbal fluency (Rosen, 1980; Huber et al., 1987; Beatty et al., 1988; Shuttleworth and Huber, 1988b). Rosen (1980) found greater impairment in controlled word association versus semantic category fluency early in the course of DAT. Just the opposite pattern has also been observed (Shuttleworth and Huber, 1988b). Patients with PD are not impaired on controlled word association but do have impairment of semantic category retrieval (Matison et al., 1982). By way of comparison, Pillon et al. (1986) found that patients with PSP had significantly greater impairment of verbal fluency (combined semantic and controlled association) compared with patients with either DAT or PD, perhaps related to the characteristically severe bradyphrenia of PSP.

Visuospatial Skills

Visuospatial skills are commonly assessed by the picture arrangement, object assembly, and the block design subtests of the Wechsler Adult Intelligence Scale (WAIS) (1955). The line orientation task (Benton et al., 1983) and copying of the Rey-Osterreith complex figure (Becker et al., 1988) are also commonly used. Impairment on these measures is seen in patients with DAT (Rosen, 1983; Becker et al., 1988), PD (Pirozzolo et al., 1982; Boller et al., 1984), HD (Caine et al., 1977; Josiassen et al., 1983), and MS (Rao et al., 1984). Reasoning utilizing visuospatial material, measured by Raven's matrices (1958), is more severely impaired in patients with DAT compared with PD (Gainotti et al., 1980; Huber et al., 1986a). Interestingly, Brouwers et al. (1984) found patients with DAT to have impaired extrapersonal but not egocentric visuospatial skills, and patients with HD had the reverse pattern.

Due to coexisting motoric impairment in many patients with subcortical syndromes, it may be best to avoid the exclusive use of visuospatial tasks that require fine manual dexterity or the drawing of complex figures (e.g., Rey-Osterrieth complex figures). Several measures of visuospatial skills including the line orientation test (Benton et al., 1983), the Visual Organization Test (Hooper, 1958), and Raven's matrices (1958) avoid such a manual component. Despite this problem, Boller et al. (1984) found patients with PD to be equally impaired on measures that did and did not involve manual manipulation.

Personality or Emotional Changes

Personality changes are common but varied in patients with different dementing disorders. Cummings and associates (1987) found that approximately one half of their patients with either DAT or MID had delusions at some point during the course of their illness, but the occurrence of hallucinations was uncommon. Patients with cortical dementias tend to have simple paranoid delusions (e.g., theft or infidelity), whereas the delusions of patients with subcortical syndromes tend to be more complicated (Cummings, 1985).

Depressive symptoms can be present in the early stages of DAT (Sim and Sussman, 1962) but are generally assumed to be replaced by increasing indifference and lack of insight with the progression of disease (Reifler et al., 1982). However, one study (Shuttleworth et al., 1987) found the severity of depressive symptoms to remain roughly constant with increasing severity of DAT. That study and another by Cummings et al. (1987) found depressive symptoms to be common but generally mild, and the occurrence of major depression to be rare in DAT.

Depressive symptoms are less severe in patients with DAT compared with those with subcortical syndromes (Gainotti et al., 1980; Mayeux et al., 1981; Huber et al., 1986a; Cummings et al., 1987). Depression in PD is probably more than a simple reaction to disability, since this symptom may antedate the onset of the movement disorder (Mindham, 1970), is generally not related to the severity of disease (Robbins, 1976; Huber et al., 1988), and is apparently related to a reduction of brain serotonin rather than to dopamine metabolism (Mayeux et al., 1984). Hallucinations and delusions are rare in PD, and when present they typically represent drug-related phenomena (Celesia and Wannamaker, 1972). Beatty et al. (1988) also found depressive symptoms to be unrelated to severity or duration of disease in patients with MS. Personality changes associated with HD include irritability, apathy, or depression (Dewhurst et al., 1969). McHugh and Folstein (1975) have also argued that episodic mood changes of mania and depression are an integral rather than a reactive feature of HD. Caine and Shoulson (1983) found that delusions can also occur in patients with HD.

Several measures of mood and personality exist. The severity of depressive symptoms can be estimated by self-rating procedures such as the Zung (1965) or Beck (1967) scales, or by the Hamilton (1960) scale, which is examiner rated. Ratings of depressive symptoms in patients with subcortical syndromes should be interpreted with caution since these ratings may be artificially elevated due to an overlap of depressive and somatic symptoms, including sleep disturbance, fatigue, appetite, and sexual dysfunction. Personality traits are most often examined formally by the Minnesota Multiphasic Personality Inventory (MMPI) (Dahlstrom and Welsh, 1960).

Language and Other Cortical Dysfunctions

Aphasia, agnosia, and apraxia are disturbances traditionally associated with cortical dysfunction, and these abnormalities are common in patients with DAT. Language disturbance in DAT is characterized by word finding difficulty in spontaneous speech, inability to name common objects (anomia), and impaired auditory verbal and reading comprehension; articulation, repetition, and oral reading abilities are generally intact (Cummings et al., 1985, 1988). This pattern of impairment is reminiscent of transcortical sensory aphasia. Both the anomia and comprehension disturbance become more severe with advancing disease (Cummings et al., 1985; Shuttleworth and Huber, 1988b).

Visual agnosia can be manifest as impaired recognition of previously familiar objects, surroundings, or faces (Shuttleworth et al., 1982; Cummings and Benson, 1983). Agnosic symptoms are probably common but are difficult to define in the demented patient. *Ideomotor apraxia* refers to the inability to perform learned movements upon verbal command in the absence of significant ataxia, weakness, sensory loss, neglect, impairment of comprehension, or unwillingness to cooperate. *Ideational apraxia* refers to the apparent loss of the conception of a motor sequence, independent of verbal command. Perceptual-motor disturbances resembling ideational apraxia often impair routine activities of daily living, such as combing hair or brushing teeth in patients with DAT.

In contrast, such disturbances are rarely encountered in subcortical disorders. Patients with PD are not impaired on measures of naming, vocabulary, or comprehension (Gainotti et al., 1980; Pirozollo et al., 1982; Matison et al., 1982; Huber et al., 1986a). Mild word finding difficulty can be present in patients with HD, but confrontation naming performance and vocabulary are relatively preserved even in the advanced stages of disease (Butters et al., 1978; Josiassen et al., 1983). Language function is also considered normal in patients with MS (Jambor, 1969; Heaton et al., 1985; Huber et al., 1987). There is no evidence of apraxia in patients with PD (Priozollo et al., 1982; Huber et al., 1986a), MS (Huber et al., 1987), HD (Cummings and Benson, 1984), or patients with depressive dementia (Caine, 1981).

General Neurologic Abnormalities

Striking differences are readily apparent between cortical and subcortical dementias in the category of general neurologic abnormalities. Patients with subcortical syndromes often have difficulty with verbal output, characterized either by a decrease in volume (hypophonia), impaired articulation (dysarthria), or both. A recent study showed patients with PD to be impaired on all measures of articulation, a problem not encountered in patients with DAT regardless of dementia severity (Cummings et al., 1988). Posture can be stooped or dystonic, and the gait is often ataxic or apraxic. The presence of tremor, chorea, or athetosis is also common. This is in sharp contrast to patients with the cortical syndrome (DAT) who tend to have essentially normal general neurologic exams (Paulson, 1985). Posture is erect, gait is usually crisp and unaffected, the patient is alert and retains social graces. Family members often report that, aside from the serious intellectual impairment, the patient appears to be in better health and may even look younger than was true prior to disease onset. The lack of general neurologic manifestations tends to be maintained until the end stages of disease, when mutism, extrapyramidal signs, and pelvicrural contractures may appear.

STUDIES CONTRASTING SUBCORTICAL AND CORTICAL DEMENTIAS

There have been few objective studies directly examining the pattern of neuropsychological differences between cortical and subcortical dementias. Mayeux and associates (1981) compared the performance of patients with DAT, PD, and HD on a lengthened version of the MMSE. Results indicated that patients with DAT had significantly lower MMSE scores compared with patients with either PD or HD. This finding supports the suggestion that cortical dementias are generally more severe compared with subcortical dementias (Benson, 1983). Patient groups were then divided into three stages of functional disability defined as mild, moderate, and severe. Results indicated that the pattern of impairments that contributed to this decline distinguished the patient groups. For patients with DAT, the decline was of a generalized nature. In contrast, patients with PD and HD showed decline mostly in memory and visuospatial function and, unlike patients with DAT, there was no significant decline in language abilities. Depression was also more common in patients with PD and HD compared with those with DAT.

A second paper by the same group (Mayeux et al., 1983) attempted to match the patient groups for overall intellectual deterioration as determined by total score on the modified MMSE and to examine whether there was a distinct pattern of performance on subtest measures. The results indicated that qualitative differences were not seen between the patient groups, and the authors suggested that the concept of subcortical dementia was of dubious validity.

These papers have methodological shortcomings. First, the assessment of qualitative differences was made by the modified MMSE, a tool designed to detect the presence and to assess the severity of dementia. Standardized neuropsychological procedures (e.g., MMSE and WAIS) provide little if any discriminating value among dementing disorders simply because they were not designed to do so (Benson, 1983; Cummings and Benson, 1984; Rao, 1986). Second, matching the patient groups in terms of dementia severity as defined by total scores on the MMSE may reduce the likelihood of detecting differences among groups on any of the subtests.

Gainotti et al. (1980) compared various dementia syndromes with specific neuropsychological measures of memory, visuospatial skills, language, and depression. Results indicated that all groups had impairment of memory, but involvement of visuospatial skills was more variable. Patients with cortical dementia (e.g., DAT) had significant impairment of verbal skills, while those with subcortical dementia (e.g.,

PD) did not. Those with PD also had significantly greater depressive symptoms compared with patients with DAT.

We have recently completed our own investigation of the distinction between cortical and subcortical dementias by comparing DAT and PD patients with appropriate normal controls using a neuropsychological test battery that was specifically designed to evaluate the proposed clinical differences (Huber et al., 1986a). This battery included measures of overall mental function (MMSE), memory, language, praxis, cognition, visuospatial skills, and mood. We found the severity of overall intellectual impairment, as measured by the MMSE, to be greater for patients with DAT compared with patients with PD. Both patients with DAT and PD were impaired in relation to controls on measures of visuospatial skills, cognition, and memory, but significantly more so in DAT than PD. Patients with PD had higher depression scores compared with controls and patients with DAT. Unlike the PD patients, those with DAT were significantly impaired on measures of language, and there was evidence of apraxia.

This research was criticized because the neuropsychological measures were abbreviated and the patient groups were not matched for severity of intellectual impairment (Mayeux and Stern, 1987). Pillon et al. (1986) provided a report based on a more rigorous design. Patients with PSP, PD, or DAT, matched for severity of intellectual impairment, were compared on a comprehensive battery of neuropsychological tests. Results indicated specific differences among the patient groups. Patients with DAT had significantly more severe impairment of orientation and verbal memory compared with the other two groups. Patients with PSP were significantly more impaired on both the digit-span and verbal fluency tests. Finally, PSP and PD patients, unlike patients with DAT, had impaired performance on the Wisconsin Card Sorting Task.

RECENT RESEARCH

To assess the differences between cortical and subcortical dementias more effectively, we have extended our evaluation battery and tested patients with PD and DAT who had dementia of comparable severity. The primary contribution of this research was the addition of a proposed method to standardize and objectively evaluate the presence or absence of a dementia syndrome in patients with a subcortical syndrome.

Determination of Dementia

Only a portion of patients with subcortical syndromes develop dementia, and estimates of dementia prevalence vary considerably. Most of this inconsistency can be attributed to the lack of both standardized criteria to define dementia and objective methods of assessment. For research purposes this is crucial in order to expand our knowledge of subcortical dementias.

Two sets of criteria to define dementia are popular. One is described in the third edition of the *Diagnostic and Statistical Manual of Mental Disorders* (DSM-III) (1980). In order to meet these criteria, there must be significant loss of social or occupational function. Such losses can be related to intellectual function in patients with DAT but could be caused by either loss of intellect, a movement disorder, or both in patients with subcortical syndromes (Mayeux et al., 1983; Growdon and Corkin, 1986).

Cummings and Benson (1983) define dementia as an acquired and persistent impairment of the intellect with compromise of at least three of the following five areas: memory, visuospatial skills, emotional or personality change, cognition, and language. These criteria are similar to those used in the DSM-III in that multiple impairments of the intellect must be present, but it minimizes the subjective judgment related to loss of social or occupational function. The Cummings and Benson (1983) definition can therefore be utilized in a more straightforward manner, using objective neuropsychological procedures related to each of the five areas of mentation. If a patient's score on a neuropsychological measure is two standard deviations or more below mean normal control performance, significant impairment can be inferred. If a patient accumulates three or more significant impairments, the criteria for dementia are met.

Preliminary Data

39 normal controls, 68 patients with PD and 14 with DAT, were included in the study. Of the patients with PD, 23 (34%) met the Cummings and Benson (1983) criteria for dementia. The severity of dementia, as measured by the MMSE, was greater in patients with DAT (mean = 14.3) compared with patients with PD and dementia (mean = 22.9, $t(35)$ = 5.1, $p < .0001$). In order to examine whether qualitative differences are present in these two dementing disorders, we matched the patient groups for severity of dementia, as estimated by the MMSE.

9 patients with DAT and 10 patients with PD matched for severity of dementia were compared with the normal controls on a variety of neuropsychological measures. Auditory verbal immediate memory was assessed by the digits-forward procedure (Wechsler, 1945). Auditory verbal recent memory was examined by both the paired-associates (Wechsler, 1945) and the distractor procedure (Peterson and Peterson, 1959). Remote memory was evaluated by Albert's test (1979). Apraxia was evaluated as described by Christensen (1975). Visuospatial skills were assessed by both Raven's matrices (1958) and the block design task of the WAIS (Wechsler, 1955). Language was examined by ascertaining vocabulary (pointing to pictures named by the examiner), confrontation naming of object drawings, and auditory verbal comprehension (comprehension and commands subtests of the Western Aphasia Battery; Kertesz, 1982). Verbal fluency was determined for the letters S and P (Rosen, 1980). Cognition was assessed by the calculation subtest of the MMSE (Folstein et al., 1975) and the similarities and differences test listed in both Cummings and Benson (1983, p.30) and Strub and Black (1977, p.112). Finally, the severity of depressive symptoms was estimated by the Beck scale (1967). An abbreviated version of this scale, excluding questions related to appearance, ability to work, preoccupation with health, disturbances of sleep and sex drive, and outlook for the future was also employed due to the likelihood of confounding depressive and somatic symptoms in patients with PD. The three groups were compared on each of the neuropsychological measures using one-way analysis of variance (ANOVA) and post hoc comparisons (Neuman-Keuls) where appropriate. The data are presented in Table 6-1.

Results indicated that both measures of cognition, the calculation subtest of the

Table 6-1 Neuropsychological Measures in Healthy Elderly Control Subjects, Patients with Dementia of the Alzheimer Type (DAT), and Patients with Parkinson's Disease (PD) and Dementia

	Controls (N = 39)		DAT (N = 9)		PD (N = 10)	F Value
Age	64.8 (1.2)	=	67.0 (3.5)	=	70.4 (2.0)	2.1, n.s.
Education	13.9 (0.4)	=	14.0 (0.7)	=	14.3 (0.9)	0.1, n.s.
MMSE	28.2 (0.2)	>	17.1 (1.5)	=	19.7 (1.3)	86.7, $p<.0001$
Orientation	9.9 (.04)	>	5.0 (1.1)	<	7.5 (0.8)	38.7, $p<.0001$
Registration	3.0 (0.0)	=	2.8 (0.2)	=	3.0 (0.0)	2.9, n.s.
Calculation	4.5 (0.1)	>	1.3 (0.5)	=	0.7 (0.2)	77.3, $p<.0001$
Recall	1.8 (0.2)	>	0.2 (0.1)	=	0.3 (0.2)	18.7, $p<.0001$
Language	9.0 (0.0)	>	7.7 (0.6)	=	8.1 (0.5)	9.7, $p<.001$
Similarities	6.3 (0.3)	>	3.0 (0.8)	=	3.1 (0.7)	19.0, $p<.0001$
Verbal fluency	13.6 (0.6)	>	7.4 (1.8)	>	4.3 (0.9)	26.4, $p<.0001$
Vocabulary	9.9 (.03)	>	9.4 (0.3)	=	9.0 (0.3)	13.1, $p<.0001$
Naming	19.2 (0.1)	>	15.8 (1.0)	<	17.8 (0.7)	15.3, $p<.0001$
Comprehension	5.0 (0.0)	=	4.9 (0.1)	=	5.0 (0.0)	2.9, n.s.
Commands	5.0 (0.0)	=	4.7 (0.2)	=	4.6 (0.4)	2.1, n.s.
Digits-forward	6.7 (0.2)	>	5.6 (0.7)	<	6.9 (0.2)	3.7, $p<.03$
Distractor task	19.2 (0.9)	>	1.7 (1.3)	=	0.8 (0.4)	82.4, $p<.0001$
Paired-associates	14.6 (0.5)	>	5.3 (0.5)	=	6.8 (0.7)	55.7, $p<.0001$
Easy items	8.5 (0.1)	>	5.2 (0.5)	=	5.9 (0.5)	43.8, $p<.0001$
Hard items	6.1 (2.7)	>	0.1 (0.1)	=	0.9 (0.3)	39.1, $p<.0001$
Remote memory	25.0 (1.4)	>	3.7 (1.3)	<	13.8 (3.2)	25.6, $p<.0001$
Raven's matrices	10.6 (0.2)	>	8.2 (0.6)	>	6.4 (0.8)	32.9, $p<.0001$
Block design	5.9 (.04)	>	1.8 (0.5)	<	3.1 (0.9)	50.6, $p<.0001$
Depression	4.8 (0.8)	=	3.9 (1.6)	<	14.4 (1.5)	17.9, $p<.0001$
Abbreviated scale	2.4 (0.5)	=	3.1 (1.1)	<	8.0 (1.0)	11.5, $p<.0001$
Apraxia	5.0 (0.0)	>	4.6 (0.4)	=	4.7 (0.2)	4.9, $p<.01$

MMSE and judgment of similarities and differences, were impaired in both patient groups to a similar extent. There was also similar impairment of vocabulary in both patient groups, but impairment of naming was more severe in patients with DAT. In contrast, verbal fluency was more severely impaired in patients with PD compared with those with DAT. The pattern of memory impairment was also different in the two patient groups. Unlike patients with PD, there was impairment of immediate memory or attentiveness (digits-forward) for patients with DAT. There was equal impairment on both measures of recent memory (paired-associates and the distractor task), but impairment of remote memory was more severe in patients with DAT. Performance on visuospatial tasks also differentiated the two patient groups. Patients with PD were more severely impaired on the reasoning task (Raven's matrices), and conversely patients with DAT had greater impairment on the measure of constructional ability (block design). Patients with DAT had more severe disturbance of orientation compared with those with PD and also had evidence of apraxia, unlike patients with PD. Depressive symptoms were significantly greater in patients with PD on both the full and abbreviated Beck scales, while patients with DAT had no significant disturbance of mood.

SUMMARY AND FUTURE RESEARCH DIRECTIONS

Subcortical dementias are characterized by a unique and identifiable pattern of intellectual disturbance. Subcortical syndromes are associated with slowed information processing, impairment of memory, poor visuospatial skills, disturbances of executive function, and abnormal mood. There is a conspicuous absence of language disturbance. More than a decade ago Albert et al. (1974) and McHugh and Folstein (1975) provided the modern description of this syndrome. Subsequently, their clinical descriptions have been confirmed through formal neuropsychological testing. Examples of procedures appropriate to the study of subcortical syndromes are summarized in Table 6-2.

At present, two research issues related to subcortical dementia remain controversial. One is the question of whether specific neuropsychological differences exist among subcortical syndromes, and the other relates to the development of objective procedures with which to delineate differences between cortical and subcortical syndromes. Two methodological problems must be resolved in order to address these questions adequately. The first concerns standardization of both criteria and procedures

Table 6-2 Neuropsychological Procedures Appropriate for the Assessment of Subcortical Dementia Syndromes

Memory
    (A) Immediate verbal (digits-forward; Wechsler, 1945)
    (B) Recent verbal (Peterson and Peterson, 1959)
    (C) Procedural (Cohen and Squire, 1980)
    (D) Remote (Albert et al., 1979)

Cognition
    (A) Calculation (Folstein et al., 1975)
    (B) Similarities/differences (Cummings and Benson, 1983, p. 30; Strub and Black, 1977, p. 112)
    (C) Executive function
        1. Wisconsin Card Sorting Task (Nelson, 1976)
        2. Odd Man Out Task (Flowers and Robertson, 1985)

Bradyphrenia
    (A) Mid- and long-latency evoked potentials (Goodin and Aminoff, 1986)
    (B) Symbol-Digit Modalities Test (Beatty et al., 1988)
    (C) Verbal fluency (Rosen, 1980)

Emotion and personality
    (A) Depressive symptoms (Beck, 1967; Hamilton, 1960)
    (B) Personality (MMPI; Dahlstrom and Welsh, 1960)

Visuospatial skills
    (A) Perceptual (line orientation; Benton et al., 1983)
    (B) Constructional (block design; Wechsler, 1945)
    (C) Copy skills (Rey-Osterreith figure; Becker et al., 1988)
    (D) Reasoning (Raven, 1958)

to establish the presence or absence of dementia. DSM-III criteria for dementia can be complicated in the evaluation of subcortical syndromes, since the subjective impression of the presence of significant impairment of social or occupational function can result from intellectual dysfunction, a movement disorder, or both. In contrast, most of the criteria defined by Cummings and Benson (1983) can be evaluated by objective neuropsychological procedures and statistical comparison with normal controls. The second methodological problem concerns matching patient groups for dementia severity prior to examination of possible qualitative differences. The MMSE (Folstein et al., 1975) provides a brief quantifiable measure that can be used to equate dementing patients for overall intellectual severity, but it is more sensitive to cortical than subcortical deficits.

As progress is made in definitional and measurement domains, the concept of subcortical dementia and the neuropsychological functions mediated by subcortical structures will be clarified.

REFERENCES

Albert, M.L. Subcortical dementia. In *Alzheimer's Disease: Senile Dementia and Related Disorders.* Katzman, R., Terry, R.D., and Bick, K.L. (eds.). Raven Press, New York, 1978 pp. 173–80.

Albert, M.S., Butters, N., and Brandt, J. Patterns of remote memory in amnesic and demented patients. *Arch Neurol* 1981a; 38:495–500.

Albert, M.S., Butters, N., and Brandt, J. Development of remote memory loss in patients with Huntington's disease. *J. Clin Exp Neuropsychol* 1981b; 13:1–12.

Albert, M.S., Butters, N., and Levin, J. Temporal gradients in the retrograde amnesia of patients with alcoholic Korsakoff's disease. *Arch Neurol* 1979; 36:211–6.

Albert, M.L., Feldman, R.G., and Willis, A.L. The subcortical dementia of progressive supranuclear palsy. *J Neurol Neurosurg Psychiatry* 1974; 37:121–30.

Beatty, W.W., Goodkin, D.E., Monson, N., Beatty, P.A., and Hertsgaard, D. Anterograde and retrograde amnesia in patients with chronic progressive multiple sclerosis. *Arch Neurol* 1988; 45:611–9.

Beck, A.T. *Depression.* University of Pennsylvania Press, Philadelphia, 1967.

Becker, J.T., Huff, J., Nebes, R.D., Holland, A., and Boller, F. Neuropsychological function in Alzheimer disease: Pattern of impairment and rates of progression. *Arch Neurol* 1988; 45:263–8.

Benson, D.F. Subcortical dementia: A clinical approach. In *The Dementias: Advances in Neurology, Vol. 38.* Mayeux, R., and Rosen, W.G., (eds.). Raven Press, New York, 1983, pp. 185–94.

Benton, A.L., Hamsher, K., Varney, N.R., and Spreen, O. *Contributions to neuropsychological assessment.* Oxford University Press, New York, 1983.

Boller, F., Passatiume, D., Keefe, N.C., Rogers, K., Morrow, L., and Kim, Y. Visuospatial impairments in Parkinson's disease. *Arch Neurol* 1984; 41:485–90.

Brouwers, P., Cox, C., Martin, A., Chase, T., and Fedio, P. Differential perceptual-spatial impairment in Huntington's and Alzheimer's dementias. *Arch Neurol* 1984; 41:1073–6.

Butters, N., Sax, D., Montgomery, K., and Tarlow, S. Comparison of the neuropsychological deficits associated with early and advanced Huntington's Disease. *Arch Neurol* 1978; 35:585–9.

Caine, E.D. Pseudodementia: Current concepts and future directions. *Arch Gen Psychiatry* 1981; 38:1359–64.

Caine, E.D., Ebert, M.H., and Weingartner, H. An outline for the analysis of dementia: The memory disorder of Huntington's disease. *Neurology* 1977; 27:1087–92.

Caine, E.D., and Shoulson, I. Psychiatric syndromes in Huntington's disease. *Am J Psychiatry* 1983; 140:728–33.

Celesia, G.G., and Wanamaker, W.M. Psychiatric disturbances in Parkinson's disease. *Dis Nerv Syst* 1972; 33:577–83.

Christensen, A.L. *Luria's Neuropsychological Investigation: Text, Manual and Tests Cards.* Spectrum, Inc., Jamaica, New York, 1975.

Cohen, N.J., and Squire, L.R. Preserved learning and retention of pattern-analyzing skill in amnesia: Dissociation of knowing how and knowing that. *Science* 1980; 210:207–10.

Cummings, J.L. Organic delusions: phenomenology, anatomical correlation, and review. *Br J Psychiatry* 1985; 146:184–97.

Cummings, J.L., and Benson, D.F. *Dementia: A Clinical Approach.* Butterworths, Woburn, Massachusetts, 1983.

Cummings, J.L., and Benson, D.F. Subcortical dementia: Review of an emerging concept. *Arch Neurol* 1984; 41:874–9.

Cummings, J.L., Benson, D.F., Hill, M.A., and Read, S. Aphasia in dementia of the Alzheimer type. *Neurology* 1985; 35:394–7.

Cummings, J.L., Darkins, A., Mendez, M., Hill, M.A., and Benson, D.F. Alzheimer's disease and Parkinson's disease: Comparison of speech and language alteration. *Neurology* 1988; 38:680–4.

Cummings, J.L., Miller, B., Hill, M.A., and Neshkes, R. Neuropsychiatric aspects of multi-infarct dementia and dementia of the Alzheimer type. *Arch Neurol* 1987; 44:389–93.

Dahlstrom, W.G., and Welsh, G.S. *An MMPI Handbook: A Guide to Use in Clinical Practice and Research.* University of Minnesota Press, Minneapolis, 1960.

Dewhurst, K., Oliver, J., Trick, K.L.K., and McKnight, A.L. Neuropsychiatric aspects of Huntington's disease. *Conf in Neurol* 1969; 31:258–68.

Diagnostic and Statistical Manual of Mental Disorders, Third edition. Williams, J. (ed.). American Psychiatric Association, Washington, DC, 1980.

Evarts, E.V., Teravainen, H., and Calne, D.B. Reaction time in Parkinson's disease. *Brain* 1981; 104:167–86.

Flowers, K.A., and Robertson, C. The effect of Parkinson's disease on the ability to maintain a mental test set. *J Neurol Neurosurg Psychiatry* 1985; 48:517–29.

Folstein, M.F., Folstein, S.E., and McHugh, P.R. Mini-mental state: A practical guide for grading the mental state of patients for the clinician. *J Psychiatr Res* 1975; 12:189–98.

Folstein, M.F., and McHugh, P.R. Dementia syndrome of depression. In *Alzheimer's Disease: Senile Dementia and Related Disorders.* Katzman, R., Terry, R.D., and Bick, K.L. (eds.). Raven Press, New York, 1978, pp. 87–93.

Gainotti, G., Caltagirone, C., Massullo, C., and Miceli, G. Patterns of neuropsychologic impairment in various diagnostic groups of dementia. In *Aging of brain and dementia.* Amaducci, L., Davison, A.N., and Antvono, P. (eds.). Raven Press, New York, 1980, pp. 245–50.

Goodin, D.S., and Aminoff, M.J. Electrophysiologic differences between subtypes of dementia. *Brain* 1986; 109:1103–13.

Growdon, J.H., and Corkin, S. Cognitive impairments in Parkinson's disease. In *Parkinson's Disease.* Yahr, M.D., and Bergmann, K.J. (eds.). *Advances in Neurology, Vol. 45.* Raven Press, New York, 1986, pp. 383–92.

Hamilton, M. A rating scale for depression. *J Neurol Neurosurg Psychiatry* 1960; 23:56–61.

Heaton, R.K., Nelson, L.M., Thompson, D.S., Burks, J.S., and Franklin, G.M. Neuropsychological findings in relapsing—remitting and chronic—progressive multiple sclerosis. *J of Consult and Clin Psychol* 1985; 49:807–21.

Hooper, H.E. *The Hooper Visual Organization Test.* Western Psychological Services, Los Angeles, 1958.

Huber, S.J., and Paulson, G.W. Memory impairment associated with progression of Huntington's disease. *Cortex* 1987; 23:275–83.

Huber, S.J., Paulson, G.W., and Shuttleworth, E.C. Relationship of motor symptoms, intellectual impairment, and depression in Parkinson's disease. *J Neurol Neurosurg Psychiatry* 1988; 51:855–8.

Huber, S.J., Paulson, G.W., Shuttleworth, E.C., Chakeres, D., Clapp, L.E., Pakalnis, A., Weiss, K., and Rammohon, K. Magnetic resonance imaging correlates of dementia in multiple sclerosis. *Arch Neurol* 1987; 44:732–6.

Huber, S.J., Shuttleworth, E.C., Paulson, G.W., Bellchambers, M.J.B., and Clapp, L.E. Cortical vs subcortical dementia: Neuropsychological differences. *Arch Neurol* 1986a; 43:392–4.

Huber, S.J., Shuttleworth, E.C., and Paulson, G.W. Dementia in Parkinson's disease. *Arch Neurol* 1986b; 43:987–90.

Jambor, K.L. Cognitive functioning in multiple sclerosis. *Br J Psychiatry* 1969; 115:765–75.

Josiassen, R., Curry, L., and Mancall, E. Development of neuropsychological deficits in Huntington's disease. Neuropsychologia 1983; 40:791–6.

Kertesz, A. *The Western Aphasia Battery.* Grune and Stratton, New York, 1982.

Lees, A.J., and Smith, E. Cognitive deficits in the early stages of Parkinson's disease. *Brain* 1983; 106:257–70.

Maher, E.R., Smith, E.R., and Lees, A.J. Cognitive deficits in the Steel-Richardson-Olszewski syndrome (progressive supranuclear palsy). *J Neurol Neurosurg Psychiatry* 1985; 48:1234–9.

Marsden, C.D. The diagnosis of dementia. In *Studies in Geriatric Psychiatry.* Issacs, A.D., and Post, F. (eds.). Wiley, New York, 1978, pp. 95–118.

Martone, M., Butters, N., and Payne, M. Dissociations between skill learning and verbal recognition in amnesia and dementia. *Arch Neurol* 1984; 41:965–70.

Matison, R., Mayeux, R., Rosen, J., and Fahn, S. "Tip-of-the-tongue" phenomenon in Parkinson's disease. *Neurology* 1982; 32:567–70.

Mayeux, R., and Stern, Y. Subcortical dementia. *Arch Neurol* 1987; 44:130–1.

Mayeux, R., Stern, Y., Cote, L., and Williams, B.W. Altered serotonin metabolism in depressed patients with Parkinson's disease. *Neurology* 1984; 34:642–8.

Mayeux, R., Stern, Y., Rosen, J., and Benson, D.F. Subcortical dementia: A recognizable clinical entity. *Trans Am Neurol Assoc* 1981; 106:313–6.

Mayeux, R., Stern, Y., Rosen, J., and Benson, D.F. Is subcortical dementia a recognizable clinical entity? *Ann Neurol* 1983; 14:278–83.

McHugh, P.R., and Folstein, M.F. Psychiatric syndromes of Huntington's chorea: a clinical and phenomenological study. In *Psychiatric Aspects of Neurological Disease.* Benson, D.F., and Blumer, D., (eds.). Grune & Stratton, New York, 1975:267–85.

Miller, G.S. The magical number seven, plus or minus two: Some limits on our capacity for processing information. *Psychol Rev* 1956; 63:81–97.

Mindham, R.H.S. Psychiatric symptoms in parkinsonism. *J Neurol Neurosurg Psychiatry* 1970; 33: 181–91.

Moscovitch, M., Moscovitch, J., and Crapper-Maclochlan, D. Memory disorder in patients with Alzheimer's disease, abstracted. *Neurology* 1981; 31:62.

Navia, B.A., Jordan, B.D., and Price, R.W. The AIDS dementia complex: I. Clinical features. *Ann Neurol* 1986; 19:517–24.

Nelson, N.E. A modified card sorting task sensitive to frontal lobe defects. *Cortex* 1976; 12:313–24.

Paulson, G.W. Early Alzheimer's disease or dementia from another cause. *Postgrad Med* 1985; 78:223–7.

Peterson, L.R., and Peterson, M.J. Short-term retention of individual verbal items. *J Exp Psychol* 1959; 58:193–8.

Pillon, B., Dubois, B., Lhermitte, F., and Agid, Y. Heterogeneity of cognitive impairment in progressive supranuclear palsy, Parkinson's disease, and Alzheimer's disease. *Neurology* 1986; 36:1179–85.

Pirozzolo, F.J., Hansch, E.C., Mortimer, J.A., Webster, D.D., and Kuschowski, M.A. Dementia in Parkinson's disease: A neuropsychological analysis. *Brain Cogn* 1982; 1:71–83.

Rafal, R.D., and Grimm, R.J. Progressive supranuclear palsy: functional analysis and response to methsergide and antiparkinsonian agents. *Neurology* 1981; 31:1507–18.

Rao, S.M. Neuropsychology of multiple sclerosis: A critical review. *J Clin Exp Neuropsychol* 1986; 8:503–42.

Rao, S.M., Hammeke, T.A., McQuillen, M.P., Khatri, B.O., Rhodes, A.M., and Pollard, S. Memory disturbance in chronic progressive multiple sclerosis. *Arch Neurol* 1984; 41:625–31.

Raven, J.C. *Standard Progressive Matrices*. Psychological Corp., New York, 1958.

Reifler, B., Larson, E., and Hanley,, R. Coexistence of cognitive impairment and depression in geriatric outpatients. *Am J Psychiatry* 1982; 139:623–6.

Robbins, A.H. Depression in patients with parkinsonism. *Br J Psychiatry* 1976; 128:141–5.

Rosen, W.G. Verbal fluency in aging and dementia. *J Clin Neuropsychol* 1980; 2:135–46.

Rosen, W.G. Neuropsychological investigation of memory, visuoconstructional, visuoperceptual, and language abilities in senile dementia of the Alzheimer type. In *The Dementias*. Mayeux, R., and Rosen, W.G. (eds.) Raven Press, New York, 1983, pp. 65–73.

Shuttleworth, E.C., and Huber, S.J. The picture absurdities task in the evaluation of dementia. 1988a, unpublished data.

Shuttleworth, E.C., and Huber, S.J. The naming disorders of dementia of Alzheimer type. *Brain Lang* 1988b; 34:222–34.

Shuttleworth, E.C., Huber, S.J., and Paulson, G.W. Depression in patients with dementia of the Alzheimer type. *J of Natl Med Assoc* 1987; 79:733–6.

Shuttleworth, E.C., Syring, V., and Allen, N. Further observations on the nature of progopagnosia. *Brain Cogn* 1982; 1:307–22.

Sim, M., and Sussman, I. Alzheimer's disease: Its natural history and differential diagnosis. *J Nerv Ment Dis* 1962; 135:489–99.

Smith, A. The serial sevens subtraction test. *Arch Neurol* 1967; 17:78–80.

Squire, L.R. The neuropsychology of human memory. *Annu Rev Neurosci* 1982; 5:241–73.

Storandt, M., Botwinich, J., Danziger, W.L., Berg, L., and Hughes, C.P. Psychometic differentiation of mild senile dementia of the Alzheimer's type. *Arch Neurol* 1984; 41:497–9.

Strub, R.L., and Black, F.W. *The mental status examination in neurology*. F.A. Davis, Philadelphia, 1977.

Taylor, A.E., Saint-Cyr, J.A., and Lang, A.E. Frontal lobe dysfunction in Parkinson's disease. *Brain* 1986; 109:845–83.

Tweedy, J.R., Langer, K.G., and McDowell, F.H. The effect of semantic relations on the memory deficits associated with Parkinson's disease. *J Clin Neuropsychol* 1982; 4:235–47.

Wechsler, D.A. A standardized memory scale for clinical use. *J Psychol* 1945; 19:85–95.

Wechsler, D. *Wechsler Adult Intelligence Scale*. The Psychological Corp., New York, 1955.

Wells, F.L., and Ruesch, J. *Mental Examiner's Handbook, Second Edition* The Psychological Corp., New York, 1972, pp. 166–72.

Wilson, R.S., Kaszniak, A.W., Klawans, H.L., and Garron, D.C. High speed memory scanning in parkinsonism. *Cortex* 1980; 16:67–72.

Zung, W.W.K. A self-rating depression scale. *Arch Gen Psychiatry* 1965; 12:63–70.

7

Huntington's Disease

SUSAN E. FOLSTEIN, JASON BRANDT,
AND MARSHAL F. FOLSTEIN

The bygone era in psychiatry, when patients could be observed in the hospital for many months, provided opportunities to follow patients' daily behavior in both unstructured settings (the psychiatric ward) and in structured settings (psychological testing). Prolonged clinical observations of severe hospitalized cases revealed similarities among patients with Huntington's disease, hydrocephalus, parkinsonism, depression, and some cases of schizophrenia, which contrasted with the mental state and behavior of patients with Alzheimer's disease observed in the same hospital. In this setting, the concept of subcortical dementia was formulated by P.R. McHugh and presented to the Academy of Neurology in 1973. It was subsequently incorporated into a chapter on Huntington's disease in *Psychiatric Aspects of Neurological Disease* by D.F. Benson and D. Blumer (McHugh and Folstein, 1975). Since that time, the concept of subcortical dementia has undergone study and review by many individuals, including the authors of other chapters of this book (Albert, Feldman, and Willis, 1974; Cummings and Benson, 1984; Mayeux et al., 1981; Whitehouse, 1986).

The patients with Huntington's disease (HD) and dementia of the Alzheimer type (DAT), upon whom the original concept of subcortical dementia was based, were subject to the selection bias for being admitted to a long-term psychiatric hospital. The validation of the concept required the study of a more representative sample of patients at varying stages of illness. In Baltimore, this opportunity arose for the authors of this chapter. Between 1980 and 1983, S. Folstein conducted a statewide survey of community dwelling and institutionalized cases of HD (Folstein et al., 1986, 1987). This representative sample is being followed with regular neurologic and psychiatric examinations until death and autopsy. A large sample of volunteers at 50% risk for HD is also being followed longitudinally. Simultaneously, M. Folstein has been following an outpatient clinic sample of patients with DAT using similar methods of examination; J. Brandt has extensively studied both patient groups neuropsychologically. It is from this collective experience that our ideas about the subcortical dementia of HD have evolved.

THE DEFINING FEATURES OF SUBCORTICAL DEMENTIA

From its conception, subcortical dementia has been defined by both cognitive and noncognitive components. Cognitively, the patients suffer from deficits in memory, visuospatial skills, sustained attention, and ability to change from one mental set to another. However, while HD patients tend to be verbally unproductive, they rarely suffer from aphasia, agnosia, or apraxia—the defining features of DAT. The associated noncognitive abnormalities originally included apathy and, in some patients, irritability and have been extended to other mood disorders.

We now propose that the definition of subcortical dementia be expanded to include abnormalities of mood, particularly depression but occasionally mania, and abnormalities of movement. Both depression and abnormal movements are prominent features of other neurologic illnesses associated with subcortical lesions, most notably Parkinson's disease and subcortical stroke. Furthermore, many of the cognitive, behavioral, and motor features of subcortical dementia are frequent accompaniments of manic-depressive disorder and of schizophrenia.

Important advances in our understanding of striatal anatomy and physiology have begun to illuminate the neuropathology and pathophysiology of HD. These new discoveries will provide the basis for understanding the mechanisms of the subcortical dementia of HD and might shed light on other similar conditions. Thus, the subcortical dementia syndrome may provide a conceptual link between those conditions with well-defined subcortical neuropathology (e.g., HD and Parkinson's disease) and mental disorders whose pathophysiologies are still unknown (e.g., schizophrenia and affective disorder).

THE CLINICAL FEATURES OF HUNTINGTON'S DISEASE

HD is characterized by the insidious onset, usually during adulthood, of chorea and subcortical dementia. The age of onset varies from childhood to old age, with an average of about 40 years. The illness begins somewhat earlier in the offspring of affected fathers (Merritt et al., 1969) and in black patients (Hayden et al., 1980; Folstein et al., 1987). The disorder gradually progresses over many years, ending in death an average of 17 years after onset. Many patients also suffer from episodes of depression and sometimes from mania, and the reported suicide rate is as high as 7% (Folstein et al., 1983). The most prominent neuropathologic features are atrophy and neuronal loss in the striatum, which begins in the medial caudate nucleus and progresses laterally to involve other areas of the caudate and the putamen (Vonsattel et al., 1985).

HD is transmitted as an autosomal dominant trait with complete lifetime penetrance. The genetic defect has been mapped by genetic linkage analysis to the distal end of the short arm of chromosome 4 (Gusella, 1983), but, at this writing, the gene itself has not yet been identified. Estimates of the prevalence of HD vary between 5 and 7 per 100,000 population. HD is more common in the adult population, found in 12 per 100,000 adults between 40 and 55 years of age (S. Folstein, 1989).

DETECTION OF COGNITIVE DEFICITS

The cognitive features of HD can be observed and assessed for clinical purposes while taking a history and by using brief but formal tests of cognition.

In order to obtain an accurate history, both at an initial evaluation or during the course of care of HD patients, a spouse or another informant will be needed. This allows the examiner to assess informally the patient's memory for remote and recent events of personal life, compared with the spouse's memory for the same events. The patient may turn to his spouse to provide information about dates of children's birth, employment, or episodes of depression. He may be vague in recalling signs or symptoms, particularly their duration and the circumstances surrounding them. During conversation, the patient may have difficulty with word finding and offer little spontaneous speech. The paucity of conversation may be a sign of depression but often indicates cognitive slowing. At the same time, it will be apparent that the patient's understanding of the questions is relatively unimpaired and that his answers, when he can give them, are reasonable.

Mini-Mental Status Examination

The Mini-Mental Status Examination (MMSE), or some other structured cognitive screening test, may be used to assess the type and variety of cognitive deficits and to follow the patient longitudinally (Folstein et al., 1975). In our experience, all patients show a gradual cognitive decline when followed over time (Figure 7-1). Nevertheless, they vary tremendously in the severity and rate of progression of their cognitive deficits

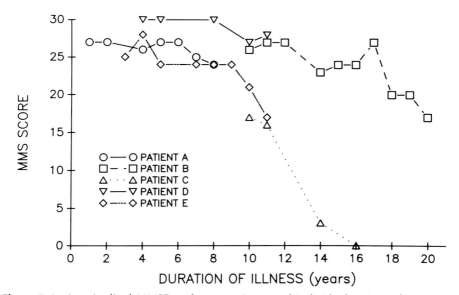

Figure 7-1 Longitudinal MMSE performance in several individual patients demonstrates the variability in rate and extent of cognitive decline.

Table 7-1   HD Patients Grouped by Total MMSE Score Vary Widely in Their Duration of Illness[a]

Score	26–30	21–25	16–20	10–15	< 10
N	41	49	35	10	46
Duration of illness					
Range (yrs)	0–15	0–36	0–31	5–25	2–29
Mean	4.7	8.3	8.8	14.0	13.7
(S.D.)	(4.0)	(6.8)	(6.8)	(6.9)	(6.0)

[a]For HD patients with scores on the MMSE within a given range, the duration of illness varied widely, although the mean duration of illness increased steadily as MMSE scores declined. Some of the variation was attributable to years of education (see text).

(Table 7-1). This variation is largely accounted for by years of education. In a multiple regression analysis, education and duration of illness were equally strong predictors of MMSE score (S. Folstein et al., unpublished data). The explanation for this association is unknown. One possibility is that early onset of disease might limit education and thus, at the time of testing, those patients with less education will appear to have more severe cognitive impairment. Another possibility is that individuals with greater pre-morbid capacity might not manifest impairment in cognition on the MMSE until some threshold number of neurons have been lost to the disease.

While failure on cognitive screening tests is associated with failure at work, *successful* MMSE performance is not a sensitive indicator of the patient's ability to work. Some patients who score in the normal range on the MMSE (and on IQ tests) are unable to function at a job because of their difficulty in initiating and sustaining performance and difficulty with more complex tasks than are covered by the MMSE, such as the capacity to change mental sets. Since the ability to perform on the MMSE is usually better than actual functional capacity, low MMSE scores are virtually always associated with inability to work.

Performance on Individual MMSE Items

While all the MMSE items gradually decline over time, the pattern of deficit is not uniform. This can best be demonstrated by comparing HD patients with DAT patients matched for overall MMSE scores (Figure 7-2) (Brandt, Folstein, and Folstein, 1988). The cognitive tasks represented by these items are discussed according to the order in which their performance becomes impaired, beginning with those affected early in the course of illness.

Serial Sevens

The first item on the MMSE to be affected in HD patients is usually Serial Sevens, a task of calculation and concentration. The patient is asked to start from 100, subtract seven, and keep subtracting seven from each remainder until five substractions are performed. In the general population, performance on Serial Sevens is related to education (Anthony et al., 1982). In HD, however, Serial Sevens is difficult even for affected in persons who have worked in jobs requiring frequent computation. It is significantly worse in HD than DAT patients matched for MMSE total scores from 24 down to 10. No HD patient with an MMSE score of 10 or less scored any points on the Serial Sevens (Figure 7-2A) item.

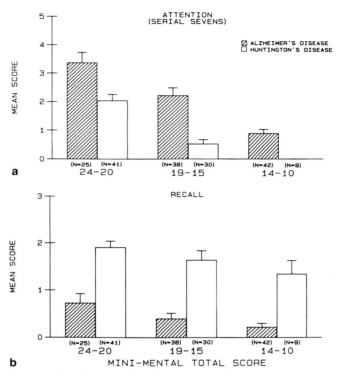

DIFFERENTIAL COGNITIVE IMPAIRMENT IN
ALZHEIMER'S DISEASE AND HUNTINGTON'S DISEASE

Figure 7-2 Patterns of performance on the Mini-Mental State Examination as a function of level of dementia in Alzheimer's disease (striped bars) and Huntington's disease (open bars).

Recall of Three Words

Recall of three words (Figure 7-2B) following a brief distraction is affected early in the course of HD, although not so severely as in DAT. Most HD patients will usually recall one or two of the three words, and many will remember all three. There are exceptional patients who continue to perform normally on this and more difficult memory tasks, and whose memory is reported by family members to be unimpaired for many years after the onset of symptoms.

Orientation and Copying Designs

Somewhat later in the course of illness, the more difficult orientation items will be missed (e.g., the date, floor of the clinic). However, orientation is better preserved than in DAT patients at the same MMSE level (Brandt et al., 1988). About the same time, patients begin to have difficulty copying the interlocking pentagons. This item is also performed poorly by normals with less than an eighth-grade education. In HD the failure is one of perception of the shape and organizing the graphomotor production. Copying the interlocking pentagons is unrelated to the severity of involuntary movements, as assessed by many observations of the performance of HD patients. HD patients who can adequately hold a pencil and execute the drawing make serious errors in the number of sides, angles, and position of the interlocking angles. They sometimes look at the example several times and attempt to make corrections in their copy, realizing that they have drawn it incorrectly, but they are usually unable to appreciate why.

Writing a Coherent Sentence

Some patients are able to write a sentence for as long as they can effectively move their hands to accomplish it. However, the sentences become shorter and less complex in grammatical structure. Most persons with MMSE scores below 14 are unable to write a sentence, usually because of cognitive failure, but sometimes because of motor disability. In this regard, HD patients perform more poorly than DAT patients.

Registration, Naming, Reading, and Easy Orientation Items

At moderate levels of dementia (MMSE 10–14), most items of the MMSE are at least partially missed, but most patients retain the ability to repeat three words spoken by the examiner and name objects visually presented. They remain partially oriented and can read a sentence. At more advanced stages performance is so impaired by motor difficulties that only the items that require simple verbal utterances are successfully performed. Even patients with severe dysarthria can be understood if the examiner is expecting a limited range of responses. Some can spell their responses, as their spoken letters are more easily understood than their words. However, when the total MMSE is as low as 10–14, orientation items, which can be successfully tested by simple speech, are typically failed. Naming is the last skill lost. Even when patients have great difficulty in initiation of speech, they can sometimes, with great expenditure of energy, name simple objects such as a pen or a watch.

Other MMSE Items

A few of the language items on the MMSE are difficult to interpret because of motor or education effects. Failure to repeat a phrase ("no ifs, ands, or buts") appears to be more dependent on dysarthria than dementia. Executing a three-stage command is impaired by a mixture of motor and cognitive deficits.

Intelligence Tests In Huntington's Disease

Full scale IQ as measured by the Wechsler Adult Intelligence Scale (WAIS or WAIS-R) drops modestly during the first years of illness, the performance scale accounting for most of the decline (Lyle and Gottesman, 1977; Brandt et al., 1984; Josiassen et al., 1982). As the illness progresses, scores continue to fall slightly, but patients rarely score in the mentally retarded range (below 70) until 10 or more years after onset. Longitudinal data on a few individual patients demonstrate the gradual decline in IQ (Figure 7-3).

The various subtests of the WAIS are not all equally affected (Figure 7-4). Vocabulary (defining words) and Information (general knowledge) are relatively spared until late in the illness, while Arithmetic (mental calculation), Digit Symbol (matching numbers with symbols as quickly as possible), Picture Arrangement (arranging pictures in a logical sequence), and Digit Span (repeating a series of numbers) are impaired early

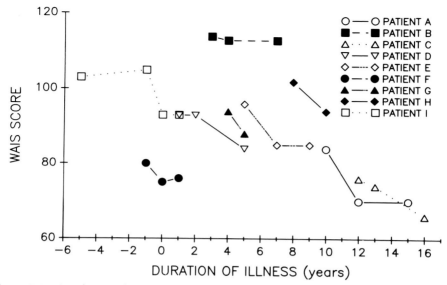

Figure 7-3   Serial IQ performance of several individual patients demonstrates that the IQ of HD patients' plateaus after an initial decline.

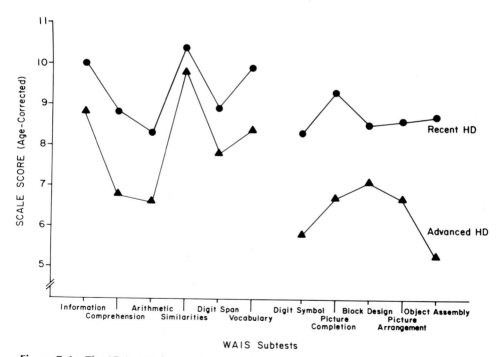

WAIS Subtests

Figure 7-4   The IQ in HD has a characteristic sawtooth pattern that is similar in patients tested early in the illness and later in the course.

in the illness (Norton, 1975; Butters et al., 1978; Josiassen et al., 1982; Brandt et al., 1984). These vulnerable subtests make sense in light of the clinical observations of impairments in memory, arithmetic, rapid performance of complex tasks, and sequential task performance.

The existence of a pattern of IQ test performance seen early in the illness has led several investigators to explore the WAIS as a method for presymptomatic testing in at-risk individuals (Lyle and Gottesman, 1977; Josiassen et al., 1982; Strauss and Brandt, 1986). However, because of the individual variability in premorbid subtest patterns, IQ tests are not useful predictors of illness for individual cases despite consistent group differences between at-risk persons who later become affected and those who escape HD. It may be possible to utilize IQ tests longitudinally as indicators of onset among individual at-risk persons who are in long-term follow-up and who can thus serve as their own controls.

SPECIFIC COGNITIVE DEFICITS IN HD

Attention and Concentration

HD patients are noted in everyday life to have difficulty sustaining performance on a wide variety of tasks—both motor and cognitive—suggesting difficulties in concentration. Most tests of attention and concentration require additional cognitive skills and are, therefore, difficult to measure in isolation. Over a wide range of tasks that require sustained concentration, such as mental arithmetic, digit-symbol coding, and reaction time, HD patients perform below the expected level for their overall cognitive ability (Fedio et al., 1979; Fisher et al., 1983).

Memory

Memory has been studied more than any other aspect of cognition in HD. Experiments have often contrasted the performance of HD patients with patients suffering from Korsakoff's syndrome or DAT. The pattern of memory and other cognitive deficits in HD varies depending on the severity of illness, which more recent studies have taken into account. Not all investigators use the same method of estimating disease duration or severity, making exact comparisons difficult. However, the bulk of evidence suggests that, although there is some difficulty with encoding new memories, the major problem is that newly acquired information cannot be recalled upon demand. Similarly, many old memories are retained but cannot be efficiently retrieved.

Studies of new learning in HD have revealed impairments in the elaboration of incoming stimuli, resulting in faulty storage of information (Caine et al., 1977; Weingartner et al., 1979). They have also demonstrated that the anterograde memory disorder of HD is qualitatively unlike that found in patients with amnesia due to alcoholic Korsakoff's syndrome, despite evidence that these patients also fail to analyze fully to-be-remembered information. Although Korsakoff patients benefit from procedures that increase the opportunity for encoding and those that decrease interitem interference, HD patients do not improve under these conditions (Butters, 1984). In contrast,

HD patients, but not amnesic Korsakoff patients, can employ successfully verbal mediators to improve their memory for pictorial materials (Butters et al., 1983). Considered together, these findings suggest that the HD patients' encoding deficits are not central to their memory disorder and that their intact language processing (Josiassen et al., 1982) can be used to facilitate mnestic processes.

Martone and her collaborators (1984) have reported that HD patients are impaired in the acquisition of a skill-based (i.e., procedural) task. HD and alcoholic Korsakoff patients were administered a mirror-reading task with word triads (e.g., doof, riahc, erif) as the experimental stimuli on each of 3 successive days. The time required to read each triad served as the dependent variable. Following the third day of skill learning, a recognition test was given to determine whether patients could remember the words from the mirror-reading task. The results revealed a double dissociation between the two patient groups on the skill learning and recognition memory tests. The amnesic Korsakoff patients evidenced a normal rate of skill learning (i.e., mirror reading) combined with severely impaired recognition memory for the verbal stimuli, while the HD patients showed normal recognition performance despite a significant retardation in their rate of skill acquisition. Fedio's earlier observation (Fedio et al., 1979) that HD patients display little improvement in learning a stylus maze despite substantial practice, and in fact violate the rules of the maze learning task, support Martone's finding. It appears then that the basal ganglia, especially the caudate nucleus, may play a major role in the acquisition of skill.

Other studies of memory failures in HD have also reported relatively normal recognition memory (Butters et al., 1985; Caine et al., 1978; Moss et al., 1986). Although HD patients are often as severely impaired as are amnesic patients on recall measures of new verbal learning, their recognition of recently presented verbal material is consistently superior to that of their amnesic counterparts. This difference between performance on recall and recognition tests has led to the proposal that the HD patient's verbal memory impairment reflects an inability to initiate systematic search strategies for the retrieval of stored information (Butters, 1984; Butters et al., 1985; Caine et al., 1978). An explicit test of this hypothesis was made by Brandt (1985). Patients with HD and normal controls attempted to recall items of general factual information. For those items for which recall failed, subjects were asked to make feeling-of-knowing judgments; that is, they were asked to estimate the likelihood that the unrecalled fact would be correctly recognized from among several alternatives. Finally, a multiple-choice recognition test was given for those items. The HD patients were as able as the normals in giving accurate feeling-of-knowing judgments. There was, as in the normals, a positive correlation between the feeling-of-knowing estimate given to an item and its likelihood of being recognized. However, the HD patient's response times during the recall test did not reflect their confidence estimates (see Figure 7-5). While normals take longer to answer an item which they have a strong feeling that they know, no such relationship was found for the HD patients. HD patients took as long to search their memories for answers to questions about which they had a strong feeling of knowing, as the ones that had little confidence in recalling. Thus there is the strong suggestion that, while HD patients' knowledge about their memory stores is relatively intact, their ability to make use of this information in allocating memory search time is faulty.

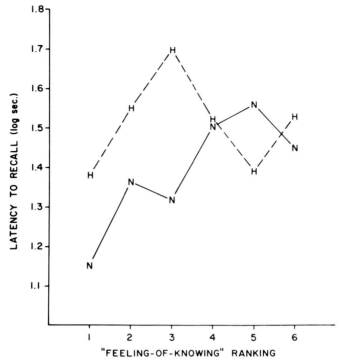

Figure 7-5 Latency to response on recall test for general information as a function of feeling-of-knowing. H, Huntington's disease; N, normal controls. (From Brandt, 1986.)

Memory for past events in HD is also qualitatively different from that in Korsakoff's disease. Patients with Korsakoff's disease display a marked temporal gradient of retrograde amnesia with events of the recent past more severely affected than events of the distant past. Patients with HD, even early in the course of the disease, are equally impaired in remembering public events from all periods of time (Albert et al., 1981a, 1981b) (Figure 7-6). This, like the verbal recognition data, suggests that failure to retrieve memories, rather than inefficient encoding, underlies memory failure in HD.

Most of the memory studies of HD patients have been limited to verbally presented material. However, one study by Moss et al. (1986) compared recognition memory for written words, colors, position of markers on a board, simple linear designs, and faces. Each test used the same paradigm, so that test difficulty across categories of stimuli was comparable. The HD patients performed as well as normal controls *only* on recognition of written words (Figure 7-7). Their recognition memory in all other test situations was severely impaired and did not differ from that of patients with DAT or Korsakoff's syndrome, suggesting that verbal memory may be relatively spared in HD (Josiassen, Curry, and Mancall, 1983). Alternatively, the general visuospatial deficits seen in HD (see following material) may interfere with testing of memory for nonverbal material.

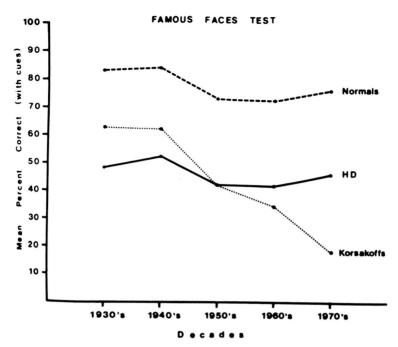

Figure 7-6 Performance of patients with Huntington's disease, alcoholic Korsakoff's syndrome, and normal controls on the Famous Faces Test of the Boston Retrograde Amnesia Battery. (From Albert et al., 1981a.)

Speech and Language

Patients with HD do not have clinically significant language disorders such as would be seen in patients with cortical lesions of the dominant hemisphere or those with cortical dementias (e.g., DAT). However, HD patients do have impairments in speech. Ludlow, Connor, and Bassich (1987) have recently studied speech planning, initiation, and production in patients with Parkinson's disease and HD. In the HD patients there were impairments in the control of syllable duration, duration of pauses between phrases, and duration of sentences, as well as a reduced rate of syllable repetition. The authors suggest that the caudate nucleus may play a major role in controlling speech movement time.

In the Controlled Oral Word Association Test (FAS Test) (Borkowski, Benton, and Spreen, 1967), the patient is asked to say as many words as possible that begin with the letters F, A, and S. One minute is allowed for each letter. Early in the illness, HD patients score well below education-, sex-, and age-based norms. They say a few words and then fall silent even if prompted to continue the task, and they seldom remember additional words within the allowed minute. Later in the testing session, however, they may spontaneously mention some other words.

Poor performance on the FAS Test is in sharp contrast to performance on the Boston Naming Test (BNT), a test of picture recognition (Butters et al., 1978). The BNT

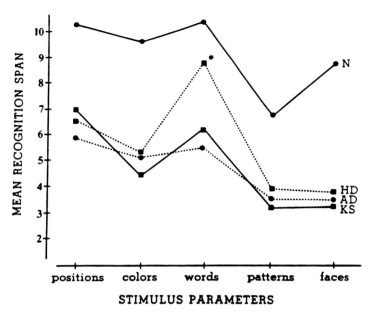

DELAYED RECOGNITION SPAN TEST

Figure 7-7 Performance on the Delayed Recognition Span Test in normals (N), patients with Huntington's disease (HD), Alzheimer's disease (AD), and Korsakoff's syndrome (KS). (From Moss et al., 1986.)

consists of a series of line drawings of common objects that patients are asked to name. Most HD patients usually achieve high scores, even in the more advanced stages of illness, if points are not deducted for slow performance.

A recent study by Smith et al. (1988) examined semantic relations in patients with mild to moderate HD. Compared with normal controls, patients with mild HD were impaired on WAIS-R Vocabulary and BNT performance, as well as on measures of verbal fluency (FAS and animal naming). While this finding is in contrast with some of Butters' previous studies, it should be noted that the naming impairment was relatively mild compared with the language deficits found in cortical dementias (e.g., DAT). Nonetheless, the data are consistent with the notion that HD patients are impaired on certain tasks that require access to lexical (word) information. In a set of experiments involving semantic priming, Smith and co-workers found that, the more severely impaired an HD patient was, the less likely it was that his semantic priming performance would reflect a sensitivity to the degree of semantic association between word pairs. Although the HD patients, as a group, showed no impairment in the ability to demonstrate a priming effect, there was a progressive decline among the HD patients in the degree to which association strength of word pairs affected the priming of semantic relations. Thus, while HD apparently does not involve the loss of semantic representations (as has been suggested of DAT), there is apparently some disruption in the activation of those relations that becomes progressively more severe as the disease advances.

Visuospatial Cognition

Although HD patients usually do not have apraxia, as measured by their ability to dress themselves or mimic motor acts, their visuospatial skills are clearly abnormal. This is so even early in the illness when failures cannot be attributed to general cognitive decline or difficulties with motor coordination (Josiassen, Curry, and Mancall, 1983). Early deficits have been documented with the WAIS subtests measuring constructional ability and visuomotor skill, such as Object Assembly (jigsawlike puzzles) and Block Design (constructing a geometric pattern using colored cubes). In addition, deficits are detected on tests that do not require motor acts (Moses et al., 1981; Fedio et al., 1979). Fedio demonstrated this using the Mosaic Comparisons task. Subjects observed two grids of 9, 16, or 25 squares each and were asked to identify the one square that differed in the two grids. HD patients, as well as some at-risk individuals, performed more poorly than controls.

HD patients also have difficulty identifying their position in space, relative to some fixed point, if their own position in space is altered. In a study by Potegal (1971), patients observed a target and were then blindfolded and asked to point with a stylus to the position where the target had been. Patients were able to do this accurately unless they were moved one step to the side, after which they could no longer accurately localize the target. Potegal suggested that patients have difficulty in updating their position in space after a self-produced movement; he had previously identified a similar phenomenon in rats with caudate lesions. This deficit in updating egocentric spatial localization was also found by Brouwers et al. (1984) using different tasks. Their study also showed that patients with DAT retained egocentric spatial orientation but lost the ability to perceive extrapersonal spatial relationships on a task performed normally by HD patients. HD patients also have trouble with tasks involving left–right discrimination, especially when the positions are not consonant with their own, as for example in a road map (Fedio et al., 1979).

"Executive" Functions in Huntington's Disease

Since the head of the caudate nucleus receives its major cortical innervation from the prefrontal cortex (Goldman and Nauta, 1977; DeLong and Georgopoulos, 1979), it would be reasonable to expect HD patients to display features of a "frontal lobe syndrome." In fact, mildly demented patients complain regularly of difficulty planning, organizing, and scheduling activities—all well-recognized aspects of frontal lobe pathology (Caine et al., 1978; Fedio et al., 1979). Objective testing confirms that many behavioral characteristics of patients with lesions confined to the frontal cortex, such as diminished verbal fluency (Butters et al., 1978; Wexler, 1979), poor maze performance (Fedio et al., 1979), inability to compensate for postural adjustments (Potegal, 1971), loss of mental flexibility (Josiassen et al., 1982; Wexler, 1979), and perseverative tendencies (Josiassen et al., 1982) are regularly seen in HD. However, studies comparing HD, DAT, and alcoholic Korsakoff patients on "frontal" perseverative tendencies have shown that HD patients are less prone to these errors of commission than are the other two patient groups (Butters et al., 1983; Butters, 1985). For example, on a verbal fluency task that assesses patients' ability to search their long-term semantic memories, both DAT and Korsakoff patients generate more perseverative responses than do patients with HD. Similarly, DAT and Korsakoff patients produce more intra-test intrusion errors on a picture-context recognition task (Butters et al., 1983) and in the immediate recall of a series of short passages (Butters, 1985). Thus, while HD patients may display some "frontal" cognitive and behavioral abnormalities, such symptoms may be more severe in other dementias and amnesic conditions, especially on nonmotor, verbal tasks.

Families often report that patients become rigid in their behavior, unable to change easily from one activity to another or to change their routines. This may be analogous to the great difficulty they have on cognitive tasks that require a change in set (Josiassen, Curry, and Mancall, 1983; Fedio et al., 1979). On Part B of the Trail Making Test, for example, subjects are asked to draw a line connecting numbered and lettered circles by alternating between numbers and letters (1-A-2-B-3-C, etc.). HD patients perform this much more slowly than would be expected from their scores on part A, where they must connect the same number of circles in numerical order (Starkstein et al., 1988). The difficulty in changing sets is also demonstrated by the Wisconsin Card Sorting Test. Subjects are asked to sort cards by pattern, color, or number but must discern the rules only by the examiner saying "right" or "wrong" as the subject sorts each card. Once the subject discerns the correct strategy, the examiner switches to a different one. HD patients quickly figure out the initial strategy but are typically not able to switch to others, persistently returning to the original one.

In fact, any task that is complex, that requires frequent set changes, that requires more than one abstraction at once (Wexler, 1979), or that uses rules not previously known to the subject (Fedio et al., 1979) will be difficult even for mildly affected HD patients.

STUDIES OF PERSONS AT-RISK

Each offspring of a person with HD has a 50% chance of having the gene and, hence, of developing the illness. Individuals at risk for HD, as a group, perform more poorly than normals on tasks that HD patients perform poorly. These include learning spatial paths, visuoperceptual analysis, and directional sense (Fedio et al., 1979). Wexler (1979) reported that, while at-risk individuals, as a group, were unimpaired in any of the cognitive domains she examined, a subgroup of them (defined by cluster analysis) had particularly low scores on tests of memory, digit-symbol coding, and response competition. Since these are tasks on which HD patients consistently perform very poorly, Wexler cautiously raised the possibility that this subgroup was composed largely of presymptomatic gene carriers.

There have been several attempts to use neuropsychological tests to determine which at-risk individuals actually carry the HD gene. Lyle and Quast (1976) performed follow-up psychological assessments of at-risk individuals 10–20 years after their initial assessments. They found that the 22 people who became ill in the interim (out of 156) had lower recall scores on the Bender Gestalt Test on initial assessment. It was later reported that lower scores on tests of abstraction and general intelligence also discriminated at-risks who later developed HD from those who did not (Lyle and Gottesman, 1977). Wexler (1979) has suggested that persons who go on to develop the HD phenotype are deficient in the "capacity to recognize and mentally encode incoming stimuli," and that prediction or very early detection of illness should be possible through examination of the patterning of a number of cognitive performances. A study by Strauss and Brandt (1986) revealed that, while HD patients and normal subjects have different profile patterns on the WAIS (ignoring overall level of performance), these differences are not sufficiently robust to segregate at-risk subjects into normal and HD groups with any reliability.

A recent study of at-risk individuals compared the neuropsychological characteristics of those individuals who were shown to have the recently discovered DNA marker for HD with those who do not have the marker. Jason et al. (1988) gave a comprehensive battery of cognitive tests to 10 asymptomatic at-risk individuals, 7 of whom had the HD marker and 3 of whom did not. While none of the three subjects in the marker-negative group had any neuropsychological impairments, 5 of the 7 in the marker-positive group did have impairments. The deficits, however, were extremely mild, and of the 41 statistical comparisons between the marker-positive and marker-negative groups, only four yielded differences significant at the $p < .05$ level. Studies underway in our center, with larger subject groups and a more selective set of neurocognitive measures, will help reveal whether asymptomatic individuals who are very likely to have the Huntington's gene display subtle impairments in mental functioning.

NONCOGNITIVE ASPECTS OF THE SUBCORTICAL DEMENTIA OF HD

Mood and Other Psychiatric Features

Huntington (1872) described insanity with a tendency to suicide as one of the characteristic features of the disease. In the Maryland survey, affective disorder was present in 38 percent of cases at some time in the course (Folstein et al., 1987); 9 percent of cases had bipolar disorder. Furthermore, the mood disorder is aggregated in affected members of some families and is uncommon in other families. The mechanism of the mood disorder is not known but is not likely to be simply a reaction to disease onset, although this certainly occurs. The mood disorder often precedes any motor or cognitive signs, occurring episodically for as long as 20 years before the onset of chorea. Furthermore, affective changes may be manic as well as depressive.

Another mood disorder that occurs frequently is described in DSM-III as "intermittent explosive disorder." This may also be a presenting symptom, causing the family to request psychiatric consultation or creating difficulties for the patient with his family or his employer. In some patients it worsens to the point of aggression toward others. More usually, patients become irritable in response to some environmental event that might reasonably cause irritation, but the response is more severe and prolonged than warranted.

This disease-associated irritability is to be distinguished from antisocial behavior that occurs in the children of affected parents. Antisocial behavior is probably related to family disruption caused by an ill and irrational parent, rather than as a consequence of the neuropathology in a young person at-risk (Folstein et al., 1983b). While many at-risk individuals with episodic depression later become affected, antisocial behavior in an at-risk individual does not predict the subsequent onset of disease.

Schizophrenialike disorders occur in about 4 percent of cases, a rate slightly higher than expected in the general population, but far less than the rates described in early studies of psychopathology in HD. HD patients do share many of the so-called negative symptoms of schizophrenia, but first-rank symptoms or even delusions and hallucinations of any type are unusual in HD patients.

Some HD patients are afflicted with an inert, apathetic state much like some patients with schizophrenia and other subcortical disorders such as Parkinson's disease or hydrocephalus. This is very common in patients after 7–10 years of illness, but some patients become apathetic almost immediately. The patient will remain in a chair watching television or doing nothing for hours. Many such patients are willing to participate in activities initiated and sustained by others but revert to inertia as soon as outside stimulation is withdrawn. In addition to this lack of activity, apathetic patients do not seem to appreciate the severity of their functional disability. They often deny even the most obvious difficulties with managing their affairs as well as physical disabilities. It is this constellation of inertia and apparent lack of concern for the gravity of the symptoms that have led us to describe the dementia of HD as an apathetic dementia.

Movement Disorders

Movement disorders always occur in HD but may begin well after the onset of mood and cognitive disorder. There are at least two types of movement disorder found in HD—voluntary and involuntary types. The involuntary movement disorder includes the typical choreiform movements, which are unpredictable, and jerking movements of the face, limbs, and trunk that happen at rest or in the midst of other movements such as walking. When severe, chorea can interfere with sequential activities such as speaking, eating, or walking. The fusion of chorea with gait leads to the dancelike or drunken movements, from which chorea drives its name. Patients can suppress choreic movements for short periods, and chorea is usually, but not always, absent during sleep. Other types of involuntary movements may also occur, including a general motor restlessness early in the course, as well as tremor and myoclonic jerks in patients whose symptoms begin early in life (S. Folstein, 1989).

The voluntary motor disorder is characterized by delayed initiation, slowing of eye movements (Leigh et al., 1983), limb movements, and general clumsiness. Voluntary motor abnormalities are seen in isolation (i.e., without chorea) in patients with the Westphal variant (common in children and young adult black patients) and in patients late in the course when chorea often subsides. Both types of motor disorder progress with the duration of illness, but the voluntary disorder correlates best with cognitive impairment (Brandt et al., 1984).

NEUROPATHOLOGIC CORRELATES

The caudate nucleus, the striatal nucleus most severely and consistently affected in HD, is not connected to the motor cortex. Instead, it receives much of its cortical input from the parietal and prefrontal lobes, especially those areas serving to integrate cognitive functions. Therefore, it is not surprising that the cognitive functions affected in HD—ability to plan and organize, verbal fluency, mental flexibility (changing sets), and some aspects of memory search and retrieval—are similar to those found in patients with frontal lobe disease (Stuss and Benson, 1984). Several investigators, using a variety of methods, have now demonstrated the relationship of caudate pathology to cognitive changes in HD. Sax et al. (1983) reported that IQ and scores on the Wechsler Memory Scale were significantly correlated with caudate atrophy as measured on a CT scan. Furthermore, SAX reported that adding chorea to a multiple regression analysis did not add to the variance in caudate atrophy, once the influence of cognitive variables was considered. Bamford et al. (1986) reported similar findings. Richfield, Twyman, and Berent (1987) reported cognitive and behavioral abnormalities (but not motor signs) similar to those seen in HD in a patient with bilateral caudate damage.

Starkstein et al. (1988) demonstrated a strong relationship between caudate atrophy, as measured by CT, and performance on several cognitive tests (Table 7-2). He found no significant correlation between scores on cognitive tests and CT measures of cortical atrophy, nor did he find any relationship between motor abnormalities and caudate or cortical atrophy.

In a recent positron emission tomography (PET) scan study, Berent et al. (1988) found that HD patients have lower cerebral metabolism in both the caudate nucleus

Table 7-2 Correlations between CT Measures in HD Patients and Neuropsychological Test Scores, N = 18[a]

Test	BCR	BFR	FFR	4CSR
Minimental status				
R	−.49	.03	−.02	.06
p value	.002	NS	NS	NS
Symbol digit modalities (written)				
R	−.65	−.30	−.04	−.48
p value	.002	NS	NS	NS
Symbol digit modalities (oral)				
R	−.67	−.41	−.12	−.47
p value	.001	NS	NS	NS
Trails A (time)				
R	.72	.32	−.18	.43
p value	.001	NS	NS	NS
Trails B (time)				
R	.80	.48	−.29	.48
p value	.0001	NS	NS	NS

[a]18 patients whose severity of illness varied were administered computed tomographic scans and a series of cognitive tests. All the cognitive tests correlated highly with a measure of caudate atrophy (bicaudate ratio, BCR) but not at all with measures of cortical atrophy: frontal horn size as measured by bifrontal ratio (BFR), the size of the frontal fissure (frontal fissure ratio, FFR), and a sum of the size of four cortical sulci (SSR). (From Starkstein et al., 1988.)

and putamen compared with normal control subjects. There was no difference between the groups in cerebral metabolic rate for glucose in the thalamus. The cerebral metabolic rate for glucose in the caudate correlated highly with verbal memory as well as total memory score (Memory Quotient) in HD patients. Much weaker correlation between these aspects of memory and metabolic rate were observed in the putamen. Very weak and nonsignificant correlations were found with PET activity in the thalamus. Within the normal control group, there were no significant relationships between cerebral metabolic rate for glucose and cognitive functioning (with the single exception of digit-symbol substitution and activity in the putamen). This study provides further evidence that, of the subcortical nuclei that can be imaged and quantified with PET, the caudate nucleus shows the strongest relationship with memory functioning in HD.

Evidence is, therefore, accumulating that cognitive features in HD are related specifically to dysfunction in the caudate nucleus, and that the cognitive functions involved are those served by the prefrontal cortex, which provides the major cortical input to the caudate. The other subcortical dementias, such as those seen in Parkinson's disease (Mortimer et al., 1987), supranuclear palsy, and the dementia of frontal lobe disease (Taylor et al., 1986; Salazar et al., 1986) have many features in common with the dementia of HD and also have neuropathologies that interrupt the connections between the prefrontal cortex and its output to the caudate nucleus (Geshwind, 1965).

SUMMARY AND CONCLUSIONS

HD provides a clear example of subcortical dementia. Patients have manifest cognitive deficits affecting attention and calculation, verbal fluency, cognitive speed, retrieval of memories, the ability to persist at a task, and the ability to change cognitive sets. They do not evidence the aphasia, amnesia, apraxis, or agnosia characteristic of patients with cortical dementia. Studies of primates (reviewed by Alexander, DeLong, and Strick, 1986) and human disease (reviewed by Stuss and Benson, 1984) have demonstrated that these functions are served by those parts of the frontal lobe that provide the major cortical input to the caudate nucleus. In x-ray computed tomography and PET studies of HD patients, measures of caudate atrophy, but not cortical measures, correlate with the severity of cognitive deficit. Disorders characterized by subcortical dementia also include abnormalities of movement and mood, and we propose that the definition of subcortical dementia be expanded to include these noncognitive features.

ACKNOWLEDGMENTS

The authors have received support from the Alzheimer's Disease Research Center - NIA AG-05146, the John Douglas French Foundation, Meridian Healthcare Systems, Huntington's Disease Center Without Walls - NINCDS-1637, Genetic Testing for Huntington's Disease - 1 R01 NS24841-01, the Consolidated Gift Fund for Dementia Research, and Research Training in the Dementias of Aging - T32 AG00149.

REFERENCES

Albert, M.S., Butters, N., and Brandt, J. Patterns of remote memory in amnesic and demented patients. *Arch Neurol* 1981a; 38:495–500.

Albert, M.S., Butters, N., and Brandt, J. Development of remote memory loss in patients with Huntington's Disease. *J Clin Exp Neuropsychol* 1981b; 3:1–12.

Albert, M.L., Feldman, R.G., and Willis, A.L. The subcortical dementia of progressive supranuclear palsy. *J Neurol Neurosurg Psychiatry* 1974; 37:121–30.

Alexander, G.E., Delong, M.R., and Strick, P.L. Parallel organization of functionally segregated circuits linking basal ganglia and cortex. *Am Rev Neurosci* 1986; 9:357–81.

Anthony, J.C. et al. Limits of the "mini-mental state" as a screening test for dementia and delirium among hospital patients. *Psychol Med* 1982; 12:397–408.

Bamford, K. et al. Neuropsychological impairment in early HD: Functional and CT correlates. *Neurology* 1986; 36 (Suppl. 1):102–3.

Berent, S. et al. Positron emission tomographic investigations of Huntington's disease: Cerebral metabolic correlates of cognitive function. *Ann Neurol* 1988; 23:541–6.

Borkowski, J.G., Genton, A.L., and Spreen, O. Word fluency and brain damage. *Neuropsychologica* 1967; 5:135–40.

Brandt, J. Access to knowledge in the dementia of Huntington's disease. *Dev Neuropsychol* 1985; 1:335–8.

Brandt, J. et al. Clinical correlates of dementia and disability in Huntington's disease. *J Clin Exp Neuropsychol* 1984; 6:401–12.

Brandt, J., Folstein, S.E., and Folstein, M.F. Differential cognitive impairment in Alzheimer's and Huntington's disease. *Ann Neurol* 1988; 23:555–61.

Brouwers, P. et al. Differential perceptual-spatial impairment in Huntington's and Alzheimer's dementia. *Arch Neurol* 1984; 41:1073–6.

Butters, N. The clinical aspects of memory disorders: Contributions from experimental studies of amnesia and dementia. *J Clin Exp Neuropsychol* 1984; 6:17–36.

Butters, N. Alcoholic Korsakoff's Syndrome: Some unresolved issues concerning etiology, neuropathology, and cognitive deficits. *J Clin Exp Neuropsychol* 1985; 7:179–208.

Butters, N. et al. The effect of verbal elaborators on the pictorial memory of brain-damaged patients. *Neuropsychologia* 1983; 21:307–23.

Butters, N. et al. Comparison of the neuropsychological deficits associated with early and advanced Huntington's Disease. *Arch Neurol* 1978; 35:585–9.

Butters, N. et al. Memory disorders associated with Huntington's disease: Verbal recall, verbal recognition, and procedural memory. *Neuropsychologia* 1985; 23:729–43.

Caine, E.D., Ebert, M., and Weingartner, H. An outline for the analysis of dementia: The memory disorder of Huntington's disease. *Neurology* 1977; 27:1087–92.

Caine, E.D. et al. Huntington's dementia: Clinical and neuropsychological features. *Arch Gen Psychiatry* 1978; 35:378–84.

Cummings, J.L., and Benson, D.F. Subcortical dementia: Review of an emerging concept. *Arch Neurol* 1984; 41:874–9.

DeLong, M.R., and Georgopoulos, A.P. Physiology of the basal ganglia—A brief overview. In *Advances in Neurology, Vol. 23: Huntington's Disease*. Chase, T.N., Wexler, N.S., and Barbeau, A. (eds.). Raven Press, New York, 1979, pp. 137–53.

Fedio, P. et al. Neuropsychological profile in Huntington's disease: Patients and those at risk. In *Advances in Neurology, Vol. 23: Huntington's Disease*. Chase, T.N., Wexler, N.S., and Barbeau, A. (eds.). Raven Press, New York, 1979, pp. 239–55.

Fisher, J.M. et al. Dementia in Huntington's disease: A cross-sectional analysis of intellectual decline. In *The Dementias.* Mayeux, R. and Rosen, W.G. (eds.). Raven Press, New York, 1983, pp. 229–38.

Folstein, M.F., Folstein, S.E., and McHugh, P.R. "Mini-Mental State": A practical method for grading the cognitive state of patients for the clinician. *J Psychiatr Res* 1975; 12:189–98.

Folstein, S.E. *Huntington's Disease: A Disorder of Families* The Johns Hopkins University Press, Baltimore, 1989.

Folstein, S.E. Unpublished data.

Folstein, S.E. et al. The association of affective disorder with Huntington disease in a case series and in families. *Psychol Med* 1983a; 13:537–42.

Folstein, S.E. et al. Conduct disorder and affective disorder among the offspring of patients with Huntington's disease. In *Childhood Psychopathology and Development* Guze, S.B., Earls, F.J., and Barrett, J.E. (eds.). 1983b, pp. 231–45.

Folstein, S.E. et al. Huntington disease in Maryland: Clinical aspects of racial variation. *Am J Hum Genet* 1987; 41:168–79.

Folstein, S.E. et al. The diagnosis of Huntington's disease. *Neurology* 1986; 36:1279–83.

Geshwind, N. Disconnexion syndromes in animals and man. *Brain* 1965; 88:237–94; 88:585–644.

Goldman, P.S., and Nauta, W.J.H. An intricately pattered prefronto-caudate projection in the rhesus monkey. *J Comp Neurol* 1977; 171:369–86.

Gusella, J.F. et al. A polymorphic DNA marker genetically linked to Huntington's disease. *Nature* 1983; 306:234–8.

Hayden, M.R., MacGregor, J.M., and Beighton, P.H. The prevalence of Huntington's chorea in South Africa. *S Afr Med J* 1980; 58:193–6.

Huntington, G. On chorea. *Med Surg Rep* 1872; 26:317–21.

Jason, G.W. et al. Presymptomatic Neuropsychological Impairment in Huntington's Disease. *Arch Neurol* 1988; 45:769–73.

Josiassen, R.C., Curry, L.M., and Mancall, E.L. Development of neuropsychological deficits in Huntington's disease. *Arch Neurol* 1983; 40:791–96.

Josiassen, R.C. et al. Patterns of intellectual deficit in Huntington's Disease. *J Clin Exp Neuropsychol* 1982; 4:173–83.

Josiassen, R.C. et al. Auditory and visual evoked potentials in Huntington's disease. *Electroencephalogr Clin Neurophysiol* 1984; 57:113–8.

Leigh, R.J. et al. Abnormal ocular motor control in Huntington's disease. *Neurology* 1983; 33:1268–75.

Ludlow, C.L., Connor, N.P., and Bassich, C.J. Speech timing in Parkinson's and Huntington's disease. *Brain Lang* 1987; 32:195–214.

Lyle, O., and Gottesman, I. Premorbid psychometric indicators of the gene for Huntington's disease. *J Consult Clin Psychol* 1977; 45:1011–22.

Lyle, O., and Quast, W. The Bender Gestalt: Use of clinical judgement versus recall in the prediction of Huntington's disease. *J Consult Clin Psychol* 1976; 44:229–32.

Martone, M. et al. Dissociation between skill learning and verbal recognition in amnesia and dementia. *Arch Neurol* 1984; 42:965–70.

Mayeux, R. et al. Is "subcortical dementia" a recognizable clinical entity? *An* 1981; 14:278–83.

McHugh, P.R., and Folstein, M.F. Psychiatric symptoms of Huntington's chorea: A clinical and phenomenologic study. In *Psychiatric Aspects of Neurological Disease.* Benson, D.F., and Blumer, D. (eds.). Raven Press, New York, 1975, pp. 267–85.

Merritt, A.D. et al. Juvenile Huntington's chorea. In *Progress of Neurogenetics.* Barbeau, A., and Brunette, T.R. (eds.). Excerpta Medica Foundation, Amsterdam, 1969, pp. 645–50.

Mortimer, J.A. et al. Cognitive and behavioral disorders in Parkinson's disease. *An International Conference on the Basal Ganglia,* abstract 14.15. The University of Leeds, England, 1987.

Moses, J. et al. Neuropsychological deficits in early, middle, and late stages of Huntington's disease as measured by the Luria-Nebraska Neuropsychological Battery. *Int J Neurosci* 1981; 14:95–100.

Moss, M. et al. Differential patterns of memory loss among patients with Alzheimer's disease, Huntington's disease, and alcoholic Korsakoff's syndrome. *Arch Neurol* 1986; 43:239–46.

Norton, J.C. Patterns of neuropsychological performance in Huntington's disease. *J Nerv Ment Dis* 1975; 161:276–9.

Potegal, M. A note on spatial-motor deficits in patients with Huntington's disease: Test of a hypothesis. *Neuropsychologia* 1971; 9:233–5.

Richfield, E.K., Twyman, R., and Berent, S. Neurological syndrome following bilateral damage to the head of the caudate nuclei. *Ann Neurol* 1987; 22:768–71.

Salazar, A.M. et al. Penetrating war injuries of the basal forebrain: Neurology and cognition. *Neurology* 1986; 36:459–65.

Sax, D. et al. Computer tomographic, neurologic, and neuropsychological correlates of Huntington's disease. *Int J Neurosci* 1983; 18:21–36.

Smith, S. et al. Priming semantic relations in patients with Huntington's disease. *Brain Lang* 1988; 33:27–40.

Starkstein, S.E. et al. Neuropsychologic and neuroradiologic correlates in Huntington's disease. *J Neurol Neurosurg Psychiatry* 1988; 51:1259–63.

Strauss, M.E., and Brandt, J. An attempt at presymptomatic identification of Huntington's disease with the WAIS. *J Clin Exp Neuropsychol* 1986; 8:210–8.

Stuss, D.T., and Benson, D.F. Neuropsychological studies of the frontal lobes. *Psychol Bull* 1984; 95:3–28.

Taylor, A.E., Saint-Cyr, J.A., and Lang, A.E. Frontal lobe dysfunction in Parkinson's disease. *Brain* 1986; 109:845–83.

Vonsattel, J.P. et al. Neuropathological classification of Huntington's disease. *J Neuropathol Exp Neurol* 1985; 44:559–77.

Weingartner, H., Caine, E.D., and Ebert, M.H. Encoding processes, learning, and recall in Huntington's disease. In *Advances in Neurology, Vol. 23: Huntington's Disease.* Chase, T.N., Wexler, N.S., and Barbeau, A. (eds.). Raven Press, New York, 1979, pp. 215–26.

Wexler, N.S. Perceptual-motor, cognitive, and emotional characteristics of persons at-risk for Huntington's disease. In *Advances in Neurology, Vol. 23: Huntington's Disease.* Chase, T.N., Wexler, N.S., and Barbeau, A. (eds.). Raven Press, New York, pp. 1979:257–71.

Whitehouse, P.J. The concept of subcortical and cortical dementia: Another look. *Ann Neurol* 1986; 19:1–6.

8

Parkinson's Disease

MORRIS FREEDMAN

Idiopathic Parkinson's disease (PD) is a degenerative brain disorder of unknown etiology initially described by James Parkinson in 1817. Approximately 0.1 percent of the population (i.e., one per thousand) suffer from this condition. Although both genetic and environmental factors have been implicated in the pathogenesis of PD (McDowell et al., 1978; Ward et al., 1983), it is of interest that the prevalence rate is uniform throughout the world (McDowell et al., 1978). The age of onset is usually between 40 and 70 years, with a peak onset in the sixth decade. Hoehn and Yahr (1967) studied 802 patients with PD and found that the mean duration of illness varied with the age of onset. In patients who first developed symptoms over the age of 50, the duration was 8 years, with a range from 1 to 30 years. Patients who developed PD at a younger age had a longer course, with a mean duration of 18.4 years and a range from 2 to 40 years.

Although dementia was not originally considered to be a feature of PD (Parkinson, 1938), it is now recognized that significant cognitive deficits commonly occur (Riklan, 1973; Cummings and Benson, 1983). Prevalence rates reported in the literature range from 4 to 93 percent (Cummings, 1988). Cummings calculated a mean prevalence of 39.9 percent based upon 4,336 cases reported in the literature, whereas Brown and Marsden (1984) have suggested that 25 percent might be a more valid estimate. Prevalence rates must, however, be viewed with caution, since the figures vary with the criteria for dementia, the population of PD patients studied, and the cognitive assessment procedures used. Also, the determination of prevalence rates carries an underlying assumption that there are, in fact, distinct subgroups of PD patients with and without dementia. This assumption has been challenged by Pirozzolo et al. (1982), who suggested that there may be a continuum of intellectual impairment ranging from no deficits to severe dementia, rather than distinct subgroups.

CLINICAL CHARACTERISTICS

Parkinson's disease is readily diagnosed by the physical signs shown by affected individuals. Abnormalities include stooped posture, bradykinesia, a 4–8 c/sec resting tremor, cogwheel rigidity, and a festinating gait. Patients may also have infrequent blinking, micrographia (small handwriting), hypophonia (reduced voice volume), dysarthria, and a tendency to speak in a monotone. A small percentage of patients have a 6–12 c/sec action tremor. Eye movement abnormalities, such as limitation of upward gaze, are not uncommon (McDowell et al., 1978). Some PD patients may have difficulty swallowing, with resultant excess saliva and drooling. Patients may also develop impotence, orthostatic hypotension, and constipation due to autonomic dysfunction.

PATHOLOGY AND PATHOPHYSIOLOGY

Neuropathologic findings consist of degenerative lesions affecting primarily the pigmented cells in the substantia nigra and other pigmented nuclei in the brain stem. Lewy bodies—eosinophilic cytoplasmic inclusions in cells of the substantia nigra and locus ceruleus—are present in almost all cases (Adams and Victor, 1985). There may also be cell loss in the nucleus basalis of Meynert (Whitehouse et al., 1983), and some cases exhibit neurofibrillary tangles, senile plaques, and granulovacuolar degeneration (Alvord et al., 1974; Hakim and Mathieson, 1979; Boller et al., 1980).

The major neurochemical deficit in PD is a marked reduction in dopamine. The dopamine deficiency involves frontal cortex and striatum, and, within the head of the caudate, the most severe reduction is found in the anterodorsal sector (Kish et al., 1986; Kish et al., 1988). Cell loss also occurs in the ventral tegmental area, the source of mesolimbic–mesocortical dopaminergic fibers. Ventral tegmental fibers project to the frontal cortex, as well as to the nucleus accumbens and entorhinal cortex (Javoy-Agid and Agid, 1980; Uhl et al., 1985; Hornykiewicz and Kish, 1986). Decreased levels of norepinephrine, acetylcholine, and somatostatin, and a reduction in serotonin receptors may also occur (Cummings, 1988).

The EEG is normal or shows nonspecific slowing. Computerized tomography is normal or shows cerebral atrophy but has no predictive value for determining cognitive function in an individual case (Freedman et al., 1984a). Blood flow studies have shown reduced flow in the frontal mesocortex (Perlmutter, 1988). Positron emission tomography (PET) studies reveal abnormalities in the basal ganglia and in the cerebral cortex (Perlmutter, 1988).

Evoked potential abnormalities have also been reported. The P300 component of the auditory evoked response has an increased latency in PD and has been significantly related to performance on neuropsychological measures of visuospatial perception, perceptual organization, visual scanning speed, and response translation speed (Hansch et al., 1982). Visual evoked responses are also abnormal, showing longer latencies and reduced amplitude (Gawel et al., 1981).

DEMENTIA SYNDROME

It is controversial whether the dementia syndrome of PD is due to (1) the subcortical neurodegenerative changes, (2) superimposed dementia of the Alzheimer type (DAT), or (3) a combination of these and assorted neurochemical deficiencies (Cummings and Benson, 1983). Although nonhuman animal models have long supported a role for subcortical brain structures in a variety of cognitive functions (Battig et al., 1960; Divac et al., 1967; Oberg and Divac, 1979; Rosvold, 1972), it is only recently that parallel concepts have emerged linking subcortical brain pathology to intellectual deficits in humans with neurological disease (Albert et al., 1974; McHugh and Folstein, 1975; Olton et al., 1985). *Subcortical dementia,* the term originally applied to the constellation of cognitive deficits attributed to subcortical brain damage in humans, was initially characterized as including: (1) memory loss, (2) impaired manipulation of acquired knowledge (i.e., calculating and abstracting abilities), (3) personality changes marked by apathy and inertia, and (4) general slowness of thought processes (Albert et al., 1974). In contrast, cortical dementias, of which DAT is the prototypical example, are distinguished by the presence of aphasia, apraxia, and agnosia (Albert et al., 1974; McHugh and Folstein, 1975). Although the concept of subcortical dementia was originally based on an analysis of the pattern of personality and cognitive deficits in progressive supranuclear palsy (Albert et al., 1974) and Huntington's disease (McHugh and Folstein, 1975), the majority of studies addressing the concept of subcortical dementia have used PD as a model of subcortical dementia and DAT as a model of cortical dementia. The focus of this chapter will be to review recent data from the study of PD that shed new light on the concept of subcortical dementia. The emphasis will be on studies that attempt to determine whether there are neuropsychological or neuroanatomical mechanisms that differentiate the cognitive deficits of PD from those of DAT.

STUDIES COMPARING PARKINSON'S AND ALZHEIMER'S DEMENTIA

Language Deficits

The cognitive deficit that best distinguishes the dementia associated with PD from that in DAT is the presence of aphasia in DAT. Cummings et al. (1988) studied language function in patients with PD and dementia, PD without dementia, and DAT using a battery composed of items from the Boston Diagnostic Aphasia Examination and the Western Aphasia Battery. The demented PD patients and the DAT patients were equated for severity of dementia on the Mini-Mental State Examination (Folstein et al., 1975). The demented PD patients had significantly more impairment on motoric speech functions, that is, on measures of dysarthria, phrase length, speech melody, and writing mechanics, compared with the DAT patients. The DAT patients, on the other hand, showed significantly more deficits in their ability to name visually presented objects and to generate animal names in a 1 minute period. They also had significantly greater impoverishment of information content in spontaneous speech compared with the demented PD patients. The latter, therefore, showed a speech and language profile that was distinct from that of DAT. The demented PD patients exhibited mild deficits in language ability, such as naming and narrative writing, indicating that their language function was not entirely normal. This is in keeping with the findings of Globus et al. (1985) and Freedman et al. (1984b), who found deficits in naming ability in PD patients with intellectual impairment.

Bayles and Tomoeda (1983) found that naming ability in a group of demented PD patients differed from that of a group of DAT patients who had been equated for severity of cognitive deficits on the basis of a bedside neurological examination and a short mental status inventory. Alzheimer's disease patients who were moderately demented were impaired on a naming task, whereas moderately demented PD patients performed normally. Others have also found intact naming ability in PD (Huber et al., 1986; Pirozzolo et al., 1982; Freedman et al., 1984b; El-Awar et al., 1987). Pillon et al. (1986) equated DAT and PD patients for severity of impairment using subtests of the Wechsler Adult Intelligence Scale and the Ravens Progressive Matrices and failed to find deficits in naming in either group. This lack of impairment may have been due to the presence of relatively mild disease in the patients studied.

Memory and Learning

Studies have shown deficits in short-term memory (Della Sala et al., 1986; Halgin et al., 1977; Hamel et al., 1975; Tweedy et al., 1982; Pirozollo et al., 1982; Reitan and Boll, 1971) and in long-term memory in PD (Brown and Marsden, 1988). Procedural learning, which refers to the ability to acquire a perceptual–motor or pattern-analyzing skill that is based upon rules (Cohen and Squire, 1980), was also found to be impaired in patients with early-stage PD tested with a simplified version of the Tower of Hanoi puzzle (Saint-Cyr et al., 1988). This contrasts with the relatively preserved skill learning that has been reported in DAT (Eslinger and Damasio, 1986).

Differences between DAT and PD dementia have also been documented with respect to the retrograde amnesia that occurs in these disorders. Sagar et al. (1988) studied retrograde memory in patients with DAT and patients with PD. The PD patients were, however, less impaired cognitively than the DAT patients. Since memory for different types of material may not be affected in the same way, they examined the patients on memory for public and personal events separately.

Public memory was assessed by the Famous Scenes Test and the Verbal Multiple Choice Recognition Test. The first task involves showing the subjects scenes depicting famous public events that occurred between 1940 and 1980. Subjects were then tested on whether they (1) recognized that they were looking at a famous scene, (2) recalled the event, and (3) recognized the content and date of the picture from a verbal multiple choice format. The second test consisted of multiple choice recognition of public events by decade.

Memory for personal events was tested using the Modified Crogert's Personal Remote Memory Test, which requires patients to relate personally experienced events from any remote time period in response to each of 10 high-frequency noun cues (e.g., bird). Although the PD and DAT patient groups showed a similar performance profile on several of the measures, the groups differed in their recognition of content and date of famous scenes from the past. The PD patients showed a selective deficit in the recognition of date, whereas the DAT patients were impaired on recognition of both date and content. The deficits in the PD patients were independent of degree of dementia. Sagar et al. postulated that the cognitive processes underlying the dating of past events may be different from those subserving other aspects of memory and that these processes may be disrupted early in PD.

Sagar et al. also found a temporal gradient in which remote events were affected less than recent ones. The temporal gradient was material specific and was seen for recall of public and personal events in both DAT and PD patients. There was no temporal gradient, however, on the tasks involving the dating of events or on the recognition tasks. Freedman et al. (1984b), in contrast to Sagar et al., did not find a temporal retrograde memory gradient in patients with PD dementia. They used the Famous Faces Test, however, which involves material that differs from that in the tasks used by Sagar and colleagues. The discrepancy in the results between the two reports may reflect the material-specific sensitivity of temporal gradients in memory.

Visuospatial Function

Visuoperceptual and visuoconstructional deficits have been well documented in PD. Examples include difficulty with angle matching (Boller et al., 1984), figure–ground discrimination and perception of spatial position, perception of constancy of shape and size and perception of spatial relationships (Villardita et al., 1982), judgment of the visual vertical and horizontal (Danta and Hilton, 1975; Proctor et al., 1964), route walking guided by a visual map (Bowen et al., 1972), touching personal body parts corresponding to those designated on a diagram (Bowen et al., 1976), and tracing tasks (Stern et al., 1984). The visuospatial tasks reported in the literature have, however, not generally been used to distinguish PD dementia from DAT (Brown and Marsden, 1988).

Conceptual Ability and Mental Set

Disturbances in conceptual ability and mental set (i.e., establishment, maintenance, and shifting of set) occur following damage to the frontal lobes (Stuss and Benson, 1986) and have been well described in PD (Taylor et al., 1986; Bowen et al., 1975; Flowers and Robertson, 1985; Flowers, 1982; Cools et al., 1984; Lees and Smith, 1983). Although patients with DAT may have similar problems, Pillon et al. (1986) showed that patients with PD dementia were impaired on a simplified version of the Wisconsin Card Sorting Test (Nelson, 1976), whereas an equally demented group of DAT patients showed no deficits. The Wisconsin Card Sorting Test is more sensitive to lesions in the dorsolateral frontal region (Milner, 1964) than to other frontal areas, and the finding of Pillon et al. suggests that different frontal lobe systems may be involved in PD with dementia and DAT.

Table 8-1 summarizes the differences between DAT and PD patients with dementia as revealed by conventional neuropsychological assessment.

STUDIES USING TASKS ADOPTED FROM ANIMAL MODELS

An alternative strategy to the more traditional descriptive and experimental approaches summarized above has been introduced recently to study the mechanisms underlying cognitive deficits in humans. Termed *comparative neuropsychology* (Oscar-Berman et al., 1980a; Weiskrantz, 1978), this approach is based upon techniques that are not only of proven reliability and validity in animal models but are also of established value in identifying cognitive impairment in brain-damaged humans (Freedman and Oscar-Berman, 1986a,b, 1987; Oscar-Berman and Zola-Morgan, 1980a,b; Oscar-Berman et al., 1982; Pribram et al., 1964; Witt and Goldman-Rakic, 1983).

Using experimental paradigms that have been validated for the demonstration of deficits leading to damage in two different brain systems implicated in DAT and PD,

Table 8-1 Neuropsychological Deficits Helpful in Differentiating Parkinson's from Alzheimer's Dementia

	Language	Memory and Learning	Conceptual Ability and Mental Set
Parkinson's disease	Motor speech and writing mechanisms (Cummings, 1988)	Recognition memory for past events (Sagar et al., 1988) Procedural memory (Saint-Cyr et al., 1988) Matching to sample (Sahakian et al., 1988)	WCST (Pillon et al., 1985) (i.e., perseveration due to dorsolateral frontal system deficits)
Alzheimer's disease	Confrontation naming (Cummings, 1988; Bayles and Tomoeda, 1983) Word list generation (Cummings, 1988) Impoverished speech content (Cummings, 1988)	Recognition memory for past events (Sagar et al., 1988) Visual learning and tactile learning (Freedman and Oscar-Berman, 1988) Delayed matching to sample (Sahakian et al., 1988)	Delayed alternation (Freedman and Oscar-Berman, 1986b) and object alternation (Freedman, 1988) (i.e., perseveration due to orbitofrontal system deficits)

that is, the prefrontal cortical–subcortical system and the parietal cortical–subcortical system, Freedman and Oscar-Berman (1986b, 1987) have garnered evidence for distinct neuroanatomical and neurobehavioral mechanisms differentiating PD dementia from DAT. Parkinson's disease patients with dementia were compared to a group of equally demented patients with DAT. Nondemented PD patients and normals served as controls. The tasks initially used to assess frontal system function consisted of delayed alternation and delayed response. These tasks were selected because different aspects are known to be mediated by separate cortical–subcortical neuronal networks (Brutkowski et al., 1963; Divac et al., 1967; Goldman et al., 1971; Kling and Tucker, 1968; Mishkin, 1957). The DAT patients, but not the demented PD patients, were found to be significantly impaired on the delayed alternation task, whereas both groups were impaired on delayed response. The delayed response findings suggest that the dorsolateral frontal cortex, or its related projection systems, are involved in an important way in the pathophysiology of the dementia in both DAT and PD. Since the head of the caudate nucleus is an integral component of the nigrostriatal system that is involved in Parkinson's disease (Hornykiewicz, 1979), it is reasonable to raise the question of whether the critical lesion for the delayed response deficits in PD is in the head of the caudate rather than in the prefrontal cortex itself. In fact, a critical focus may even be the anterodorsal sector of the head of the caudate, since this is the area to which the dorsolateral frontal cortex projects most prominently (Johnson et al., 1968). Within the caudate nucleus in Parkinson's patients, it is the anterior portion of the caudate head that undergoes the most severe loss of dopamine concentration (Kish et al., 1986, 1988). In DAT, on the other hand, the critical focus in the dorsolateral frontal system likely lies within the frontal cortex itself, since there are well-documented neuropathologic abnormalities at this site in this disorder (Tomlinson, 1977).

Delayed alternation and delayed response both measure spatial mnemonic factors

(Butters and Rosvold, 1968; Goldman and Rosvold, 1970). In addition, delayed alternation is sensitive to perseveration (Mishkin, 1964). Although both are most severely affected following dorsolateral frontal lesions, poor performance on delayed alternation may also be produced by orbitofrontal damage (Brutkowski et al., 1963; Mishkin, 1969). Since orbitofrontal lesions produce the most marked deficits in perseveration (Mishkin, 1964), Freedman and Oscar-Berman (1986b) postulated that orbitofrontal system damage may have produced the deficits on delayed alternation and might therefore be prominent in DAT but not in PD with dementia. Freedman (1988) therefore administered an object alternation task to patients with DAT and PD. This task is a measure of perseveration and is more sensitive to orbitofrontal than to dorsolateral frontal system lesions in nonhuman primates. Object alternation was found to be significantly impaired in patients with DAT compared with patients with PD dementia. Although the patients with PD dementia also showed impairment on object alternation compared with normals, an error analysis revealed that the performance of the DAT patients, but not the PD patients, was characterized by abnormal response perseveration. This supported the interpretation that the marked perseverative deficits in DAT were due to the presence of orbitofrontal system dysfunction, whereas the milder and qualitatively different deficits in PD may reflect dorsolateral frontal system involvement.

In another study, Freedman and Oscar-Berman (1988) used a spatial and visual learning problem, each with two components composed of (1) original learning and (2) reversals of the original learning. These paradigms have been successful in demonstrating differential deficits in humans with neurological disease following frontal and temporal systems, and they show well-documented profiles in nonhuman primates with selective lesions in the frontal lobes, temporal lobes, and fornix (Oscar-Berman and Zola-Morgan, 1980a). The original learning of a novel visual discrimination problem and reversals of this learning were found to be significantly impaired in patients with DAT, compared with patients with PD and dementia (Freedman and Oscar-Berman, 1988). An error analysis of the subjects' responses revealed that perseverative errors were significantly more common in the DAT than in the PD dementia. The performance profile on the visual tasks supports the interpretation that disturbance in orbitofrontal system function contributed to deficits in DAT. In contrast to the performance on the visual tasks, the patients with DAT and PD with dementia showed a similar performance profile on the spatial tasks. Both groups were unimpaired on the original spatial discrimination problem, whereas both groups showed significant deficits on reversals of the original learning. This profile of intact performance on spatial original learning and impaired performance on spatial reversal learning has been documented following lesions in the hippocampus, anterior inferotemporal area, and fornix (Oscar-Berman and Zola-Morgan, 1980a). Further studies are required to determine which of these lesion sites accounts for the observed deficits.

Freedman and Oscar-Berman (1987) also assessed the parietal cortical–subcortical system using a tactile discrimination learning and reversal learning paradigm. Tactile discrimination learning is sensitive to bilateral parietal lobe lesions in nonhuman primates (Wilson, 1957), and reversal learning provides a measure of perseveration, with touch as the input modality. The results showed that tactile discrimination learning was significantly impaired in the DAT patients compared with the demented PD patients. These findings support clinical as well as recent PET studies (Chase et al., 1984; Cutler et al., 1985), and neuropathologic data (Brun and Englund, 1981), suggesting that parietal lobe involvement is prominent and appears early in the progression of DAT. Both the DAT and demented PD patients were significantly impaired in their ability to learn a reversal strategy on the tactile task. However, an analysis of error patterns of the two groups showed that there was a difference in the types of errors made. As expected, perseveration was a significantly greater factor in contributing to the deficits in the DAT patients compared with all other groups. Since perseveration is associated with frontal lobe lesions (Sandson and Albert, 1984), this tendency is likely due to the known orbitofrontal pathology (Tomlinson, 1977) in this disorder.

Visuospatial memory and learning deficits that distinguish PD from DAT have also been described by others using experimental tasks adopted from animal models. Sahakian et al. (1988) administered a series of tasks that were adopted from animal models to patients with DAT and PD. The tests consisted of a matching-to-sample task, a delayed matching-to-sample task, and a delayed response task. There were two groups of PD patients: one on medication and the other off medication. For the PD patients off medication and the DAT patients, there was a double dissociation in performance profile: Only the PD patients were impaired on the matching-to-sample task, whereas only the DAT group was significantly impaired on the delayed matching-to-sample task. As discussed by Sahakian et al. (1988), impaired performance on matching-to-sample tasks in monkeys is seen following lesions in the ventral portions of the prefrontal cortex. Delayed matching-to-sample, on the other hand, is impaired following lesions in the inferotemporal cortex, hippocampus, amygdala, and projection sites related to these areas, such as the mediodorsal nucleus of the thalamus and anterior thalamic nucleus. Based on the data from animal models, the matching-to-sample deficit in PD may reflect frontal system lesions in the frontal cortex or in frontal cortical projection systems, such as the head of the caudate. In DAT, the well-documented temporal lobe lesions (Tomlinson, 1977) may account for the deficits on delayed matching-to-sample. Interestingly, alcoholic Korsakoff patients also show a pattern of intact performance on matching-to-sample combined with deficits on delayed matching-to-sample; brain damage in Korsakoff's syndrome may include mamillary bodies and medial dorsal nucleus of the thalamus (Oscar-Berman et al., 1982) and produce a syndrome similar to that seen with hippocampal lesions.

In the delayed response type of task, Sahakian et al. (1988) found that the DAT patients and the PD patients on medication were significantly impaired. In animal models the most prominent deficits on such tasks occur following dorsolateral frontal lobe lesions. Freedman and Oscar-Berman (1986b) found similar deficits in patients with PD dementia and in patients with DAT using a classical delayed response procedure. Whereas Freedman and Oscar-Berman found deficits in PD only if they were demented, Sahakian et al. observed deficits in PD patients who were not demented, suggesting that their task was more difficult than the one employed by Freedman and Oscar-Berman. (see Table 8-2.)

Thus, the pathogenesis of the intellectual deterioration in PD may not be uniform in all cases. The ubiquitous dopamine deficit may account for the subcortical–frontal dementia syndrome most commonly encountered, whereas patients with severe or atypical dementias may harbor more extensive pathologic changes. Future studies must consider the possible heterogeneity of the dementia syndromes of PD.

Table 8-2   Anatomical Projection Systems Implicated in Alzheimer's and
Parkinson's Dementia

	Dorsolateral Frontal	Orbitofrontal	Parietal	Temporal
Parkinson's disease	Delayed response Object alternation[a] Tactile reversal learning[a]	Matching-to-sample	Tactile reversal learning[a]	—
Alzheimer's disease	Delayed response	Delayed alternation Object alternation[a] Visual original learning Visual reversal learning Tactile reversal learning[a]	Tactile original learning Tactile reversal learning[a]	Delayed matching-to-sample

[a]The anatomical systems implicated by deficits on these tasks were based upon qualitative error analyses (see text for details).

PATHOPHYSIOLOGY OF THE DEMENTIA SYNDROME

The pathophysiological basis of the dementia syndrome of PD has not been determined. There may be varying contributions from subcortical lesions and their associated neurochemical deficiences, as well as changes of the Alzheimer type producing several different patterns of dementia in PD patients (Cummings, 1988).

A role for dopamine in the mental status alterations in PD is suggested by the consistent correlation between dementia and akinesia (a dopamine-dependent sign) and by the ability to reverse the intellectual loss partially with dopamine therapy (Meier and Martin, 1970; Mortimer et al., 1982). Furthermore, Stern et al. (1984) found correlations between attentional deficits in PD and altered levels of norepinephrine metabolites in the cerebrospinal fluid of PD patients, indicating that norepinephrine changes may also be involved in some aspects of the dementia syndrome. Atrophy of the nucleus basalis of Meynert has been observed in some, but not all, PD patients with dementia, suggesting that cholinergic deficits may be superimposed on the monoaminergic deficiencies in a subgroup of patients (Whitehouse et al., 1983). Thus, changes in at least three and possibly more neurotransmitters may contribute to the mental status changes in PD.

Several types of histopathologic changes have also been found in the brains of PD patients. Classic pathologic changes involving the substantia nigra, locus ceruleus, and ventral tegmental areas can produce a dementia syndrome, but most patients with obvious mental status deficits have additional alterations in the nucleus basalis. Histopathologic changes identical to those occurring in DAT have been identified in some patients with PD (Hakim and Mathieson, 1979; Boller et al., 1980), and the dementia syndrome in these cases likely results from combined cortical and subcortical dysfunction. Heston (1981), however, has shown that these two disorders do not commonly co-occur in unselected samples, and DAT is unlikely to account for all of the cases of PD with dementia (Cummings, 1988).

Thus, the pathogenesis of the intellectual deterioration in PD may not be uniform in all cases. The ubiquitous dopamine deficit and nigrostriatal and ventral–tegmental–frontal pathology may account for the subcortical–frontal dementia syndrome most commonly encountered, whereas patients with severe or atypical dementias may harbor more extensive pathological and neurochemical changes. Future studies must consider the possible heterogeneity of the dementia syndromes of PD.

CONCLUSIONS

The results of recent studies lend strong support to the concept that there are important differences in the cognitive deficits associated with PD and DAT. From a neurobehavioral point of view the data suggest that there are qualitative as well as quantitative differences in language, memory, learning, and different forms of perseveration (Table 8-1). The data also suggest that dorsolateral frontal, orbitofrontal, temporal, and parietal lobe systems are more prominently involved in DAT than in PD dementia, whereas dorsolateral frontal projection systems are most prominently involved in the dementia of PD (Table 8-2). In PD a critical lesion site may be the anterodorsal sector of the head of the caudate: This is the predominant region of the caudate head to which the dorsolateral frontal cortex projects (Johnson et al., 1968), and it is the region that undergoes the most severe loss of dopamine concentration (Kish et al., 1986, 1988).

The data on PD and DAT are insufficient at the present time to determine whether the labels *subcortical* and *cortical* for the cognitive deficits in these disorders reflect a completely accurate neuroanatomical emphasis. The growing body of evidence suggests that the concepts underlying these labels remain viable (i.e., that they represent distinct patterns of dementia).

ACKNOWLEDGMENTS

I gratefully acknowledge Dr. Marlene Oscar-Berman and Stephanie P. Bernstein for reviewing the manuscript and offering helpful suggestions, and Vicki Gilchrist for secretarial assistance.

Dr. Freedman is supported by a research grant from the Medical Research Council of Canada and a Career Scientist Award from the Ministry of Health of Ontario.

REFERENCES

Adams, R.D., and Victor, M. *Principles of Neurology*, Third Edition, McGraw-Hill, New York, 1985, pp. 874–80.

Albert, M.L., Feldman, R.G., and Willis, A.L. "The subcortical dementia" of progressive supranuclear palsy. *J Neurol Neurosurg Psychiatry* 1974; 37:121–30.

Alvord, E.C., Forno, L.S., Kusske, J.A., Kauffman, R.J., Rhodes, J.S., and Goetowski, C.R. The pathology of Parkinsonism: A comparison of degenerations in cerebral cortex and brainstem. *Adv Neurol* 1974; 5:175–93.

Battig, K., Rosvold, H.E., and Mishkin, M. Comparison of the effects of frontal and caudate lesions on delayed response and alternation in monkeys. *J Comp Psychol* 1960; 53:400–4.

Bayles, K.A., Tomoeda, C.K. Confrontation naming impairment in dementia. *Brain Lang* 1983; 19:98–114.

Boller, F., Mizutani, T., Roessmann, U., and Gambetti, P. Parkinson disease, dementia, and Alzheimer disease: Clinicopathological correlations. *Ann Neurol* 1980; 7:329–35.

Boller, F., Passafiume, D., Keefe, N.C., Rogers, K., Morrow, L., and Kim, Y. Visuospatial impairments in Parkinson's disease: Role of perceptual and motor factors. *Arch Neurol* 1984; 41:485–90.

Bowen, F.P., Burns, M.M., Brady, E.M., and Yahr, M.D. A note on alterations of personal orientation in Parkinsonism. *Neuropsychologia* 1976; 14:425–9.

Bowen, F.P., Hoehn, M.M., and Yahr, M.D. Parkinsonism: Alterations and spatial orientation as determined by a route-walking test. *Neuropsychologia* 1972; 10:355–61.

Bowen, F.P., Kamienny, R.S., Burns, M.M., and Yahr, M.D. Parkinsonism: Effects of levodopa treatment on concept formation. *Neurology* 1975; 25:701–4.

Brown, R.G., and Marsden, C.D. How common is dementia in Parkinson's disease? *Lancet* 1984; ii:1262–5.

Brown, R.G., and Marsden, C.D. "Subcortical dementia": The neuropsychological evidence. *Neuroscience* 1988; 25:363–87.

Brun, A., and Englund, E. Regional pattern of degeneration in Alzheimer's disease: Neuronal loss and histopathological grading. *Histopathology* 1981; 5:549–64.

Brutkowski, S., Mishkin, M., and Rosvold, H.E. In *Central and Peripheral Mechanisms of Motor Function*. Gutmann, E. and Hnik, P. (eds.). Czechoslovak Academy of Sciences, Prague, 1963, pp. 133–41.

Butters, N., and Rosvold, H.E. Effect of septal lesions on resistance to extinction and delayed alternation in monkeys. *J Comp Physiol Psychol* 1968; 66:389–95.

Chase, T.N., Foster, N.J., Fedio, P., Brooks, R., Mansi, L., and Dichiro, G. Regional Cortical Dysfunction in Alzheimer's disease as determined by positron emission tomography. *Ann Neurol* 1984; 15 (suppl.): S170–4.

Cohen, N.J., and Squire, L.R. Preserved Learning and Retention of Pattern-Analyzing Skill in Amnesia: Dissociation of Knowing How and Knowing That. *Science* 1980; 210:207–10.

Cools, A.R., Van Der Bercken, J.H.L., Horstink, M.W.T., Van Spaendonck, K.P.M., and Berger, H.J.C. Cognitive and motor shifting aptitude disorder in Parkinson's disease. *J Neurol Neurosurg Psychiatry* 1984; 47:443–53.

Cummings, J.L. Intellectual impairment in Parkinson's disease: Clinical, pathologic and biochemical correlates. *J Geriatr Psychiatry Neurol* 1988; 1:24–36.

Cummings, J.L., and Benson, D.F., (eds.). *Dementia: A Clinical Approach*. Butterworths, Boston, 1983, pp. 89–99.

Cummings, J.L., Darkins, A., Mendez, M., Hill, M.A., and Benson, D.F. Alzheimer's disease and Parkinson's disease: Comparison of speech and language alterations. *Neurology* 1988; 38:680–4.

Cutler, N.R., Haxby, J.V., Duara, R., Grady, C.L., Moore, A.M., Parisi, J.E., White, J., Heston, L., Margolin, R.M., and Rapoport, S.I. Brain metabolism as measured with positron emission tomography: Serial assessment in a patient with familial Alzheimer's disease. *Neurology* 1985; 35:1556–61.

Danta, G., and Hilton, R.C. Judgement of the visual vertical and horizontal in patients with Parkinsonism. *Neurology* 1975; 25:43–7.

Della Sala, S., Di Lorenzo, G., Giordano, A., and Spinnler, H. Is there a specific visuo-spatial impairment in Parkinsonians? *J Neurol Neurosurg Psychiatry* 1986; 49:1258–65.

Divac, I., Rosvold, H.E., and Szwarcbart, M.K. Behavioral effects of selective ablation of the caudate nucleus. *J Comp Physiol Psychol* 1967; 63:184–90.

El-Awar, M., Becker, J.T., Hammond, K.M., Nebes, R.D., and Boller, F. Learning Deficit in Parkinson's disease: Comparison with Alzheimer's disease and normal aging. *Arch Neurol* 1987; 44:180–4.

Eslinger, J., and Damasio, A.R. Preserved motor learning in Alzheimer's disease: Implications for anatomy and behaviour. *J Neurosci* 1986; 6:3006–9.

Flowers, K.A. Frontal lobe signs as a component of Parkinsonism. *Neurobehav Brain Res* 1982; 5:100–1.

Flowers, K.A., and Robertson, C. The effects of Parkinson's disease on the ability to maintain a mental set. *J Neurol Neurosurg Psychiatry* 1985; 48:517–29.

Folstein, M.F., Folstein, S.E., and McHugh, P.R. Mini-mental state. *J Psychiatr Res* 1975; 12:189–98.

Freedman, M. Object alternation in orbitofrontal system dysfunction in Alzheimer's and Parkinson's disease. *Submitted*. 1988.

Freedman, M., Knoefel, J., Naeser, M., and Levine, H. Computerized axial tomography in aging. In *Clinical Neurology of Aging*. Albert, M.L. (ed.). Oxford University Press, New York, 1984a, pp. 139–48.

Freedman, M., Rivoira, P., Butters, N., Sax, D.S., and Robert, G. Retrograde amnesia in Parkinson's disease. *Can J Neurol Sci* 1984b; 11:297–301.

Freedman, M., and Oscar-Berman, M. Bilateral frontal lobe disease and selective delayed response deficits in humans. *Behav Neurosci* 1986a; 100:337–42.

Freedman, M., and Oscar-Berman, M. Selective delayed response deficits in Alzheimer's and Parkinson's disease. *Arch Neurol* 1986b; 43:886–90.

Freedman, M., and Oscar-Berman, M. Tactile discrimination learning deficits in Alzheimer's and Parkinson's disease. *Arch Neurol* 1987; 44:394–8.

Freedman, M., and Oscar-Berman, M. Spatial and visual learning deficits in Alzheimer's and Parkinson's disease. *Brain Cognition* 1989; 11:114–26.

Gawel, M.J., Das, P., Vincent, S., and Clifford Rose, F. Visual and auditory evoked responses in patients with Parkinson's disease. *J Neurol Neurosurg Psychiatry* 1981; 227–32.

Globus, M., Mildworf, B., and Melamed, E. Cerebral blood flow and cognitive impairment in Parkinson's disease. *Neurology* 1985; 35:1135–9.

Goldman, P.S., and Rosvold, H.E. Localization of function within the dorsolateral prefrontal cortex of the rhesus monkey. *Exp Neurol* 1970; 27:291–304.

Goldman, P.S., Rosvold, H.E., Vest, B., and Galkin, T.W. Analysis of delayed alternation deficits produced by dorsolateral prefrontal lesions in the rhesus monkey. *J Comp Psychol* 1971; 77:212–20.

Hakim, A.M., and Mathieson, G. Dementia in Parkinson's disease: A neurological study. *Neurology* 1979; 29:1209–14.

Halgin, R., Riklan, M., and Mistak, H. Levodopa, Parkinsonism, and recent memory. *J Nerv Ment Dis* 1977; 164:268–72.

Hamel, A.R., and Riklan, M. Cognitive and perceptual effects of long-range L-dopa therapy in Parkinsonism. *J Clin Psychol* 1975; 31:321–3.

Hansch, E.C., Syndulko, K., Cohne, S.N., Goldberg, Z.I., Potvin, A.R., and Tourtellotte, W.W. Cognition in Parkinson disease: An event-related potential perspective. *Ann Neurol* 1982; 11:599–607.

Heston, L.L. Genetic studies of dementia with emphasis on Parkinson's disease and Alzheimer's neuropathology. In *The Epidemiology of Dementia*. Mortimer, J.A., and Schuman, L.M. (eds.). Oxford University Press, New York, 1981, pp. 101–14.

Hoehn, M.M., and Yahr, M.D. Parkinsonism: Onset, progression and mortality. *Neurology* 1967; 17:427–42.

Hornykiewicz, O. Brain dopamine in Parkinson's disease and other neurological disturbances. In *The Neurobiology of Dopamine*. Horn, A.S., Korf, J., and Westerink, B.H.C. (eds.). Academic Press, New York, 1979, pp. 633–54.

Hornykiewicz, O., and Kish, S.J. Biochemical pathophysiology of Parkinson's disease. In *Advances in Neurology*. Yahr, M.D., and Bergmann, K.J. (eds.). Raven Press, New York, 1986, pp. 19–34.

Huber, S.J., Shuttleworth, E.C., Paulson, G.W., Bellchambers, M.J.G., and Clapp, L.E. Cortical vs subcortical dementia: Neuropsychological differences. *Arch Neurol* 1986; 43:392–4.

Javoy-Agid, F., and Agid, Y. Is the mesocortical dopaminergic system involved in Parkinson's disease? *Neurology* 1980; 30:1326–30.

Johnson, T.N., Rosvold, H.E., and Mishkin, M. Projections of behaviorally defined sectors of the prefrontal cortex to the basal ganglia, septum and diencephalon of the monkey. *Exp Neurol* 1968; 21:20–34.

Kish, S.J., Rajput, A., Gilbert, J., Rozdilsky, B., Chang, L.J., Shannak, K., and Hornykiewicz, O. Elevated GABA level in striatal but not extrastriatal brain regions in Parkinson's disease: correlation with striatal dopamine loss. *Ann Neurol* 1986; 20:26–31.

Kish, S.J., Shannak, K., and Hornykiewicz, O. Uneven pattern of dopamine loss in the striatum of patients with idiopathic Parkinson's disease: Pathophysiologic and clinical implications. *N Engl J Med* 1988; 318:876–80.

Kling, A., and Tucker, T.J. Sparing of function following localized brain lesions in neonatal monkeys. In *The Neuropsychology of Development*. Isaacson, R.L. (ed.). John Wiley & Sons Inc., New York, 1968, pp. 121–45.

Lees, A.J., and Smith, E. Cognitive deficits in early stages of Parkinson's disease. *Brain* 1983; 106:257–70.

McDowell, F.H., Lee, J.E., and Sweet, R.D. Extrapyramidal disease. In *Clinical Neurology, Vol. 3*, Chapter 38. Baker, A.B., and Baker, L.H. (eds.). Harper and Rowe, New York, 1978, pp. 19–27.

McHugh, P.R., and Folstein, M.F. Psychiatric syndromes of Huntington's disease: A clinical and phenomenological study. In *Psychiatric Aspects of Neurological Disease*. Benson, D.F., and Blumer, D. (eds.). Grune and Stratton, New York, 1975, pp. 267–86.

Meier, M.J., and Martin, W.E. Intellectual changes associated with levodopa therapy. *JAMA* 1970; 213:465–6.

Milner, B. Some effects of frontal lobectomy in man. In *The Frontal Granular Cortex and Behavior*. Warren, J.M., and Akert, K. (eds.). McGraw-Hill Book Company, New York, 1964, pp. 313–34.

Mishkin, M. Effects of small frontal lesions on delayed alternation in monkeys. *J Neurophysiol* 1957; 20:615–22.

Mishkin, M. Perseveration of central sets after frontal lesions in monkeys. In *The Frontal Granular Cortex and Behavior*. Warren, J.M., and Akert, K. (eds.). McGraw-Hill Book Company, New York, 1964, pp. 219–41.

Mishkin, M. A re-examination of the effects of frontal lesions on object alternation. *Neuropsychologia* 1969; 7:357–63.

Mortimer, J.A., Pirozzolo, F.J., Hansch, E.C., and Webster, D.D. Relationship of motor symptoms to intellectual deficits in Parkinson disease. *Neurology* 1982; 32:133–7.

Nelson, H.E. A modified card sorting test sensitive to frontal lobe defects. *Cortex* 1976; 12:313–24.

Oberg, R.E., and Divac, I. "Cognitive" functions of the neostriatum. In *The Neostriatum*. Divac, I., and Oberg, R.E. (eds.). Pergamon Press, Oxford, 1979, pp. 291–313.

Olton, D.S., Gamzu, E., and Corkin, S. (eds.). Memory dysfunction: An integration of animal and human research from preclinical and clinical perspectives. *Ann NY Acad Sci* 1985; 444:1–553.

Oscar-Berman, M., and Zola-Morgan, S.M. Comparative neuropsychology and Korsakoff's syndrome. I. Spatial and visual reversal learning. *Neuropsychologia* 1980a; 18:499–512.

Oscar-Berman, M., and Zola-Morgan, S.M. Comparative neuropsychology and Korsakoff's syndrome. II. Two-choice visual discrimination learning. *Neuropsychologia* 1980b; 18:513–26.

Oscar-Berman, M., Zola-Morgan, S.M., Oberg, R.G.E., and Bonner, R.T. Comparative neuropsychology and Korsakoff's syndrome. III. Delayed response, delayed alternation and DRL performance. *Neuropsychologia* 1982; 20:187–202.

Parkinson, J.An essay on the shaking palsy. *Medical Classics* 1938; 2:964–97.

Perlmutter, J.S. New insights into the pathophysiology of Parkinson's disease: The challenge of positron emission tomography. *Trends Neurosci* 1988; 11:203–8.

Pillon, B., Dubois, B., Lhermitte, F., and Agid, Y. Heterogeneity of cognitive impairment in progressive supranuclear palsy, Parkinson's disease, and Alzheimer's disease. *Neurology* 1986; 36:1179–85.

Pirozzolo, F.J., Hansch, E.C., Mortimer, J.A., Webster, D.D., and Kuskowski, M.A. Dementia in Parkinson's disease: A neuropsychological analysis. *Brain Cogn* 1982; 1:71–83.

Pribram, K.H., Ahumada, A., and Hartog, J. A progress report on the neurological processes disturbed by frontal lesions in primates. In *The Frontal Granular Cortex and Behavior.* Warren, J.M., and Akert, K. (eds.). McGraw Hill International Book Company, New York, 1964, pp. 28–55.

Proctor, F., Riklan, M., Cooper, I.S., and Teuver, H.L. Judgement of visual and postural vertical by parkinsonian patients. *Neurology* 1964; 14:287–93.

Reitan, R.M., and Boll, T.J. Intellectual and cognitive functions in Parkinson's disease. *J Consult Clin Psychol* 1971; 37:364–9.

Riklan, M. *L-Dopa and Parkinsonism. A Psychological Assessment.* Charles C. Thomas, Springfield, Illinois, 1973, pp. 80–145.

Rosvold, H.E. The frontal lobe system: Cortical–subcortical interrelationships. *Acta Neurobiol Exp (Warsz)* 1972; 32:439–60.

Sagar, H.J., Cohen, N.J., Sullivan, E.V., Corkin, S., and Growdon, J.H. Remote memory function in Alzheimer's disease and Parkinson's disease. *Brain* 1988; 111:185–206.

Sahakian, B.J., Morris, R.G., Evenden, J.L., Heald, A., Levy, R., Philpot, M., and Robbins, T.W. A comparative study of visuospatial memory and learning in Alzheimer-type dementia and Parkinson's disease. *Brain* 1988; 111:695–718.

Saint-Cyr, J.A., Taylor, A.E., and Lang, A.E. Procedural learning and neostriatal dysfunction in man. *Brain* 1988; 111:941–59.

Sandson, J.S., and Albert, M.L. Varieties of perseveration. *Neuropsychologia* 1984; 6:715–32.

Stern, Y., Mayeux, R., and Rosen, J. Contribution of perceptual motor dysfunction to construction and tracing disturbances in Parkinson's disease. *J Neurol Neurosurg Psychiatry* 1984; 47:983–9.

Stuss, D.T., and Benson, D.F. (eds.). *The Frontal Lobes.* Raven Press, New York, 1986, pp. 194–216.

Taylor, A.E., Saint-Cyr, J.A., and Lang, A.E. Frontal lobe dysfunction in Parkinson's disease. *Brain* 1986; 109:845–83.

Tomlinson, B.E. The pathology of dementia. In *Dementia.* Wells, C.E. (ed.). F.A. Davis, Philadelphia, 1977, pp. 113–53.

Tweedy, J.R., Langer, K.G., and McDowell, F.H. The effects of semantic relations on the memory deficit associated with Parkinson's disease. *J Clin Neuropsychol* 1982; 4:235–47.

Uhl, G.R., Hedreen, J.C., and Price, D.L. Parkinson's disease: Loss of neurons from the ventral tegmental area contralateral to therapeutic surgical lesions. *Neurology* 1985; 35:1215–8.

Villardita, C., Smirni, P., Le Pira, F., Zappala, G., and Nicoletti, F. Mental deterioration, visuoperceptive disabilities and constructional apraxia in Parkinson's disease. *Acta Neurol Scand* 1982; 66:112–20.

Ward, C.D., Duvoisin, R.C., and Nutt, J.D. Parkinson's disease in 65 pairs of twins and in a set of quadruplets. *Neurology* 1983; 33:815–24.

Weiskrantz, L.A. (ed.). A comparison of hippocampal pathology in man and in other animals. In *Functions of the Septo-Hippocampal System*. Ciba Foundation Symposium 58. Elsevier, New York, 1978, pp. 373–406.

Whitehouse, P.J., Price, D.L., Struble, R.G., Clarke, A.W., Coyle, J.T., and DeLong, M.R. Alzheimer's disease and senile dementia: Loss of neurons in the basal forebrain. *Science* 1982; 215:1237–9.

Wilson, M. Effects of circumscribed cortical lesions upon somesthetic and visual discrimination in the monkey. *J Comp Physiol Psychol* 1957; 50:630–5.

Witt, E.D., and Goldman-Rakic, P.S. Intermittent thiamine deficiency in the rhesus monkey. II. Evidence for memory loss. *Ann Neurol* 1983; 13:396–401.

9

Progressive Supranuclear Palsy
(Steele-Richardson-Olszewski Syndrome)

A.J. LEES

The fully established clinical picture of the Steele-Richardson-Olszewski syndrome or progressive supranuclear palsy (PSP) is so distinctive that one can scarcely comprehend that it was not recognized as a distinct clinico-pathologic entity until 1963, when a paper was presented by the late J.C. Richardson at the American Neurological Association describing the semeiology of eight patients with a progressive nonfamilial degenerative nervous disease with defects of ocular gaze, extensor rigidity of the neck, spasticity of the face, and neuropsychological impairment (Richardson, Steele and Olszewski, 1963). Six of these patients were examined pathologically, and marked nerve cell loss was found in a large number of brain-stem structures, but there was a predilection for the subthalamic nucleus, the globus pallidus, substantia nigra, periaqueductal grey matter, superior colliculus, locus coeruleus, and the dentate, pontine, and raphe nuclei. Globose neurofibrillary tangles were noted in abundance in the affected areas together with gliosis. The cerebral cortex appeared to be spared (Steele, Richardson, and Olszewski, 1964). More recent pathological studies have highlighted cell loss in other brain-stem nuclei, including the interstitial nucleus of Cajal (Fukushima-Kudo et al., 1987) and the cholinergic pedunculo-pontine tegmental nucleus (Zweig et al., 1985). The etiology remains unknown, but either a toxin or a slow virus seems the most promising option to pursue. Piecemeal descriptions of the syndrome are available in the earlier literature; so it is unlikely to be a new disorder.

DEMOGRAPHY

The prevalence of PSP is unknown, but even if one adheres to relatively rigid diagnostic criteria (see Table 9-1) it is by no means a rare condition, and series of more than 50 patients are being collected and described in the literature (Maher and Lees, 1986). Altogether there are now more than 500 cases in medical reports. Using the records of neurologists, nursing homes, and a movement disorder center, Golbe et al. found the prevalence in two central New Jersey counties to be 1.39 per 100,000 members of the population, without significant sex differences. Mastaglia and colleagues (1973) estimated the incidence to be 4 per million in Western Australia. These figures are almost certainly underestimates, although errors of commission as well as omission

Table 9-1   Diagnostic Criteria for the Clinical Diagnosis of Steele-Richardson-Olszewski Syndrome

Definition

A progressive nonfamilial disorder beginning in middle or old age with a supranuclear ophthalmoplegia including down-gaze abnormalities and at least two or more of the following five cardinal features:

   1. Axial dystonia and rigidity
   2. Pseudobulbar palsy
   3. Bradykinesia and rigidity
   4. Frontal lobe signs (bradyphrenia, perseveration, forced grasping, and utilization behavior)
   5. Postural instability with falls backward

Other signs
   Rest tremor
   Chorea
   Dystonia of the limbs and face
   Cerebellar ataxia
   Muscle wasting, fasciculation, and weakness
   Respiratory dyskinesias (inspiratory gasps, tachypnoea)
   Depression
   Schizophreniform psychoses
   Echolalia and palilalia
   Myoclonus
   Perceptive deafness
   Sleep disturbances
   Other ocular abnormalities
   Epilepsy

are possible. The median age at onset of the syndrome is 65 years, and the median survival is 6 years (Kristensen, 1985; Maher and Lees, 1986). A delay in diagnosis of at least 3 to 4 years is common, and it has been estimated that as many as 12 percent of patients diagnosed as having Parkinson's disease might in fact turn out to have PSP. Patients usually die from a respiratory arrest occurring either as a consequence of hypostatic pneumonia or of central nervous system involvement of the respiratory centers.

CLINICAL FEATURES

The early complaints are vague, nonspecific, and often frankly misleading; the early signs may involve many different neuronal systems and when present in isolation are not diagnostic. The initial symptom in most patients is a disturbance of gait, often with frequent falls. Disorders of articulation and neurobehavioral disturbances are other early features. Many patients are misdiagnosed as having Alzheimer's disease or a psychotic illness. Blurred vision, reading difficulties, problems looking down while eating, double vision, photophobia, and dry eyes are the most common ocular symptoms. Swallowing difficulties, explosive coughing, and psychomotor slowing are other early symptoms. The minimum diagnostic criteria are shown in Table 9-1. In the absence of any diagnostic laboratory test or specific appearance on neuroimaging, a supranuclear down-gaze palsy is an essential diagnostic prerequisite. However, the

Table 9-2 Multisystem Degenerative Disorders in Which a Supranuclear
Ophthalmoplegia Has Been Reported

1. Creutzfeld-Jakob disease
2. Olivo-ponto-cerebellar degeneration
3. Cortico-basal degeneration
4. Dentato-pallido-nigro-luysian atrophy
5. Subcortical gliosis of Neumann
6. Dystonoic lipidosis (adult-onset Niemann-Pick)
7. Joseph's disease (Azorean disease, Machado's disease)
8. Young-onset familial neurofibrillary tangle disorder
9. Young-onset tangle disorder in mentally retarded

ophthalmoplegia frequently appears late in the course of the illness, and, in a number of cases, typical pathology of PSP has been described without the patient having any eye movement abnormalities at all in life (Dubas, Gray, and Escourolle, 1983). The issue is further complicated by the fact that there are a number of other progressive nonfamilial nervous diseases that may have a supranuclear ophthalmoplegia as part of the clinical picture (see Table 9-2). A minimum of two of a further five cardinal features should be present before the diagnosis is considered clinically definite.

NEUROPSYCHOLOGICAL ABNORMALITIES

Cognitive impairment occurred in seven of the nine patients comprising the seminal report, but Steele in his later writings emphasized this as an inconstant finding even in the terminal phases of the malady (Steele, 1972). Some authors have suggested that neuropsychological impairments are restricted to nonverbal tasks requiring visual scanning ability (Kimura et al., 1981), and Fisk and colleagues (1982) failed to find significant differences between the verbal IQs of a small number of patients compared with controls. In keeping with the earlier report of Kimura, these authors confirmed a low score on the Performance IQ due primarily to difficulties with the Digit Symbol subtest, a task placing a high demand on visual scanning. On Picture Completion, a task that does not emphasize scanning movements, no significant differences between the patients and controls were detected. Fisk and colleagues concluded that dementia should not be considered an integral feature of PSP.

In contrast to studies failing to demonstrate substantial intellectual impairment, most investigations using comprehensive neuropsychological batteries sensitive to subortical and frontal lobe-like functions have documented the occurrence of dementia in PSP. Albert, Feldman, and Willis (1974) reviewed the available literature on 42 patients and delineated a composite behavioral profile consisting of forgetfulness, slowness of thought processes, changes in personality with apathy or depression, and occasionally irritability, forced inappropriate laughing or crying with outbursts of rage, and an impaired ability to manipulate acquired knowledge. On the basis of the available literature and studies on 5 of his own patients, Albert and colleagues speculated that this spectrum of symptoms might be due to impaired timing, alerting, and activating mechanisms resulting from damage to frontolimbic connections. This study was among the first to reintroduce the concept of subcortical dementia into contemporary neurology, and the description of the mental status changes in PSP has become the model for the intellectual deficits characteristic of subcortical dementia.

In a more recent neuropsychological investigation of 27 patients, 18 were found to be demented at the time of first hospital referral. The dementia was moderate in 9 patients and severe in the other 9. Of 10 patients tested, 7 had disproportionate difficulties with tests believed to be relatively specific for frontal lobe function (verbal fluency, Weigl's test). Frontal lobe "signs" were also seen in some patients, including forced grasping, imitation and utilization behavior, and motor perseveration (Maher, Smith, and Lees, 1985). Similar findings were reported by Cambier and colleagues (1985) in 10 patients aged 52 to 80 years with a duration of illness of 1 to 5 years. Depression and outbursts of irritability were prominent in 5 patients. Neuropsychological testing revealed slowing, impaired attention, diminished verbal fluency, simplified linguistic output, poor abstract thinking and reasoning, and mild to moderate memory loss. In addition, grasp reflexes, motor impersistence, and imitation and utilization behavior were noted. Pillon and colleagues (1986) compared the neuropsychological abnormalities in PSP with Parkinson's disease and Alzheimer's disease patients matched for age and severity of intellectual deterioration as well as with controls. The scores of the three groups of patients were significantly lower than those of controls and were comparable on tests of verbal and visuospatial function as well as global memory. The patients with PSP, and to a lesser degree those with Parkinson's disease, were more impaired on tests sensitive to frontal lobe function (verbal fluency, simplified Wisconsin Card Sorting Test), and the patients with Alzheimer's disease had more severe verbal memory disturbances. Similarly, a recent study by Dubois et al. (1988) found that PSP and Parkinson's disease patients were inferior to controls on tests of memory, Verbal IQ, speed of cognitive processing, and frontal lobe-like functions, and the PSP patients were significantly more impaired than those with Parkinson's disease on the frontal lobe tasks and speed of cognition.

Neuropsychological assessment of PSP can be extremely difficult because of the accompanying severe visual disturbances, axial dystonia, and dysarthria. Nevertheless, it can be concluded that specific neuropsychological impairments do occur, including slowness of initiation of thought and a difficulty in generating and switching smoothly from one cognitive set to another. These deficits lead to complaints of apathy, inertia, depression, and forgetfulness, sometimes combined with emotional incontinence.

NEUROIMAGING

Computer tomography (CT) scan studies in putative cases of PSP have confirmed the findings of atrophy of the midbrain tegmentum, superior colliculus, and pons. Mild cortical atrophy may also occur, particularly in prefrontal and temporal regions (Haldeman et al., 1981; Masucci et al., 1985). A CT scan will also exclude a multicerebral infarct state or hydrocephalus masquerading as PSP. Schonfeld and colleagues (1987) have recently divided the disorder into four clinical groups according to severity of disease and functional disability and assessed CT findings with 5-mm-thick sections through the brain stem in a plane parallel with the orbito-meatal line. In Grade I, patients had a decreased anteroposterior diameter of the midbrain tegmentum. As the disease progressed to Grade II, more severe atrophy of the pons and midbrain with dilatation of the quadrigeminal plate cistern was noted. In Grades III and IV there was dilatation of the aqueduct with progressive dilatation of the third and fourth ventricles and atrophy of the temporal lobes. Cortical atrophy was variable and not a prominent radiological feature. The authors concluded that these findings might be particularly helpful in distinguishing PSP from multisystem degeneration (olivo-ponto-cerebellar atrophy), where moderate to severe cerebellar and pontine atrophy occurs with negligible or mild midbrain involvement.

Magnetic resonance imaging with a high-field-strength magnet promises to be a much more powerful diagnostic tool for studying the basal ganglia degenerations. Focal atrophy of the midbrain, particularly the tectum, with dilatation of the aqueduct, quadrigeminal plate cistern, and the posterior portion of the third ventricle, have been reported in PSP (Rutledge et al., 1987; Drayer et al., 1986).

Regional brain metabolism has been investigated in two studies using positron emission tomography. D'Antona and colleagues (1985) measured brain glucose utilization in 6 patients with probable PSP and demonstrated decreased mean glucose utilization in all cortical areas, but the decrease reached statistical significance only in frontal regions. No correlation, however, was found between frontal glucose utilization and frontal lobe function. We studied 5 patients with clinically definite PSP using positron emission tomography and tracers of dopamine metabolism, blood flow, and oxygen metabolism. A global decrease in blood flow and oxygen utilization was found, but the decrease was most marked in the frontal regions. The degree of impairment in oxygen utilization in the frontal zones paralleled roughly the duration of the disease, but there was no association with psychological test scores. Blood flow was impaired to a greater extent than oxygen utilization, resulting in raised oxygen extraction, a result that could partially be explained by a lower pCO_2 in the patients. An alternative explanation for this finding would be involvement of brain vasculature in the pathophysiology of the disease, in addition to neuronal degeneration. Striatal dopamine formation and storage, as indicated by L-18(F) fluorodopa uptake, was significantly decreased in PSP compared with control values, and the severity of this decrease paralleled the degree of reduction in frontal cerebral blood flow. These results suggest that the functional impairment of cerebral function in PSP might be determined to a large extent by brain-stem pathology (Leenders, Frackowiak, and Lees, 1988).

Single photon emission tomography provides a measure of cerebral blood flow and reveals diminished activity in the frontal lobes, particularly in the medial frontal region (Figure 9-1).

PATHOPHYSIOLOGY

Three main areas of damage can be distinguished at light-microscopic level: the pallido-subthalamic complex, with particular destruction of the internal segments of the pallidum at the origin of the pallido-thalamo frontal pathway; the zona compacta of the substantia nigra, which is the source of striatal dopaminergic neurones; and finally, the superior colliculus, periaqueductal grey matter, and pretectal areas known to be involved in the control of ocular movements. The amygdala and most areas of the cerebral neocortex, with the possible exception of the frontal lobe, and the cerebellar cortex are spared. The rigidity in extension may be due to lesions in the interstitial

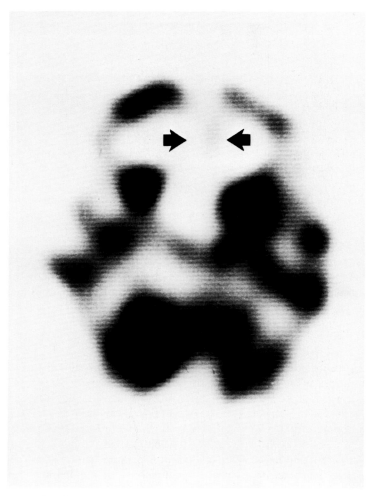

Figure 9-1 Single photon emission computed tomogram (SPECT) using iodo-amphet-amine to reveal decreased cerebral blood flow in the medial aspects of both frontal lobes. Horizontal (above) and mid-sagittal (facing) sections are shown.

nucleus of Cajal and the parkinsonian symptoms are almost certainly due to nigrostri-atal damage.

A biochemical neuropathologic study of 9 patients and 27 controls showed a marked reduction in (3H) spiperone D2 receptor binding in the putamen (42 percent), caudate nucleus (48 percent), nucleus accumbens (44 percent), frontal cortex (34 percent), and substantia innominata (67 percent). A significant negative correlation was found between the numbers of neurofibrillary tangles and the number of (3H) spipe-rone binding sites. Dopamine levels were reduced by more than 85 percent and homo-vanillic acid levels (HVA) by 50 percent in the caudate nucleus and putamen, but intriguingly, in contrast to Parkinson's disease, no reduction was observed in the nu-cleus accumbens or frontal cortex. Significant correlations were found for HVA, (3H)

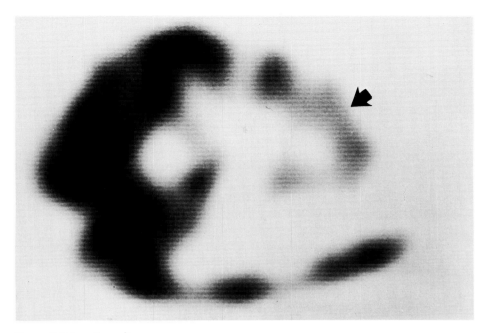

Figure 9-1 (continued)

spiperone binding, and choline acetyl transferase (ChAT) activity in both the caudate and putamen (Ruberg et al., 1985). Kish and colleagues (1985) also found 80 percent loss of dopamine and 50 percent loss of HVA, comparable to that found in Parkinson's disease, in 5 pathologically verified cases, 3 of whom had not had a supranuclear gaze palsy in life and 2 of whom had severe Alzheimer-type dementia. However, there was a slightly greater loss of dopamine in the caudate than in the putamen, the reverse of what is normally found in Parkinson's disease. Dopamine and HVA were also normal in this study in the nucleus accumbens, hypothalamus, and temporal cortex, although a 33 percent reduction of dopamine occurred in the paraolfactory cortex. Taken together, therefore, these two studies suggest that, in contrast in Parkinson's disease, the striatal cholinergic interneurons are damaged as well as the nigrostriatal dopaminergic pathway. Furthermore, it seems unlikely that the neuropsychiatric impairment in PSP can be ascribed to lesions in the dopaminergic mesocortico-limbic pathway.

Discrepant findings have been reported regarding acetylcholine function as measured by ChAT. Ruberg el al. found ChAT to be decreased slightly in the cerebral cortex (20 percent), moderately in the caudate, putamen, and nucleus accumbens (40–60 percent), and severely in the substantia innominata (70 percent). Using (3H) quinoclidinyl benzylate as an indicator of cholinergic transmission potential, no significant differences between PSP patients and controls were found. Ruberg and colleagues (1985) interpreted these findings of widespread loss of subcortical ChAT as reflecting in part loss of neurons in the cholinergic pedunculo-pontine tegmental nucleus, which has major subcortical, but only minor cortical, output connections. The neuropsychological impairments characteristic of PSP and attributed to basal ganglia damage might also bear some relation to cell loss in this nucleus. Kish and colleagues (1985) found normal ChAT levels in all neocortical areas in 4 patients and modest reductions in the striatum, temporal cortex, and hippocampus. It seems likely, therefore, that, although modest cell loss occurs in the substantia innominata in PSP, the neuropsychological abnormalities cannot be caused primarily by cortical cholinergic deficits.

Available evidence suggests, therefore, that the neuropsychological deficits in PSP are most likely due to neuronal loss in the caudate nucleus and globus pallidus with dysfunction of the complex connections with prefrontal cortical regions leading to functional frontal lobe-like impairment. It remains possible, however, that lesions in other brain-stem structures such as the pedunculo-pontine tegmental nucleus, the mesencephalic tegmental area, and the locus coeruleus may contribute to the dementia syndrome.

TREATMENT

Tricyclic antidepressants may be of modest benefit in improving the emotional incontinence and psychomotor retardation of PSP (Kvale, 1982; Newman, 1985). The intellectual deficits, however, are as refractory as the motor symptoms to any form of drug manipulation.

REFERENCES

Albert, M.L., Feldman, R.G., and Willis, A.L. The "subcortical dementia" of progressive supranuclear palsy. *J Neurol Neurosurg Psychiatry* 1974; 37:121–30.
Cambier, J., Masson, M., Viader, F., Limodin, J., and Strube, A. Le syndrome frontal de la paralysie supranucleaire progressive. *Rev Neurol (Paris)* 1985; 141:528–36.
D'Antona, R., Baron, J.C., Samson, Y., Serdaru, M., Viader, F., Agid, Y., and Cambier, J. Subcortical dementia: frontal cortex hypometabolism detected by positron tomography in patients with progressive supranuclear palsy. *Brain* 1985; 108:785–99.
Drayer, B.P., Olanow, W., Burger, P., Johnson, G.A., Hurfkens, R., and Riederer, S. Parkinson plus syndrome: diagnosis using high field MR imaging of brain iron. *Radiology* 1986; 159:493–8.
Dubas, F., Gray, F., and Escourolle, R. Maladie de Steele-Richardson-Olszewski sans ophthalmoplegie. *Rev Neurol (Paris)* 1983; 139:407–16.
Dubois, B., Pillon, B., Legault, F., Agid, Y., and Lhermitte, F. Slowing of cognitive processing in progressive supranuclear palsy. *Arch Neurol* 1985; 45:1194–9.
Fisk, J.D., Goodale, M.Z., Burkhart, G., and Barnett, H.J.M. Progressive supranuclear palsy: The relationship between ocular motor dysfunction and psychological test performance. *Neurology* 1982; 32:698–705.
Fukushima-Kudo, J., Fukushima, K., and Tashiro, K. Rigidity and dorsiflexion of the neck in progressive supranuclear palsy and the interstitial nucleus of Cajal. *J Neurol Neurosurg Psychiatry* 1987; 50:1197–203.
Haldeman, S., Goldman, J.W., Hyde, J., Pribram, H.F.W. Progressive supranuclear palsy. Computed tomography and response to anti-parkinsonian drugs. *Neurology* 1981; 31:442–5.
Kimura, D., Barnett, H.J.M., and Burkhart, G. The psychological test pattern in progressive supranuclear palsy. *Neuropsychologia* 1981; 19:301–6.

Kish, S.J., Chang, L.J., Mirchandani, L., Shannak, K., and Hornykiewicz, O. Progressive supranuclear palsy: relationship between extrapyramidal disturbances, dementia and brain neurotransmitter markers. *Neurology* 1985; 26:764–8.

Kristensen, M.O. Progressive supranuclear palsy—20 years later. *Acta Neurol Scand* 1985; 71:177–89.

Kvale, J.N. Amitriptyline in the management of progressive supranuclear palsy. *Arch Neurol* 1982; 39:387–8.

Leenders, K.L., Frackowiak, R.S.J., and Lees, A.J. Progressive supranuclear palsy: brain energy metabolism, blood flow and fluorodopa uptake measured by positron emission tomography. *Brain* 1988; 111:615–30.

Maher, E.R., and Lees, A.J. The clinical features and natural history of the Steele-Richardson-Olszewski syndrome (progressive supranuclear palsy). *Neurology* 1986; 36:1005–8.

Maher, E.R., Smith, E.M., and Lees, A.J. Cognitive defects in the Steele-Richardson-Olszewski syndrome (progressive supranuclear palsy). *J Neurol Neurosurg Psychiatry* 1985; 48:1234–9.

Mastaglia, F.L., Grainger, K., Kee, F., Sadka, M., and Lefory, R. Progressive supranuclear palsy: the Steele-Richardson-Olszewski syndrome: Clinical and electrophysiological observations in eleven cases. *Proc Aust Assoc Neurol* 1973; 10:35–44.

Masucci, E.F., Borts, F.T., Smirniotopoulos, J.G., and Kurtzke, J.F. Thin section CT of midbrain abnormalities in progressive supranuclear palsy. *Am J Neuroradiol* 1985; 6:767–72.

Newman, G.C. Treatment of progressive supranuclear palsy with tricyclic antidepressants. *Neurology* 1985; 35:1189–93.

Pillon, B., Dubois, B., L'Hermitte, F., and Agid, Y. Heterogeneity of intellectual impairment in progressive supranuclear palsy, Parkinson's disease and Alzheimer's disease. *Neurology* 1986; 36:1179–85.

Richardson, J.C., Steele, J., and Olszewski, J. Supranuclear ophthalmoplegia, pseudobulbar palsy, nuchal dystonia and dementia. *Trans Am Neurol Assoc* 1963; 88:25-7.

Ruberg, M., Javoy-Agid, F., Hirsch, E., and Scatton, B. Dopaminergic and cholinergic lesions in progressive supranuclear palsy. *Ann Neurol* 1985; 18:523–9.

Rutledge, J.N., Hilal, S.K., Schallert, T., Silver, A.J., Defendini, R.D., and Fahn, S. Magnetic resonance imaging of parkinsonians. In *Recent Developments in Parkinson's Disease, Vol. 2,* Fahn, S. et al. (eds.). Macmillan Healthcare, New Jersey, 1987, pp. 123–34.

Schonfield, S.M., Golbe, L.I., Sage, J.I., Safer, J.N., and Duvoisin, R.C. Computed tomography findings in progressive supranuclear palsy: Correlation with clinical grade. *Movement Disorders* 1987; 2:263–78.

Steele, J.C. Progressive supranuclear palsy. *Brain* 1972; 95:693–704.

Steele, J.C., Richardson, J.C., and Olszewski, J. Progressive supranuclear palsy. A heterogeneous degeneration involving the brain stem, basal ganglia and cerebellum with vertical gaze and pseudobulbar palsy, nuchal dystonia and dementia. *Arch Neurol* 1964; 10:333–58.

Zweig, R.M., Whitehouse, P.J., Casanova, M.F., Walker, L.C., Jankel, W.R., and Price, D.L. Loss of putative cholinergic neurones of the pedunculopontine nucleus in progressive supranuclear palsy. *Ann Neurol* 1985; 18:144.

10

Thalamic Degeneration

KEITH D. McDANIEL

Thalamic degeneration may occur as an associated feature of some of the multisystem atrophies, or, less frequently, may be the major component of the inadequately studied degenerative syndrome called *thalamic dementia*. In 1939 Stern published a report of a case "for which no analogy could be found in the literature" (Stern, 1939). He described a 41-year-old male with symptoms of drowsiness, apathy, hypophonia, memory loss, and rigidity. The symptoms rapidly progressed to mutism, and death occurred within 11 months of onset. Pathologically, marked neuronal loss and severe gliosis were found in many of the thalamic nuclei; there were only minimal changes in other regions of the brain. Stern suggested a correlation between the dementia and the thalamic degeneration based upon thalamo-cortical connections.

Although selective thalamic degeneration is rare, a sufficient number of clinico-pathologic studies have been published to suggest the existence of a relatively discrete thalamic degenerative disease that invariably leads to dementia. This chapter will focus primarily on the characteristics of those cases with "pure" thalamic degeneration and will briefly discuss the multisystem atrophies that have concomitant thalamic involvement.

DEMOGRAPHY

Selective thalamic degeneration is extremely rare. After eliminating cases associated with multiple systems degeneration and those with limited neuropathologic data, there are only 21 cases in the literature (Tables 10-1 and 10-2).

Approximately one half of the cases reported are familial (Lugaresi et al., 1986; Martin et al., 1983; Oda, 1976/1977). Little et al. (1986) have described an entire kindred with seven confirmed and two probable cases of thalamic degeneration. The age of onset is variable with a range of 18 to 72 years; the majority of cases have presented with symptoms between the fourth and sixth decade. Patients frequently have a rapidly progressive course with the interval between initial symptoms to death being measured in months to a few years.

Thalamic degeneration may be a component of some of the multisystem degenerative disorders (Martin et al., 1974). It has been reported in cases of spinocerebellar degeneration (Martin et al., 1974; Poser et al., 1957), familial multisystems atrophy (Katz et al., 1984), and reticulo-pallido-dentato-rubral multisystem atrophy (Kosaka et al., 1977). In these cases the age of onset is also relatively young; however, the course is more variable and may be prolonged for several years or even for decades.

CLINICAL CHARACTERISTICS

Abnormal neurologic signs are minimal in patients with selective thalamic degeneration (Table 10-1). The most common finding is a mixed movement disorder that is frequently difficult to characterize. Abnormal limb and trunk movements have been described as "grotesque" (Stern, 1939) and "bizarre" (Little et al., 1986). Tremor (Lugaresi et al., 1986; Moossy et al., 1987), choreoathetosis (Schulman, 1957), and myoclonus (Little et al., 1986; Schulman, 1957; Stern, 1939) have all been reported, sometimes occurring simultaneously in the same patient. Primitive reflexes such as suck, snout, and grasp are the second most frequently cited class of neurologic findings (Martin et al., 1983; Moossy et al., 1987; Oda, 1976/1977; Stern, 1939). The autonomic nervous system is found to be dysfunctional in a small percentage of patients. Fixed or poorly reactive pupils (Lugaresi et al., 1986; Oda, 1976/1977), abnormal sweating and hypersalivation (Hori et al., 1981; Lugaresi et al., 1986; Martin et al., 1983; Oda, 1976/1977) have been reported. Alterations in sleep–wake cycle may manifest as hypersomnolence (Little et al., 1986; Stern, 1939) or insomnia (Lugaresi, 1986). Infrequently described abnormalities have included hyperreflexia (Moossy et al., 1987; Oda, 1976/1977), dysarthria (Lugaresi et al., 1986; Oda, 1976/1977), and limited upward gaze (Lugaresi et al., 1986).

Abnormalities on elementary neurologic examination are usually dramatic in the multisystem degenerations that have associated thalamic involvement. Ataxia, paraparesis, spasticity, blindness, optic atrophy, nystagmus, dysarthria, and movement disorders may be present in varying degree.

DEMENTIA SYNDROME

There have been no systematic studies of the salient features of the dementia associated with thalamic degeneration. Because of the rarity of the disorder, insufficient numbers of patients have been subjected to standardized neuropsychological assessment. A further difficulty in studying this patient population is the rapidity with which the disorder progresses, frequently leaving the patient mute, immobile, and nearly comatose within a short period of time. Consequently, few patients are examined in detail early in their course. Despite these limitations, clinical descriptions of such patients contain many overlapping features. Similarly, there is a conspicuous absence of some abnormalities, particularly aphasia, agnosia, and apraxia. Table 10-1 summarizes the primary clinical findings of all cases described to date. The most prevalent and consistent of the abnormalities of mental status will be discussed in the following.

Table 10-1 Clinical Features of Thalamic Degeneration

Author Year	No. of Cases	Age (Years)	Duration	Clinical Features				Neurodiagnostic	
				Psychiatric and Neurovegetative	Neurobehavioral	Neurologic	Movement Disorder	Radiology/ EEG	CSF
Stern (1939)	1	41	11 mo	"Run down," apathy, loss of initiative, "sullen," drowsy, loss of insight	Poor memory, decreased verbal output, writing and reading impaired	Pupils fixed to light and convergence + suck, + grasp	"Unusual hand movements," "grotesque pointing"	Skull films: normal	Normal
Grunthal (1942)	1	35	26 yrs	Psychosis	Slowly progressive dementia				
Schulman et al. (1957)	1	50	6 mo	"Run down," tired, irritable, apathy, violent temper, inappropriate laughter	Inattentive, poor memory, decreased verbal output		Choreoathetosis, ataxia, myoclonus	Ventriculogram: mild dilitation EEG: Slow waves	Normal
Garcin et al. (1963)	1	56	9 mo	Apathy	Memory loss, dementia	Dysarthria	Choreoathetosis, myoclonus		
Oda (1976)	4	18–43	9–19 mo	Apathy (1), personality change (1), excitability (1), hypersomnia (1)	Delirium (2), amnestic (4), akinetic-mute (1), dementia (2), opticospatial agnosia (1)	Loss of pupillary reflexes (2), pyramidal signs (3), dysarthria (2), rigidity (2)	Tremor (1), ataxia (2), unusual movements (2)		

Reference	N	Age	Duration	Behavioral/Psychiatric	Cognitive	Neurological signs	Movement	Imaging/EEG	CSF
Hori et al. (1981)	1	43	9 mo	Apathy, personality change, disinhibited, visual hallucinations	Disorientation, confabulation, memory loss	Dysphagia, mydriasis	Oculogyric crisis	Pneumoencephalogram and angiogram: normal	Normal
Pilz and Erhart (1981)	1	61	20 yrs	Apathy, inertia, emotional lability, delusions, visual hallucinations	Disoriented, memory loss, decreased writing, geographical disorientation		"Atactic gait"	EEG: Slightly abnormal	Pandy +
Martin et al. (1983)	1	21	3 yrs	"Strange behavior," staring, lack of insight	Memory loss, temporal disorientation, poor abstractions and calculating abilities	Snout reflex, mumbling speech	Tremulous	CT: normal	Normal
Little et al. (1986)	7	25–72	6–24 mo	Psychosis (2), somnolence (3), hallucinations (2), "slowness" (1)	"Dementia" (1), memory loss (2), confusion (1), disorientation (1)	Mumbling speech (1), gait disturbance (2)	Myoclonus (1), bizarre hand movements (1)	Pneumoencephalogram and angiogram: normal (1), EEG: slow wave abnormality (?#)	Normal (?#)
Lugaresi et al. (1986)	1	53	9 mo	Slowness, motor agitation, dreamlike state, insomnia	Confusion and disorientation in late stages	Dysarthria, limited upward gaze, miosis	Tremor, myoclonus	EEG: Diffuse slowing	Mildly elevated protein
Moossy et al. (1987)	2	31; 67	1 yr; 4 yrs	"Depression" (2), slow (2), blunted (2), decreased insight (2)	Disoriented (2), memory loss (2), poor visuospatial skills (2), poor calculations (2)	Decreased verbal output (1) or mute (1), brisk reflexes (2), rigidity (1)	Tremor (1), rhythmic jaw chewing movements (1)	CT: normal (1) atrophy (1) Xenon CT: decreased thalamic blood flow (1) EEG: generalized slowing (1)	Moderately elevated protein (1)

Behavior

Depression is the most common diagnosis received by these patients during their initial evaluations. The constellation of symptoms reported by patients and family members is indicative of a mood disorder. Patients are described as apathetic, disinterested, and depressed. The histories of these patients also consistently refer to personality changes, particularly lack of initiative, inertia, irritability, sulleness, and a loss of emotional reactivity. Examination reveals an individual with psychomotor retardation, blunted or inappropriate affect, masked facies, and lack of insight. This appearance, coupled with the paucity of verbal behavior, led one investigator to refer to such a patient as "akinetic and mute" (Oda, 1976/1977). Less frequently, psychotic symptoms and bizarre behavior may emerge as a component of the psychiatric presentation (Little et al., 1986). Schulman (1957) described a case with inappropriate laughter, irritability, and violent temper outbursts. The case reported by Hori et al. (1981) also demonstrated disinhibited behavior and rage attacks. Visual hallucinations (Hori et al., 1981; Pilz and Erhart, 1981) and somatic delusions (Pilz and Erhart, 1981) have also been reported.

Arousal and Attention

Hypersomnolence is not an uncommon complaint in patients with thalamic degeneration. With such a profound disturbance in arousal, attention span and concentrating abilities are necessarily compromised. The case reported by Lugaresi et al. (1986) presented with insomnia. Daytime observations revealed the patient to be in a "dream-like state"; later in the course the patient became drowsy and stuporous. Other investigators have used terms such as "dreamy state" and "delirious" to describe patients, suggesting significant impairment in the domains of arousal and attention (Hori et al., 1981; Oda, 1976/1977). In two publications in which quantitative testing of attention was reported, forward digit span was found to be diminished to 3–4 digits (Schulman, 1957) and 5 digits (Martin et al., 1983), respectively. Patients are virtually always described as "disoriented," but it is difficult to determine if this finding is secondary to their disturbance of arousal and attention or represents a primary memory disorder.

Memory

Memory impairment is consistently reported as a prominent feature in patients with thalamic degeneration. they are described as demonstrating "poor memory," "forgetfulness," or "amnesia." Objective testing is rarely reported in detail other than to note that these patients are frequently temporally and at times spacially disoriented. Additionally, they are found to have extreme difficulty learning new information and to a lesser degree retrieving old information. Based upon the published clinical descriptions, it is unclear whether the memory disorder falls more into the realm of amnesia (an inability to learn new material) or forgetfulness (an inability to retrieve material that is substantially improved with cueing).

Language and Speech

Classic aphasic disturbances are not reported in patients with thalamic degeneration, although complete language examinations using aphasia batteries have not been conducted. Spontaneous verbal output is characterized in some patients as incomprehensible (Martin et al., 1983), unintelligible (Lugaresi et al., 1986), or incoherent (Little et al., 1986). In each of these cases the speech itself was noted to be "mumbly," and an articulatory disturbance may have confounded the language examination. A specific comprehension defect has been suggested in at least one case (Moossy et al., 1987). The most consistent findings pertain to aspects of speech rather than language. Virtually all cases reported have had diminished verbal output with associated hypophonic, monotonous speech. As the paucity of verbal output progresses, a mumbly quality supersedes. In the middle to late stages of the disease process, patients are commonly mute. Many reports claim that writing is impaired, sometimes early in the course of the illness (Stern, 1939; Oda, 1976/1977; Pilz and Erhart, 1981; Little et al., 1986).

Cognition

Reasoning, insight, and calculating abilities are impaired relatively early in the course of thalamic degeneration. Deterioration of job performance is a frequent reason for referral to the physician. Virtually all patients are described as having diminished or no insight into the nature of their difficulties. Abstract reasoning and proverb interpretation is impaired, and, when specifically tested, calculating abilities are markedly diminished from premorbid levels (Schulman, 1957; Martin et al., 1983; Moossy et al., 1987).

Visuospatial Skills

Geographic orientation and visuospatial constructional abilities are usually not commented upon in the literature. Oda (1976/1977) characterized one patient as having an "optico-spatial agnosia" but did not discuss the specific finding that led to this conclusion. Pilz and Erhart's case (1981) was reported to have difficulty finding his way back home from his customary walks early in the illness. Marked difficulty with design copying and block construction were noted in one case (Moossy et al., 1987).

PATHOPHYSIOLOGY

Electrophysiology

Electroencephalograms were performed on approximately one half of all reported cases of thalamic degeneration. All were abnormal, usually demonstrating a generalized slow-wave abnormality of mild to moderate severity. Notably, none of the patients' recordings revealed evidence of periodicity or high-voltage synchronous sharp waves.

Radiology

Ventriculograms and/or angiograms were sometimes performed in patients in the pre-computerized tomography (CT) era and revealed either normal findings or mild ventricular enlargement. Similarly, CT scans have shown either no abnormalities or generalized atrophy with mild dilatation of the ventricular system. A xenon-enhanced CT scan was utilized in one case report and demonstrated significantly decreased blood flow within the thalamus with normal blood flow in the cortex, white matter, and caudate nucleus (Moossy et al., 1987).

Recently, Grossman et al. (1988) studied two patients with atypical dementia syndromes and found no diagnostic changes on serial CT scans or magnetic resonance imaging, but left thalamic hypometabolism was demonstrated using F-fluorodeoxyglucose positron emission tomography. At the time of reporting, neither of these patients had come to post mortem examination for neuropathologic confirmation of the suspected thalamic degeneration.

Cerebrospinal Fluid

Cerebrospinal fluid examination usually reveals no abnormalities. Two reported cases have had moderately elevated protein levels in the range of 76–135 mg per deciliter (Lugaresi et al., 1986; Moossy et al., 1987).

NEUROPATHOLOGY

As previously noted, the most marked neuropathologic changes are found in the thalamus. It should be noted, however, that in no case has the thalamus been the unique site of involvement. Minimal cell loss and gliosis frequently occurs in such structures as inferior olivary nuclei, red nuclei, vestibular nuclei, and cerebellum. Mild gliosis and vacuolization of white matter is a common associated finding. Finally, cortical neurons may be slightly reduced in number or may show mild swelling and chromatolysis.

Despite the minimal changes noted elsewhere, the thalamic pathology is dramatic and frequently widespread within the thalamic nuclei. The changes include severe astrogliosis and neuronal loss (Figure 10-1). Although much of the thalamus is atrophic and gliotic, several thalamic nuclei are preferentially involved. Table 10-2 classifies the thalamic nuclei according to functional organization. As is readily apparent from the table, the limbic projection nuclei are consistently the most severely affected. Diffuse reticular nuclei and cortical association nuclei are less consistently involved. With the exception of a few cases, the specific projection nuclei are minimally involved or spared altogether. The implications of this hierarchical pattern of involvement will be discussed in the final section of the chapter.

As previously noted, thalamic nuclei may be involved in multiple system atrophies and heredito-degenerative syndromes. Degeneration of pulvinar, anterior thalamus, and dorsal medial thalamus may be associated with the heredofamilial ataxias in which there is also prominent involvement of spinocerebellar tracts, posterior columns, pyramidal tracts, optic pathways, dentato-rubral tracts, and the pallido-nigral-luysian sys-

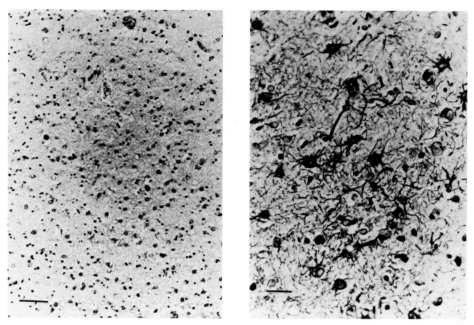

Figure 10-1   Sections from dorsomedial thalamus of a patient with thalamic degeneration. (A) Hematoxyline-eosin stain. (B) Holzer method stain. Note the nearly complete loss of neurons (A) and marked fibrillary gliosis (B). (Reprinted by permission of the publisher from Little, B.W., Brown, P.W., Rodgers-Johnson, P., Perl, D.P., and Gadjusek, D.C. *Ann Neurol* 1986; 20:231–9. Copyright 1986, Little, Brown & Company, Boston, Massachusetts.)

tem (Kosaka et al., 1977; Martin et al., 1974; Poser et al., 1957). Katz et al (1984) reported anterior, dorsal medial, and ventral lateral thalamic nuclear degeneration in a case of familial spastic paraparesis with optic atrophy and dementia. Thalamic cortical association nuclei and specific relay nuclei are sometimes affected in Friedreich's ataxia, spinocerebellar degenerations, dyssynergia cerebellaris myoclonia, and Werdnig-Hoffmann disease (Martin, 1975).

DIFFERENTIAL DIAGNOSIS OF THALAMIC DEMENTIA

Pick's disease Type II (Moossy et al., 1987), a term initially introduced by Neumann (1949) and later modified to *progressive subcortical* gliosis (Neumann and Cohn, 1967), shares clinical and pathologic features with thalamic dementia. Patients with progressive subcortical gliosis have similar neuropsychological deficits to those with selective thalamic degeneration; however, their course is generally much more prolonged, frequently persisting for 5–10 years. Neuropathologic examination reveals subcortical gliosis involving white matter, basal ganglia, thalamus, brain stem, and ventral horns of the spinal cord.

   The diagnosis of Creutzfeldt-Jakob disease is often entertained in patients later found to have thalamic degeneration. Clinically the presentation and course may ap-

Table 10-2 Pathologic Features of Thalamic Degeneration[a]

Author Year	Stern[b] 1939	Grunthal[c] 1942	Schulman et al.[d] 1957	Garcin et al.[e] 1963	Oda[f] 1976	Hori et al.[g] 1981	Pilz and Erhart[h] 1981	Martin et al.[i] 1983	Little et al.[j] 1986	Lugaresi et al.[k] 1986	Moossy et al.[l] 1987
Thalamic Pathology											
Limbic Projection nn.											
Dorsal Medial	+++	+++	+++	+++	+++	+++	+++	+++	+++	+++	+++
Anterior	++	−	++	++	++	+++	+++	++	+	+++	+
Diffuse Reticular nn.											
Centromedian	+++	−	−			+	++	−	+++	−	++
Intralaminar	++		−			−	−	++	+++		+
Reticular	−		+++		+	−					+
Cortical Association nn.											
Pulvinar				++	++	++	++	++			
Lateral Posterior	+++	−	+++		++	+++	++	−			+++
Lateral Dorsal	+++	−	+++	++	++	+++	++	++	++		+++
Specific Projection nn.											
Lateral Geniculate	−	−			−	−	++	−	−		
Medial Geniculate	−	−			−	+		−	−		
Ventral Posterior			+		−	+	+	−			
Medial											
Ventral Posterior			+		−	+	+	−			
Lateral											
Ventral Lateral	−	−	−			+	+	−		−	
Ventral Anterior	−	−	−	+	+	++	+	++			

[a]Key: degree of involvement: +++, severe; ++, moderate; +, mild; −, none; if left blank, information unavailable. Neuronal loss and/or gliosis in other CNS structures:

[b]Inferior olivary nuclei; frontal and parietal cortex; white matter.

[c]Red nuclei.

[d]Minimal cortical and white matter gliosis.

[e]Frontal cortex; insula; medial occipital cortex.

[f]Inferior olivary nuclei; vestibular nuclei; pretectum; substantia nigra; Purkinje cell loss.

[g]Cingulate gyrus; superior colliculi; inferior olivary nuclei; cerebellar vermis.

[h]Lateral amygdala; inferior olivary nuclei; vestibular nuclei; third and fourth cortical layers of frontal and occipital lobes.

[i]Vestibular nuclei; inferior olivary nuclei; bulbar reticular formation.

[j]Inferior olivary nuclei.

[k]Inferior olivary nuclei.

[l]Basal nucleus of Meynert; caudate; putamen; globus pallidus; amygdala; subthalamus.

pear identical. A rapidly progressive dementia syndrome with myoclonus occurring in a kindred or sporadically are characteristics shared by the two disorders. Because cerebral spongiosis was found in the cases reported by Schulman (1957) and Garcin et al. (1963), Martin (1975) considered these cases as examples of the "thalamic form" of Creutzfeldt-Jakob disease. Creutzfeldt-Jakob disease and selective thalamic degeneration, however, can be distinguished by at least three features. First, the spongiform findings of Creutzfeldt-Jakob disease are not limited to the extracellular changes associated with thalamic degeneration (Little et al., 1986). In Creutzfeldt-Jakob disease the vacuoles are intracellular within astrocytes and neurons (Masters and Richardson, 1978). Second, the characteristic electroencephalographic patterns of Creutzfeldt-Jakob disease (periodic bursts with a slow background) are seen in 75–90 percent of patients at some time during their disease (Cummings and Benson, 1983) and have never been reported in patients with pathologically proven thalamic degeneration. Finally, human-to-primate transmission has not been successful in any of the reported cases of thalamic degeneration, whereas this can be achieved in many cases of Creutzfeldt-Jakob disease.

FUNCTIONAL CONSIDERATIONS

The clinical characteristics of the dementia associated with thalamic degeneration have been delineated in this chapter. Previous investigators have made little effort to classify the type of dementia precisely, especially with regard to the subcortical–cortical dichotomy (Cummings and Benson, 1984). Most authors have, however, emphasized the common findings of psychomotor retardation, inertia, loss of initiative, diminished speech output, and disturbances in attention, concentration, and memory, without the classic cortical signs of aphasia, apraxia, and agnosia. These features fit closely with the concept of subcortical dementia. Importantly, many patients do not present for a formal neurologic evaluation until the middle to late stages of the disease. Moossy et al. (1987) stated that, by the time their cases presented for assessment, it was impossible to make a distinction between a subcortical and cortical dementia pattern.

There has been little effort to draw clinico-neuroanatomic correlations in cases of thalamic degeneration. Grunthal (1942) suggested that the clinical features of his case were the equivalent of a frontal lobe dementia. This observation is consistent with what is known regarding thalamo-cortical connections and the sites of the major neuropathology in thalamic degeneration.

Table 10-2 lists the location of thalamic pathology in the thalamic degenerations and suggests some preliminary conclusions regarding clinico-anatomic relationships in the cases reported to date. The classification utilized in this table organizes nuclear groups according to functional divisions, rather than strict anatomic locations. In every reported case the most notable finding is severe involvement of the dorsal medial thalamic nucleus. There are rich reciprocal connections between dorsal medial nucleus and prefrontal cortex. Loss of dorsal medial nuclear function and/or projections to the frontal lobe may account for the affective and motivational symptoms seen in patients with thalamic dementia. The dorsal medial nucleus has also been implicated in subserving mnestic function, and degeneration of this region may be etiologically related to the memory disorder seen in this patient population. Finally, the dorsal medial nu-

cleus has extensive connections with intralaminar thalamic nuclear groups that themselves are important for maintaining wakefulness and arousal, suggesting that the hypersomnolence seen in some patients is related to interruption of this intrathalamic
system.

The anterior thalamic nucleus is the second limbic projection nucleus consistently
involved in the degenerative process. The anterior nucleus is known to be part of the
Papez circuit, receiving the mamillothalamic tract and projecting to the cingulate gyrus. Although the precise role of the anterior nucleus remains unknown, it shares with
the dorsal medial nucleus a putative role in the mediation of memory functions and
emotional–visceral responses. Taken together, dysfunction of the dorsal medial and
anterior thalamic nuclei and their respective cortical projections may be responsible
for much of the neuropsychiatric symptomatology and memory dysfunction reported
in patients with thalamic degeneration.

The diffuse reticular nuclei, including centromedian, intralaminar, and reticular,
are variably involved in thalamic degeneration. The brain-stem reticular formation is
the principal source of afferents to the intralaminar nucleus, which then sends efferents
to widespread cortical regions. One speculation is that disorders of arousal reported in
patients may be secondary to involvement of this system. Clinico-anatomic correlations for centromedian and reticular nuclei are less clear.

The thalamic cortical association nuclei are often moderately to severely degenerated in the cases reported. The lateral dorsal nucleus, the function of which is poorly
understood, projects primarily to the posterior cingulate gyrus and parietal cortex. The
lateral posterior nucleus projects to superior and inferior parietal lobules. These association cortices are important in cognitive and symbolic processes. Although never
reported in detail, there is frequent mention of difficulties with reasoning, insight, and
calculations in case studies of thalamic degeneration. Finally, the pulvinar is a large
lateral nucleus with projections primarily to the occipital cortex. Less dense efferents
project to temporal and frontal cortex.

A striking finding in nearly all reported cases is the absence or near absence of
pathologic changes in specific thalamic projection nuclei. This may account for the
sparing of primary visual, auditory, and somesthetic functions in these patients.

In addition to their dementia syndrome, many patients demonstrate a spectrum of
movement disorders from choreoathetosis to myoclonus. Of the extrathalamic structures involved in these patients, the inferior olivary nuclei and red nuclei frequently
show gliosis and neuronal loss. Degeneration of these structures may be related to the
development of the reported movement disorders.

In summary, the clinical features of the patients with selective thalamic degeneration, especially if examined relatively early in their course, are characteristic of subcortical dementia. Additionally, with the exception of minimal extrathalamic cortical,
basal ganglia, and brain-stem involvement, the neuropathology is localized to selective
thalamic nuclei. Limbic projection nuclei are consistently severely degenerated. There
is less consistent involvement of diffuse reticular and cortical association nuclei. The
specific sites of pathology correlate with the phenomenology of the dementia. Publications of future cases of thalamic degeneration should attempt to delineate more precisely the clinical features of the disorder. Correlation of the characteristics of the
subcortical dementia with the selective thalamic degeneration will provide further in-

sight into the role of specific thalamic nuclei in the maintenance of personality, mood, affective response, motivation, psychomotor speed, memory, and cognition.

REFERENCES

Cummings, J.L., and Benson, D.F. *Dementia. A Clinical Approach.* Butterworths, Boston, 1983, pp. 151–2.

Cummings, J.L., and Benson, D.F. Subcortical dementia: Review of an emerging concept. *Arch Neurol* 1984; 41:874–9.

Garcin, R., Brion, S., and Khochneiviss, A.A. Le syndrome de Creutzfeldt-Jakob et les syndromes cortico-stries du presenium. *Rev Neurol (Paris)* 1963; 109:419–41.

Grossman, M., Chawluk, J.B., Hurtig, H., Alavi, A., Gur, R.C., Saykin, A., and Reivich, M. Progressive thalamic dementia: a positron emission tomographic (PET) study. American Academy of Neurology Meeting. April, 1988. Cincinnati, Ohio.

Grunthal, E. Über thalamische demenz. *Monatsschr Psychiat Neurol* 1942; 106: 114–28.

Hori, A., Ikeda, K., Kosaka, K., Shinohara, S., and Iizuka, R. System degeneration of the thalamus. A clinico-neuropathological study. *Arch Psychiatr Nervenkr* 1981; 231:71–80.

Katz, D.A., Naseem, A., Horoupian, D.S., Rothner, A.D., and Davies, P. Familial multisystem atrophy with possible thalamic dementia. *Neurology* 1984; 34:1213–7.

Kosaka, K., Oyanagi, S., Matsushita, M., Hori, A., and Iwase, S. Multiple system degeneration involving thalamus, reticular formation, pallido-nigral, pallido-luysian and dentato-rubral systems. *Acta Neuropathol (Berl)* 1977; 39:89–95.

Little, B.W., Brown, P.W., Rodgers-Johnson, P., Perl, D.P., and Gadjusek, D.C. Familial myoclonic dementia masquerading as Creutzfeldt-Jakob disease. *Ann Neurol* 1986; 20:231–9.

Lugaresi, E., Medori, R., Montagna, P., Baruzzi, A., Cortelli, P., Lugaresi, A., Tinuper, D., Zucconi, M., and Gambetti, P. Fatal familial insomnia and dysautonomia with selective degeneration of thalamic nuclei. *N Engl J Med* 1986; 315:997–1003.

Martin, J.J. Thalamic degenerations. In *Handbook of Clinical Neurology.* Vinken, P.J., and Bruyn, G.W. (eds.). North Holland Publishing Co., Amsterdam, 1975, pp. 587–664.

Martin, J.J., van Dessel, G., Lagrou, A., de Barsy, A.M., and Dierick, W. Multiple system atrophies. A neuropathological and neurochemical study. *J Neurol Sci* 1974; 21:251–72.

Martin, J.J., Yap, M., Wei, I.P., and Tan, T.E. Selective thalamic degeneration—report of a case with memory and mental disturbances. *Clin Neuropathol* 1983; 2:156–62.

Masters, C.L., and Richardson, E.P., Jr. Subacute spongiform encephalopathy (Creutzfeldt-Jakob disease). *Brain* 1978; 101:333–44.

Moossy, J., Martinez, A.J., Hanin, I., Rao, G., Yonas, H., and Boller, J. Thalamic and subcortical gliosis with dementia. *Arch Neurol* 1987; 44:510–3.

Neumann, M.A. Pick's disease. *J Neuropathol Exp Neurol* 1949; 8:255–82.

Neumann, M.A., and Cohn, R. Progressive subcortical gliosis, a rare form of senile dementia. *Brain* 1967; 90:405–18.

Oda, M. Thalamus degeneration in Japan: A review from clinical and pathological viewpoints. *Appl Neurophysiol* 1976/1977; 39:178–98.

Pilz, P., and Erhart, P. Thalamic degeneration. In Tellinger, K., Gullobta, F., Mossakowski, M. (eds.). *Experimental and clinical neuropathology.* Springer-Verlag, New York, 1981, pp. 362–64.

Poser, C.M., Dewulf, A., and van Bogdert, L. Atypical cerebellar degeneration associated with
    leucodystrophy. *J Neuropathol Exp Neurol* 1957; 16:209–37.
Stern, K. Severe dementia associated with bilateral symmetrical degeneration of the thalamus.
    Brain 1939; 62:157–71.
Schulman, S. Bilateral symmetrical degeneration of the thalamus. *J Neuropathol Exp Neurol*
    1957; 17:446–70.

11

Subcortical Vascular Dementias

DONALD T. STUSS AND JEFFREY L. CUMMINGS

Vascular dementia is common; it is second only to dementia of the Alzheimer type as a cause of chronic progressive intellectual decline. The profile of neuropsychological deficits in vascular dementia syndromes is determined by the location, multiplicity, and extent of ischemic tissue injury (Cummings, 1987; Cummings and Benson, 1983). Table 11-1 summarizes the principal types of vascular dementia. Occlusion of the carotid arteries will result in infarctions located at the border zones between the anterior and middle or between the middle and posterior cerebral arteries. The resulting clinical syndrome is composed primarily of cortical-type deficits, including transcortical aphasia with preserved repetition, visuospatial deficits, and motor and sensory changes involving predominantly the proximal arm and leg. Occlusion of the middle cerebral artery, anterior cerebral artery, or posterior cerebral artery will produce hemisphere-specific cortical deficits resulting from dysfunctional tissue in the irrigated territory of the artery. Typical left-hemisphere deficits include aphasia, apraxia, alexia, agraphia, and acalculia, whereas right-hemisphere injury produces more profound visuospatial deficits, amusia, and dysprosody. Pyramidal tract dysfunction, loss of cortically mediated sensory abilities, or homonymous hemianopia may also be present contralateral to the infarction. Three types of small-vessel vascular dementia syndromes have also been described: thalamic dementia, lacunar state, and Binswanger's disease. These conditions manifest subcortical types of dementias and are presented in detail later. Involvement of the smallest arteries by inflammatory processes in collagen-vascular diseases or by ultrasmall emboli in embolic disorders produces diffuse cortical dysfunction. Thus the profile of neuropsychological deficits in vascular dementia is determined by the size of the vessel occluded, which, in turn, reflects the etiology of the vascular disease (Cummings, 1987; Erkinjuntti, 1987). In some conditions several sizes of vessels are involved, and the resulting dementia syndrome has both cortical and subcortical features.

Vascular dementias producing primarily a subcortical pattern of intellectual deterioration are presented in this chapter.

Table 11-1   Classification of Vascular Dementia

Vessel Size	Vessels Involved	Type of Dementia	Typical Neuropsychological Deficits
Large	Carotid	Cortical	Transcortical aphasia, visuospatial deficits
Large	Anterior, middle, posterior cerebral arteries	Cortical	Aphasia, apraxia, amnesia, alexia, agraphia, amusia, acalculia, dysprosody
Small	Thalamic branches of posterior cerebral artery	Subcortical	Apathy, amnesia, poor executive function
Small	Lenticulostriate branches of intracranial vessels	Subcortical	Lacunar state: depression, memory loss, poor executive function
Small	Penetrating vessels of surface cortical vessels	Subcortical	Binswanger's disease: mood changes, memory loss, poor executive function
Very small	Cortical vessels	Cortical	Confusional state
Large and small	Multiple vessels	Cortical and subcortical	Combinations of the above

THALAMIC VASCULAR DEMENTIA

Anatomic and Vascular Correlates

Understanding the neuropsychological deficits that follow thalamic lesions is dependent on a knowledge of the function of specific thalamic nuclei, the reciprocal connections between defined thalamic regions and specific cortical areas, and the vascular supply of the thalamus (Martin, 1968). The thalamus contains at least three principal types of cortical projection nuclei (specific sensory, nonspecific, association), as well as nuclear groups connecting with the limbic system and frontal lobe (Aggleton and Mishkin, 1983; Martin, 1968; Mishkin, 1982; Nauta, 1971). The neuropsychological syndromes following thalamic infarction are determined by the specific nuclear regions affected.

Neurological Features

Fisher (1959) reported three cardinal characteristics of thalamic hemorrhage: greater sensory than motor loss; oculomotor impairments, particularly disturbed vertical gaze; and moderate dysphasia, if pathology was in the dominant hemisphere. Choi and colleagues (1983) reported memory impairment as the predominant feature. A modified schema based on two recent classifications (Graff-Radford et al., 1985; Kawahara et al., 1986) relating thalamic pathology to clinical disturbances is presented in Table 11-2. In practice, some variation in presentation is expected, depending on the extent of pathology.

Neuropsychological Features

Neuropsychological alterations after thalamic vascular insult are described. These can be viewed within the general approach presented previously, but they are described as individual clinical phenomena to clarify their potential roles in subcortical thalamic vascular dementia.

Arousal, Attentional, and "Frontal" Deficits

Disorders of arousal, including loss of consciousness, are common after thalamic hemorrhage. While this is most likely with bilateral paramedian thalamic infarction, coma and extreme disturbances of consciousness can occur even with an apparent unilateral lesion (Friedman, 1985; Graff-Radford et al., 1985; Mills and Swanson, 1978; Stuss et al., 1988). Exceptions to this observation exist; there is one reported case of intact consciousness with bilateral lesions (Karabelas et al., 1985), and controversy exists about the effect of unilateral lesions on consciousness (Castaigne et al., 1981). In patients with an initial disturbance of consciousness, there is gradual improvement with time, moving from a state of apparent akinetic mutism to stupor and hypersomnia, with considerable fluctuation in the level of arousal (Archer et al., 1981; Castaigne et al., 1981; Guberman and Stuss, 1983; Katz et al., 1987). In later stages the patient may be fully alert; however, the patient will be slow to respond, apathetic, and exhibit a tendency to fall asleep if unstimulated (Katz et al., 1987; Mills and Swanson, 1978; Stuss et al., 1988).

The postulated pathology associated with hypersomnolence varies, but ascending activating systems defined anatomically or biochemically have been consistently implicated (Castaigne et al., 1981; Katz et al., 1987; Graff-Radford et al., 1984; Mills and Swanson, 1978). Recent research suggests that the thalamus has a specific role in the production and regulation of sleep and wakefulness that may be affected by thalamic pathology (Imeri et al., 1988; Lugaresi et al., 1986).

Even when the level of alertness appears normal, the patient with a thalamic lesion often continues to have attentional problems. These deficits are not observed in simple tasks such as digit span (Stuss et al., 1988; Swanson and Schmidley, 1985; Winocur et al., 1984). With less structured tasks, however, the attentional problem is readily elicited. Other deficits, particularly memory, can be affected to such a degree that it is difficult to dissociate them from the attentional deficit (Archer et al., 1981; Castaigne et al., 1966; Katz et al., 1987; Schott et al., 1980). Under certain circumstances, however, the disturbances can be differentiated. Stuss et al. (1988) were able to demonstrate an attentional problem with a simple maze learning task (see Figure 11-1). Two patients with unilateral thalamic lesions revealed learning curves with repeated trials, interspersed with trials in which the subjects made errors on the first move, indicating an attentional rather than memory disorder.

In addition to a selective attentional disorder, patients with thalamic lesions often have behavioral changes that resemble those described after focal frontal or frontal-limbic system damage (Damasio, 1985; Luria, 1973, 1980; Milner, 1964; Stuss and Benson, 1984, 1986). In the early stages confabulation and reduplicative paramnesia may be present (Brion et al., 1983; Swanson and Schmidley, 1985; Stuss et al., 1988). Perhaps the most striking disorder is an alteration in mood and concern. Patients are

Table 11-2 Thalamic Syndromes

Thalamic Group	Artery	Motor and Sensory Signs	Behavioral Changes	Prognosis
I. Anterolateral	Tuberothalamic	Facial paresis for emotional movement	Minimal disturbance of consciousness, even initially	Good
		Mild or absent Hemiparesis Sensory loss	Impaired memory and attention In initial stages, asymmetrical findings L-impairment of intellect, speech, language, all spheres of memory Improves markedly, but same pattern exists	
II. Posterolateral	Geniculo-thalamic	Dejerine-Roussy syndrome	Second most likely to have disturbed consciousness	Poorest
		Most severe sensory loss in all primary modalities	Few other behavioral deficits unless concomitant PCA occlusion	
		Hemiparesis if posterior limb of internal capsule involved Ocular disturbance miosis light reflex upward-gaze palsy convergence spasm		

III. Medial	Interpeduncular	Uncommon sensory or motor deficits	Most disturbed consciousness, particularly in early stages	Poor
	Paramedian Thalamic	Ocular disturbance common vertical gaze miosis light reflex	Impaired cognition, attention, visuospatial Language generally spared, memory disturbance most severe and lasting disability, personality change and loss of spontaneity	
IV. Lateral thalamus Posterior internal capsule (Graff-Radford et al., 1985)		Hemiparesis, dysarthria	Mild language disturbance, mild amnesia	
Anterior choroidal dorsal (Kawahara et al., 1986)			L Thalamus mixed transcortical aphasia R Thalamus constructional impairment, topographic memory disturbance	Excellent

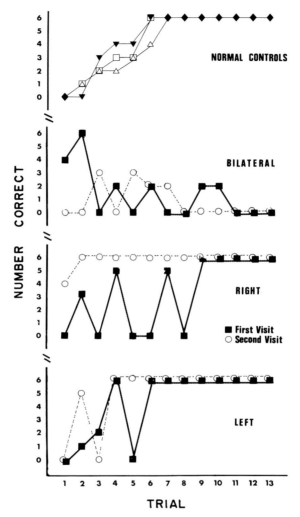

Figure 11-1 An illustration of the performance of patients with thalamic infarctions on a simplified maze learning test. A total of 6 correct moves are possible for each trial. 13 trials were given to each patient. The results of one testing of three normal control subjects are illustrated on top for comparison. The patients could be differentiated by their lesion location: bilateral, right, left. Patients were tested on two separate occasions. The "scalloping" effect, with an error occurring most often on the very first trial, suggested that motivational and/or attentional problems influenced the learning process. [Reprinted with permission from Academic Press, Stuss et al., (1988).]

frequently described as apathetic, akinetic, unconcerned, and euphoric (Katz et al., 1987; Mills and Swanson, 1978; Schott et al., 1980; Speedie and Heilman, 1983). Other "frontal" characteristics include perseveration, inability to maintain stable interests, increased susceptibility to interference, and problems in "chunking" and sequencing information.

The dorsomedial (DM) nucleus has massive projections to the prefrontal cortex, and animal research has consistently demonstrated similar deficits after either DM or focal frontal lesions (Fuster and Alexander, 1973; Schulman, 1964). Thus, lesions of the DM nucleus may be responsible for the "frontal lobe"–type behaviors observed with thalamic lesions. Pathology in nonspecific thalamic areas can also result in an arousal disturbance (Ojemann, 1977; Wallesch et al., 1983). In the chronic stage the attentional deficit can be described as an alerting, gating, sustained attention, or motivational problem similar to those occurring with frontal lobe disturbances (Mateer and Ojemann, 1983; Scheibel, 1980). The anatomic and motivational changes may be secondary to thalamic–limbic connections as well as frontal lobe dysfunction (Cummings and Benson, 1984). The emotional changes have been associated with lesions in specific locations (Graff-Radford et al., 1984); euphoric patients lacking insight had lesions in the dorsomedial thalamus, an area that projects to the orbitofrontal cortex, whereas withdrawn akinetic patients had pathology in the anterior thalamus, which projects to the cingulate.

Language Dysfunction

A role for the thalamus in language processes has been frequently described (Dejerine and Roussy, 1906; Schuell et al., 1965). While the language disturbance is difficult to characterize, the major findings of previous studies can be summarized. Attentional problems are obvious and frequently obscure recognition of a true language impairment (Castaigne et al., 1981; Graff-Radford et al., 1984). Language performance may be variable (Stuss et al., 1988). Luria (1977) labeled the deficit "quasiaphasic" secondary to vigilance mechanisms in the dominant thalamus.

Certain language changes are accepted as being characteristic of chronic thalamic lesions (Archer et al., 1981; Bogousslavsky et al., 1986; Crosson, 1984; Graff-Radford and Damasio, 1985; Speedie and Heilman, 1982; Stuss et al., 1988). Repetition is normal, with possible problems in repeating long phrases secondary to memory disturbances. Comprehension is normal or nearly normal. Mutism may occur in the initial stages. Subsequently, there is poor initiation of speech, with a general poverty of output and many pauses. Word list generation is moderately to severely impaired. Speech has diminished volume, impaired prosody, and variable dysarthria. Verbalizations are contaminated by perseverations, and there is a loss of the logical organization of discourse. Reading and writing are normal, although the latter may be impaired by motor disturbances. While phonemic and semantic paraphasias have been noted, perseverations, perceptual errors, nonaphasia misnaming, intrusions, and confabulations may be more characteristic. Naming is disturbed by many of the same influences affecting spontaneous speech. True anomia, however, is observed.

Language disorders occur almost universally after damage to the left thalamus (Barraguer-Bordas et al., 1981; Walshe et al., 1977). There is controversy about the necessary lesion within the thalamus. The majority of studies suggest necessary involvement of the pulvinar (see Crosson, 1984, for a review); others implicate the ventrolateral nucleus (Davous et al., 1984; Graff-Radford et al., 1984, 1985; McFarling et al., 1982). DM lesions, on the other hand, appear to result primarily in a memory disturbance sparing language skills. Graff-Radford and Damasio (1984) suggest two types of thalamic language disturbance based on lesion location: (1) ventrolateral and ventroanterior pathology, causing deficits similar to those described earlier; (2) pulvinar and posterolateral lesions, with normal or increased speech output and neologisms, anomia, and possible comprehension deficits.

The thalamic language disturbance is best explained as a disruption of cortical–subcortical integration (Crosson, 1984, 1985). Thus, the language disturbance after thalamic vascular insult could be attributed to multiple dysfunctions, including alterations in alerting, arousal, and monitoring.

Visuospatial Disorders

Most investigators have found that visuospatial disturbances are more apparent with bilateral or primarily right thalamic damage and absent with unilateral left pathology (Henderson, 1982; Speedie and Heilman, 1982; Stuss et al., 1988). In contrast, Graff-Radford et al. (1984) described visuospatial disturbances in four out of five thalamic patients, even in those with apparent unilateral left pathology. Differentiation again may depend on specific nuclear involvement, as well as the overlay of the "frontal" disturbance.

Memory

Amnesia secondary to focal diencephalic region pathology is now accepted. While typified by Korsakoff patients, a striking memory disorder secondary to vascular thalamic insult has been frequently reported. Anterograde memory disturbance is most striking (Markowitsch, 1982; Michel et al., 1982; Schott et al., 1980; von Cramon and Eilert, 1979; Winocur et al., 1984). Controversy exists concerning the neuropathology underlying the memory disorder. Many studies stress the importance of the mamillary bodies (MB), the anterior thalamic nuclei, and the mamillothalamic tract (bundle of Vicq d'Azyr) connecting the MB to the anterior thalamic nuclei (Barbizet et al., 1981; von Cramon et al., 1985). More frequently, following the theories concerning Korsakoff's syndrome, the DM nucleus has been implicated as the diencephalic area most directly related to memory (e.g., Ignelzi and Squire, 1976; Mills and Swanson, 1978). A third position is that, while a lesion on either system may cause some amnesia, damage to both the MB and DM nuclei are necessary for severe memory involvement (Aggleton and Mishkin, 1983; Squire, 1980). The critical lesion may involve the internal medullary lamina in conjunction with changes in the mamillothalamic tract (von Cramon et al., 1985).

The thalamic memory disturbance also appears to be hemisphere specific. While bilateral lesions result in a severe and persistent memory disorder, unilateral left and right lesions produce verbal and nonverbal memory disturbances, respectively (Speedie and Heilman, 1982, 1983; Stuss et al., 1988) (see Figure 11-2).

Thalamic Dementia Syndrome

Thalamic lesions produce subcortical dementia syndromes (Castaigne et al., 1966; Chassagnon et al., 1969). This is most likely in patients with bilateral thalamic lesions. Such patients meet the clinical criteria for dementia, being impaired in several functions: attention, language, memory, personality, and visuospatial disorders. The dementia syndrome, however, is not that proposed for dementia of the Alzheimer type (Cummings and Benson, 1983). Many of the characteristics are more typical of sub-

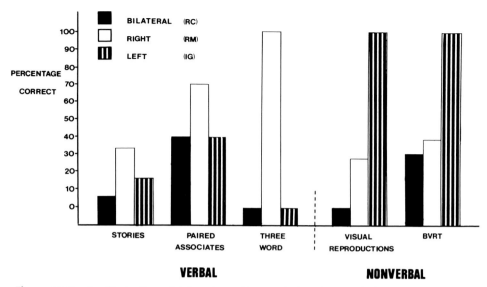

Figure 11-2 An illustration of delayed recall on verbal and nonverbal measures of memory for all three patients with thalamic lesions (bilateral, right, and left) several months after insult, demonstrating the hemispheric asymmetry of the thalamic memory disorder. Stories, paired associates, and visual reproductions were derived from the Wechsler Memory Scale. BVRT refers to the Benton Visual Retention Test, multiple choice format. For the three word test, the patient was asked to recall three words after a 5 minute delay. [Reprinted with permission from Academic Press, Stuss et al., (1988).]

cortical dementia: absence of apraxia, agnosia, or a definite aphasia; slowness in information processing speed; cognitive "dilapidation"; inertia and apathy. Many of the symptoms are typical of frontal and/or anterior limbic damage (Damasio, 1985; Poirier et al., 1983; Stuss and Benson, 1984, 1986). *Frontal–subcortical, frontal system*, or *frontal limbic syndrome* may be a more appropriate term for these cases (Albert, 1978; Freedman and Albert, 1985). The dementia syndrome associated with bilateral thalamic vascular insults differs from other subcortical dementias in combining a frontal–subcortical disturbance with a severe memory disorder (Stuss et al., 1988). Mental status changes in patients with unilateral pathology have sufficiently mild mental status changes that the term *dementia* is unwarranted.

LACUNAR STATE

Lacunes are small infarctions occurring in the deep gray nuclei of the hemispheres, cerebral and cerebellar white matter, and the brain stem (Fisher, 1982). They are most commonly the result of hypertension-related fibrinoid necrosis of arterioles, with resultant occlusion and ischemic infarction. A variety of syndromes has been ascribed to individual lacunes. *Lacunar state* refers to the occurrence of multiple lacunes, usually manifested by combined motoric and intellectual dysfunction.

Clinical Features

Historically, most patients with lacunar state present with a series of distinct episodes, each heralding a new vascular event and the appearance of new symptoms. In up to one third of patients with demonstrable lacunar infarctions, however, the deterioration is gradual, and the syndrome may be mistaken for a degenerative process (Weisberg, 1982).

The clinical syndrome associated with multiple lacunar infarctions has prominent motor dysfunction with more limited somatosensory and visual impairment. Pyramidal signs are particularly common and include spasticity, gait abnormalities, hyperreflexia, and extensor plantar responses. Pseudobulbar palsy with dysarthria, dysphagia, facial paresis, exaggerated jaw and facial reflexes, hyperactive gag response, and sham emotional displays may also occur (Hughes et al., 1954; Ishii et al., 1986). Extrapyramidal symptoms are frequently intermixed with the upper motor neuron signs. Parkinsonism, unilateral or bilateral ballismus or chorea, and syndromes resembling progressive supranuclear palsy have been described (Critchley, 1929; Dubinsky and Jankovic, 1987; Sethi et al., 1987). Loss of bladder and bowel control may result from upper motor neuron disturbances or behavioral alterations associated with frontal lobe lesions.

Computerized tomography (CT) reveals evidence of lacunar infarction in approximately one half of the patients who present with clinical syndromes associated with lacunar infarctions (Figure 11-3) (Nelson et al., 1980). In other patients the cavities are too small to be visualized by CT. Magnetic resonance imaging (MRI) reveals a higher percentage of lesions than CT.

No treatment is available to restore intellectual function in the lacunar state, but control of hypertension, abstinence from smoking, and administration of antiplatelet-aggregating agents are warranted to ameliorate progression of the disorder.

Dementia Syndrome

Most studies of vascular dementia have included mixed groups of patients with cortical and subcortical infarctions, making it difficult to deduce the neuropsychological deficits ascribable to the lacunar lesions per se. Critchley (1929) was among the first to note the existence of dementia in association with "arteriosclerotic parkinsonism." Among the characteristics he observed in affected patients were: impaired memory and disorientation, poor response to novelty, limitation of the field of interest, emotional instability, decreased ability to make associations, difficulty passing from one idea to another, inattention, and perseveration. Little of substance has been added to this description. In one of the few investigations based on patients studied pathologically as well as clinically, Ishii and co-workers (1986) found loss of spontaneity in 100 percent of 30 patients with lacunar state, dysarthria in 80 percent, urinary incontinence in 73 percent, mood changes in 67 percent, small-stepped gait in 57 percent, acute confusional episodes in 47 percent, and grasp reflexes in 33 percent. Studies of language function in patients with vascular dementia primarily of the lacunar type have shown that the patients exhibit a "Brociod"-type output with shortened phrase length, diminished lexical variety, syntactic simplification, and dysarthria (Hier et al., 1985). Language changes are less severe than in patients with dementia of the Alzheimer type

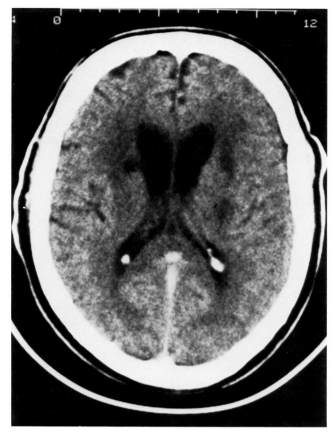

Figure 11-3 Computerized tomogram of a patient with lacunar state and several lacunar infarctions in the periventricular areas.

with equally severe intellectual impairment (Powell et al., 1988). Thus, the dementia of the lacunar state exhibits memory and frontal lobe–type deficits with relative sparing of language function, a pattern consistent with dysfunction of the frontal–subcortical axis.

Neuropathology

Lacunes are small trabeculated cavities that occur in the deeper parts of the cerebral hemispheres, cerebellum, and brain stem. They range in size from 3 mm to 2 cm in diameter. Lacunes contain a few macrophages, are surrounded by gliotic changes, and may include small amounts of hemosiderin. The lesions result from occlusion of arterioles at a site proximal to the infarction. The most common vascular change is fibrinoid necrosis associated with chronic hypertension. Embolic particles arising from the heart or a more proximal large vessel may also produce lacunar infarctions, and diabetes and other systemic disorders may contribute to the vascular pathology (Fisher, 1969, 1982). The common lacunar sites in order of decreasing frequency are: periventricular white matter anterior to the frontal horns of the lateral ventricles, nonfrontal hemispheric white matter, head of caudate nucleus, putamen, thalamus, pons, and cerebellum (Fisher, 1982; Ishii et al., 1986). The periventricular ischemic changes of Binswanger's disease frequently co-occur with lacunar state. Thalamic vascular dementia follows infarction of the thalamus.

BINSWANGER'S DISEASE

Binswanger's disease is distinguished from other vascular dementias by the predominance of ischemic injury to the periventricular areas and the white matter of the cerebral hemispheres. In most cases lacunar state and Binswanger-type changes of the white matter coexist (Roman, 1987).

Clinical Features

Unlike other vascular dementias, Binswanger's disease often has an insidious onset and progresses gradually. Thus it imitates the course of degenerative processes and may lack the stepwise progression of most multi-infarct dementias (Babikian and Ropper, 1987; Biemond, 1970; Olszewski, 1962). In some cases plateau periods or periods with symptomatic improvement and recovery of function occur (Caplan and Schoene, 1978). The usual patient with Binswanger's disease is 50–70 years old, and the typical survival after onset is 5 years. Men and women are equally likely to be affected. Hypertension is the most common predisposing medical circumstance (Babikian and Ropper, 1987).

The clinical deficits associated with Binswanger's disease vary from mild to severe, reflecting the severity and extent of axonal disruption by the white matter changes. In several cases asymmetric weakness, pyramidal signs, and pseudobulbar palsy are present. Incontinence, gait disorders, parkinsonism, and dysarthria are also common signs (Caplan and Schoene, 1978; Kinkel et al., 1985; Roman, 1987; Thompson and Marsden, 1987; Tomonaga et al., 1982).

The criteria for radiologic diagnosis of Binswanger's disease are currently being reconsidered. Periventricular lucencies on CT may be found in "normal" elderly individuals without neurological complaints. Examination of these cases, however, demonstrates that the affected patients have significantly lower levels of intellectual performance, as well as more motor signs than patients without these radiologic changes (Steingart et al., 1987). Thus, periventricular lucencies may be indicative of mild changes of the Binswanger type even in apparently asymptomatic individuals. In patients with clinical signs of Binswanger's disease, CT demonstrates cerebral cortical atrophy, dilated ventricles, and periventricular lucencies (Figure 11-4) (Rosenberg et al., 1979; Zeumer et al., 1980). MRI is considerably more sensitive to the white matter changes of Binswanger's disease and reveals extensive periventricular regions with high signal intensity in affected patients (Erkinjuntti et al., 1984).

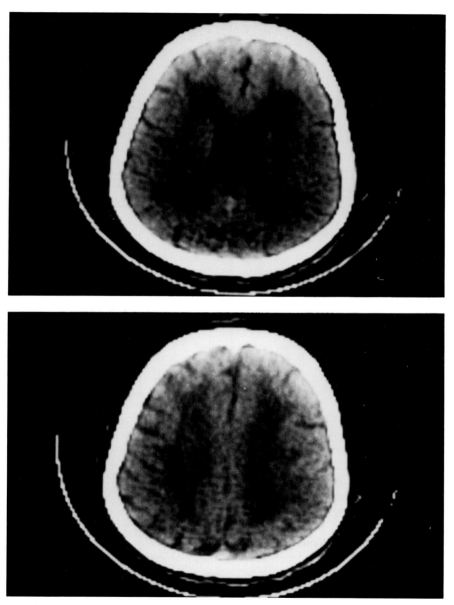

Figure 11-4   Two levels of computerized tomography from a patient with autopsy-proven Binswanger's disease, showing extensive periventricular demyelination.

Dementia Syndrome

A variety of types of mental status alterations have been observed in the course of Binswanger's disease. Mood alterations, including manic symptoms with hyperactivity, jocularity, and elated feelings, as well as depression with suicidal ideation, have been described (Babikian and Ropper, 1987). In addition, psychosis with paranoid delusions has occurred in a substantial number of patients (Tomonaga et al., 1982). Typical personality changes include apathy, irritability, and loss of interest.

The dementia of Binswanger's disease has not been fully characterized, but the usual features include characteristics of subcortical or frontal-subcortical axis dysfunction. Poor judgment, abulia (lack of spontaneity), long latencies when generating responses to queries, and perseveration are prominent, whereas memory deficits are relatively mild. These features may coexist with evidence of neglect or aphasia or other disturbances more characteristic of cerebral cortical dysfunction in patients with combined subcortical and cortical vascular lesions (Caplan and Schoene, 1978).

Neuropathology

At autopsy, the brain has widened sulci and narrowed gyri indicative of loss of cerebral substance. Coronal sections reveal ventricular enlargement, sometimes of marked degree. The white matter may be severely atrophic, or the changes may be subtle and not obvious to gross inspection. Myelin stains demonstrate loss of myelin in the periventricular regions in mild cases and extensive involvement of the hemispheric white matter in severe cases. The short arcuate fibers are spared. Loss of white matter is most severe in the frontal lobes.

Microscopically, the mildly affected regions have loss of myelin and of oligodendroglia as well as proliferation of astrocytes. In severely involved regions the lesions are ischemic infarctions with cavitation, loss of myelin and cellular elements, and reactive astrogliosis (Babikian and Ropper, 1987; Roman, 1987). Arterioles show fibrohyalin thickening with segmental occlusions. In most cases of Binswanger's disease, there are lacunes in the basal ganglia and thalamus as well as demyelination (Figure 11-5), and some patients have accompanying cortical infarctions (Loizou et al., 1981; Roman, 1987).

COMMENT

The predominant neuropsychological deficits in Binswanger's disease reflect dysfunction of the frontal–subcortical axis. The behavioral disturbances correlate with the ischemic demyelination that primarily involves the subcortical regions of the frontal lobes. Thus, Binswanger's disease joins the acquired immune deficiency syndrome (AIDS) encephalopathy and the dementia of multiple sclerosis (discussed elsewhere in this volume) as white matter syndromes in which the profile of neuropsychological dysfunction is more closely allied with the pattern of subcortical than of cortical dysfunction. The differential diagnosis of subcortical dementia should include diseases affecting the hemispheric white matter, as well as those affecting the deep gray matter structures.

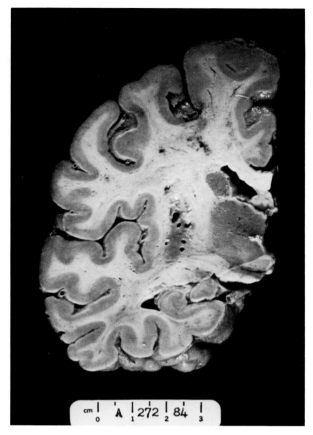

Figure 11-5 Coronal section of brain of a patient with Binswanger's disease, demonstrating marked white matter changes and coexisting lacunar infarctions.

ACKNOWLEDGMENTS

This project was supported by the Veterans Administration and the Ontario Mental Health Foundation. The manuscript was typed by M. Lecompte, Bonita Porch, and Kamela Peden.

REFERENCES

Aggleton, J.P., and Mishkin, M. Visual recognition impairment following medial thalamic lesions in monkeys. *Neuropsychologia* 1983; 21:189–97.

Albert, M.L. Subcortical dementia. In *Alzheimer's Disease: Senile Dementia and Related Disorders.* Katzman, R., Terry, R.D., and Bick, K.L. (eds.). Raven Press, New York, 1978, pp. 173–80.

Archer, C.R., Ilinsky, I.A., Goldfader, P.R., and Smith, Jr., K.R. Aphasia in thalamic stroke: CT stereotactic localization. *J Comput Assist Tomogr* 1981; 5:427–32.

Babikian, V., and Ropper, A.H. Binswanger's disease: A review. *Stroke* 1987; 18:2–12.

Barbizet, J., Degos, J.D., Louarn, F., Nguyen, J.P., and Mas, J.L. Amnesia from bilateral ischemic lesions of the thalamus. *Rev Neurol (Paris)* 1981; 137:415–24.

Barraguer-Bordas, L., Illa, I., Escartin, A., Ruscalleda, J., and Marti-Vilalta, J.L. Thalamic hemorrhage. A study of 23 patients with diagnosis by computed tomography. *Stroke* 1981; 12:524–7.

Biemond, A. On Binswanger's subcortical arteriosclerotic encephalopathy and the possibility of its clinical recognition. *Psychiatr Neurol Neurochir* 1970; 73:413–7.

Bogousslavsky, J., Miklossy, J., Deruaz, J.P., Regli, F., and Assal, G. Unilateral left paramedian infarction of thalamus and midbrain: A clinico-pathological study. *J Neuro Neurosurg Psychiatry* 1986; 49:686–94.

Brion, S., Mikol, J., and Plas, J. Memoire et specialisation fonctionelle hemispherique. Rapport anatomo-clinique. *Rev Neurol (Paris)* 1983; 139:39–43.

Caplan, L.R., and Schoene, W.C. Clinical features of subcortical arteriosclerotic encephalopathy (Binswanger disease). *Neurology* 1978; 28:1206–15.

Castaigne, P., Buge, A., Cambier, J., Escourolle, R., Brunet, P., and Degos, J.D. Demence thalamique d'origine vasculaire par ramollissement bilateral, limite au territoire du pedicule retro-mamillaire. A propos de deux observations anatomo-cliniques. *Rev Neurol (Paris)* 1966; 114:89–107.

Castaigne, P., Lhermitte, F., Buge, A., Escourolle, R., Hauw, J.J., and Lyon-Caen, O. Paramedian thalamic and midbrain infarcts: Clinical and neuropathological study. *Ann Neurol* 1981; 10:127–48.

Chassagnon, C., Boucher, M., Tommasi, M., Bianchi, G.-S., and Moene, Y. Demence thalamique d'origine vasculaire (observation anatomo-clinique). *J Med Lyon* 1969; 50:1153–66.

Choi, D., Sudarsky, L., Schachter, S., Biber, M., and Burke, P. Medial thalamic hemorrhage with amnesia. *Arch Neurol* 1983; 40:611–3.

Critchley, M. Arteriosclerotic parkinsonism. *Brain* 1929; 52:23–83.

Crosson, B. Role of the dominant thalamus in language: A review. *Psychol Bull* 1984; 96:491–517.

Crosson, B. Subcortical functions in language: A working model. *Brain Lang* 1985; 25:257–92.

Cummings, J.L. Multi-infarct dementia: Diagnosis and management. *Psychosomatics* 1987; 28:117–26.

Cummings, J.L., and Benson, D.F. *Dementia: A Clinical Approach.* Butterworths, Boston, 1983.

Cummings, J.L., and Benson, D.F. Subcortical dementia. Review of an emerging concept. *Arch Neurol* 1984; 41:874–9.

Damasio, A.R. The frontal lobes. In *Clinical Neuropsychology.* Heilman, K.M., and Valenstein, E. (eds.). Oxford University Press, New York, 1985, pp. 339–75.

Davous, P., Bianco, C., Duval-Lota, A.M., De Recondo, J., Vedrenne, C., and Rondot, P. Aphasie par infarctus thalamique paramedian gauche. Observation anatomo-clinique. *Rev Neurol (Paris)* 1984; 140:711–9.

Dejerine, J., and Roussy, G. Le syndrome thalamique. *Rev Neurol (Paris)* 1906; 14:521–32.

Dubinsky, R.M., and Jankovic, J. Progressive supranuclear palsy and a multi-infarct state. *Neurology* 1987; 37:570–6.

Erkinjuntti, T. Types of multi-infarct dementia. *Acta Neurol Scand* 1987; 75:391–9.

Erkinjuntti, T., Sipponen, J.T., Iivanainen, M., Ketonen, L., Sulkava, R., and Sepponen, R.E. Cerebral NMR and CT imaging in dementia. *J Comput Assist Tomogr* 1984; 8:614–8.

Fisher, C.M. The pathologic and clinical aspects of thalamic hemorrhage. *Trans Am Neurol Assoc* 1959; 84:56–9.

Fisher, C.M. The arterial lesions underlying lacunes. *Acta Neuropathol (Berl)* 1969; 12:1–15.

Fisher, C.M. Lacunar strokes and infarct: A review. *Neurology* 1982; 32:871–6.

Freedman, M., and Albert, M.L. Subcortical dementia. In *Handbook of Clinical Neurology. Second Edition. Vol. 46 Neurobehavioral Disorders.* Frederiks, J.A.M. (ed.). Elsevier, Amsterdam, 1985, pp. 311–6.

Friedman, J.H. Syndrome of diffuse encephalopathy due to nondominant thalamic infarction. *Neurology* 1985; 35:1524–6.

Fuster, J.M., and Alexander, G.E. Firing changes in cells of the nucleus medialis dorsalis associated with delayed response behavior. *Brain Res* 1973; 61:79–91.

Graff-Radford, N.R., and Damasio, A.R. Disturbances of speech and language associated with thalamic dysfunction. *Semin Neurol* 1985; 4:162–8.

Graff-Radford, N.R., Damasio, H., Yamada, T., Eslinger, P.J., and Damasio, A.R. Nonhemorrhagic thalamic infarction. Clinical, neuropsychological and electrophysiological findings in four anatomical groups defined by computerized tomography. *Brain* 1985; 108:485–516.

Graff-Radford, N.R., Eslinger, P.J., Damasio, A.R., and Yamada, T. Nonhemorrhagic infarction of the thalamus: Behavioral, anatomic, and physiologic correlates. *Neurology* 1984; 34:14–23.

Guberman, A., and Stuss, D. The syndrome of bilateral paramedian thalamic infarction. *Neurology* 1983; 33:540–6.

Henderson, V.W., Alexander, M.P., and Naeser, M.A. Right thalamic injury, impaired visuospatial perception, and alexia. *Neurology* 1982; 32:235–40.

Hier, D.B., Hagenlocker, K., and Shindler, A.G. Language disintegration in dementia: Effects of etiology and severity. *Brain Lang* 1985; 25:117–33.

Hughes, W., Dodgson, M.C.H., and MacLennon, D.C. Chronic cerebral hypertensive disease. Lancet 1954; 2:770–4.

Ignelzi, R.J., and Squire, L.R. Recovery from anterograde and retrograde amnesia following percutaneous drainage of a cystic craniopharyngioma. *J Neurol Neurosurg Psychiatry* 1976; 39:1231–6.

Imeri, L., Moneta, M.E., and Mancia, M. Changes in spontaneous activity of medialis dorsalis thalamic neurones during sleep and wakefulness. *Electroencephalogr Clin Neurophysiol* 1988; 69:82–4.

Ishii, N., Nishahara, Y., and Imamura, T. Why do frontal lobe symptoms predominate in vascular dementia with lacunes? *Neurology* 1986; 36:340–5.

Karabelas, G., Kalfakis, N., Kasvikis, I., and Vassilopoulos, D. Unusual features in a case of bilateral paramedian thalamic infarction. *J Neurol Neurosurg Psychiatry* 1985; 48:186.

Katz, D.I., Alexander, M.P., and Mandell, A.M. Dementia following strokes in the mesencephalon and diencephalon. *Arch Neurol* 1987; 44:1127–33.

Kawahara, N., Sato, K., Muraki, M., Tanaka, K., Kaneko, M., and Uemura, K. CT classification of small thalamic hemorrhages and their clinical implications. *Neurology* 1986; 36:165–72.

Kinkel, W.R., Jacobs, L., Polachini, H., Bates, V., and Heffner, Jr., R.R. Subcortical arteriosclerotic encephalopathy (Binswanger's disease). Computed tomographic, nuclear magnetic resonance, and clinical correlations. *Arch Neurol* 1985; 42:951–9.

Loizou, L.A., Kendall, B.E., and Marshall, J. Subcortical arteriosclerotic encephalopathy: A clinical and radiological investigation. *J Neurol Neurosurg Psychiatry* 1981; 44:294–304.

Lugaresi, E., Medori, R., Montagna, P., Baruzzi, A., Cortelli, P., Lugaresi, A., Tinuper, P., Zucconi, M., and Gambetti, P. Fatal familial insomnia and dysautonomia with selective degeneration of thalamic nuclei. *N Engl J Med* 1986; 315:997–1003.

Luria, A.R. *The Working Brain.* Basic Books, New York, 1973.

Luria, A.R. On quasi-aphasic speech disturbances in lesions of the deep structures of the brain. *Brain Lang* 1977; 4:432–59.

Luria, A.R. *Higher Cortical Functions in Man.* Basic Books, New York, 1980.

Markowitsch, H.J. Thalamic mediodorsal nucleus and memory. A critical evaluation of studies in animals and man. *Neurosci Biobehav Rev* 1982; 6:351–80.

Martin, J.J. Thalamic syndromes. In *Handbook of Clinical Neurology, Vol. 2.* Vinken, P.J., and Bruyn, G.W. (eds.). North Holland, Amsterdam, 1968, pp. 469–96.

Mateer, C.A., and Ojemann, G.A. Thalamic mechanisms in language and memory. In *Language Functions and Brain Organization.* Segalowitz, S.J. (ed.). Academic Press, New York, 1983, pp. 171–91.

McFarling, D., Rothi, L.J., and Heilman, K.M. Transcortical aphasia from ischaemic infarcts of the thalamus: A report of two cases. *J Neurol Neurosurg Psychiatry* 1982; 45:107–12.

Michel, D., Laurent, B., Foyatier, N., Blanc, A., and Portafaix, M. Infarctus thalamique paramedian gauche (etude de la memoire et du langage). *Rev Neurol (Paris)* 1982; 138:533–50.

Mills, R.P., and Swanson, P.D. Vertical oculomotor apraxia and memory loss. *Ann Neurol* 1978; 4:149–53.

Milner, B. Some effects of frontal lobectomy in man. In *The Frontal Granular Cortex and Behavior.* Warren, J.M., and Akert, K. (eds.). McGraw-Hill, New York, 1964, pp. 313–34.

Mishkin, M. A memory system in the monkey. In *The Neuropsychiatry of Cognitive Function.* Broadbent, D.E., and Weiskrantz, L. (eds.). The Royal Society, London, 1982, pp. 85–95.

Nauta, W.J.H. The problem of the frontal lobe: A reinterpretation. *J Psychiatr Res* 1971; 8:167–87.

Nelson, R.F., Pullicino, P., Kendall, B.E., and Marshall, J. Computed tomography in patients presenting with lacunar syndromes. *Stroke* 1980; 11:256–61.

Ojemann, G.A. Asymmetric function of the thalamus in man. *Ann NY Acad Sci* 1977; 299:380–96.

Olszweski, J. Subcortical arteriosclerotic encephalopathy. *World Neurol* 1962; 3:359–75.

Poirier, J., Barbizet, J., Gaston, A., and Meyrignac, C. Demence thalamique lacunes expansives du territoire thalamo-mesencephalique paramedian hydrocephalie par stenose de l'aqueduc de sylvius. *Rev Neurol (Paris)* 1983; 139:349–58.

Powell, A.L., Cummings, J.L., Hill, M.A., and Benson, D.F. Speech and language alterations in multi-infarct dementia. *Neurology* 1988; 38:717–9.

Roman, G.C. Senile dementia of the Binswanger type. *JAMA* 1987; 258:1782–8.

Rosenberg, G.A., Koenfeld, M., Stovring, J., and Bicknell, J.M. Subcortical arteriosclerotic encephalopathy (Binswanger): Computerized tomography. *Neurology* 1979; 29:1102–6.

Scheibel, A.B. Anatomical and physiological substrates of arousal: A view from the bridge. In *The Reticular Formation Revisited.* Hobson, J.A., and Brazier, M.A.B. (eds.). Raven Press, New York, 1980, pp. 55–66.

Schott, B., Mauguiere, F., Laurent, B., Serclerat, O., and Fisher, C. L'amnesie thalamique. *Rev Neurol (Paris)* 1980; 136:117–30.

Schuell, H., Jenkins, J.J., and Jiminez-Pabon, E. *Aphasia in Adults.* Harper and Row, New York, 1965.

Schulman, S. Impaired delayed response from thalamic lesions (studies in monkeys). *Arch Neurol* 1964; 11:477–99.

Sethi, K.D., Nichols, F.T., and Yaghmai, F. Generalized chorea due to basal ganglia lacunar infarcts. *Movement Disorders* 1987; 2:61–6.

Speedie, L.J., and Heilman, K.M. Amnestic disturbance following infarction of the left dor-somedial nucleus of the thalamus. *Neuropsychologia* 1982; 20:597–604.

Speedie, L.J., and Heilman, K.M. Anterograde memory deficits for visuospatial material after infarction of the right thalamus. *Arch Neurol* 1983; 40:183–6.

Squire, L.R. The anatomy of amnesia. *Trends Neurosci* 1980; 3:52–4.

Steingart, A., Hachinski, V.C., Lau, C., Fox, A.J., Diaz, F., Cape, R., Lee, D., Inzitari, D., and Merskey, H. Cognitive and neurologic findings in subjects with diffuse white matter lucencies on computed tomographic scan (leuko-araiosis). *Arch Neurol* 1987; 44:32–5.

Stuss, D.T., and Benson, D.F. Neuropsychological studies of the frontal lobes. *Psychol Bull* 1984; 95:3–28.

Stuss, D.T., and Benson, D.F. *The Frontal Lobes*. Raven Press, New York, 1986.

Stuss, D.T., Guberman, A., Nelson, R., and La Rochelle, S. The neuropsychology of para-median thalamic infarcts. *Brain Cogn* 1988; 8:348–78.

Swanson, R.A., and Schmidley, J.W. Amnestic syndrome and vertical gaze palsy: Early detec-tion of bilateral thalamic infarction by CT and NMR. *Stroke* 1985; 16:823–7.

Thompson, P.D., and Marsden, C.D. Gait disorder of subcortical arteriosclerotic encephalop-athy: Binswanger's disease. *Movement Disorders* 1987; 2:1–8.

Tomonaga, M., Yamanouchi, H., Tohgi, H., and Kameyama, M. Clinicopathologic study of progressive subcortical vascular encephalopathy (Binswanger type) in the elderly. *J Am Geriatr Soc* 1982; 30:524–9.

von Cramon, D., and Eilert, P. Ein Beitrag zum amnestischen Syndrom des Menschen. *Ner-venarzt* 1979; 50:643–8.

von Cramon, D.Y., and Hebel, N., and Schuri, U. A contribution to the anatomical basis of thalamic amnesia. *Brain* 1985; 108:993–1008.

Wallesch, C.W., Kornhuber, H.H., Kunz, T., and Brunner, R.J. Neuropsychological deficits associated with small unilateral thalamic lesions. *Brain* 1983; 106:141–52.

Walshe, T.M., Davis, K.R., and Fisher, C.M. Thalamic hemorrhage: A computed tomo-graphic–clinical correlation. *Neurology* 1977; 27:217–22.

Weisberg, L.A. Lacunar infarcts. Clinical and computed tomographic correlations. *Arch Neurol* 1982; 39:37–40.

Winocur, G., Oxbury, S., Roberts, R., Agnetti, V., and Davis, C. Amnesia in a patient with bilateral lesions to the thalamus. *Neuropsychologia* 1984; 22:123–43.

Zeumer, H., Schonsky, B., and Sturm, K.W. Predominant white matter involvement in sub-cortical arteriosclerotic encephalopathy (Binswanger disease). *J Comput Assist Tomogr* 1980; 4:14–9.

12

Multiple Sclerosis

STEPHEN M. RAO

[In] most of the patients affected by multilocular sclerosis, . . . there is marked enfeeblement of the memory; conceptions are formed slowly; the intellectual and emotional faculties
are blunted in their totality. The dominant feeling in the patients appears to be a sort of
almost stupid indifference in reference to all things (Charcot, 1877, p. 194).

As the writings of Charcot attest, dementia has been recognized as a prominent feature
of multiple sclerosis (MS) since the nineteenth century. For most of this century, however, neurological thinking has focused primarily on the wide array of sensory and
motor symptoms that produce physical disability. Dementia, on the other hand, has
been considered a rare and late manifestation of the disease (Adams and Victor, 1985;
McKhann, 1982; Walton, 1977). This viewpoint contrasts with the observation, derived from autopsy and more recent magnetic resonance studies, that the cerebrum is
commonly and widely affected in MS patients (Rao, 1986).

Neuropsychological investigations, most published within the past decade, have
provided scientific support for Charcot's perceptive clinical impressions. These studies
have consistently demonstrated that cognitive dysfunction is common, occurring in
greater than 50 percent of patients (Peyser and Poser, 1986; Rao, 1986). They also
indicate that dementia can occur in the early stages of the illness, sometimes representing the initial symptom (Lyon-Caen et al., 1986; Young et al., 1976). The present
chapter will provide a brief overview of the disease, review the relevant neurobehavioral literature, and attempt to relate the behavioral disturbance in MS to neuropathology. The thesis that MS produces a specific pattern of cognitive disruption similar to
that of other subcortical dementias will be examined.

DEMOGRAPHY OF MULTIPLE SCLEROSIS

Prevalence

Multiple sclerosis is the most common, nontraumatic, disabling neurologic illness affecting young and middle-aged adults (Johnson et al., 1979). Prevalence in the United
States is approximately 60 per 100,000 (Baum and Rothschild, 1981; Kurtzke, 1984).

Epidemiological studies indicate that the prevalence of MS varies according to latitude. For example, in a nationwide survey of the United States (Baum and Rothschild, 1981), the prevalence rate for individuals residing above the thirty-seventh parallel (69 per 100,000) was found to be nearly twice that for individuals residing below the thirty-seventh parallel (36 per 100,000). Studies of migration patterns suggest that a reduction in the risk of developing MS occurs if an individual moves from a high to low risk region prior to ages 12–15 (Kurtzke et al., 1985). These findings have spurred various environmental etiologic hypotheses, although no specific agent has been identified. The prevalence of MS is 1.5–1.9 times more common in females than males, and the rate among whites is nearly twice that among nonwhites (Baum and Rothschild, 1981).

Precise prevalence estimates are difficult to obtain in MS for several reasons. First, it is estimated that as many 5–15 percent of individuals with a presumably benign course of MS may be unaware of their diagnosis and therefore would not be included in the statistics cited above (Silberberg, 1977). Several cases of "silent," undiagnosed MS have been reported at autopsy (Gilbert and Sadler, 1983; MacKay and Hirano, 1967); it is noteworthy that, in most of these cases, the demyelinated lesions were located primarily within the cerebrum. Second, the false positive and negative rates for the diagnosis of MS are high compared with other neurologic illnesses (Poser, 1984). Finally, these statistics do not include patients with isolated symptoms, like optic neuritis, who may eventually develop MS, but who do not meet accepted diagnostic criteria (e.g., Poser et al., 1983), requiring symptoms that imply multiple lesion sites (Kinnunen, 1983).

Etiology

The exact cause of MS is unknown. As noted above from the migration studies, early exposure to an environmental agent, presumably a virus, may play an important role. A recent nationwide twin study conducted in Canada (Ebers et al., 1986) indicated that the concordance rate for 27 monozygotic pairs was 25.9 percent while the rate for 43 dizygotic pairs was 2.3 percent, thus supporting a genetic factor. There is also strong evidence that alterations in immune response are important in the pathogenesis of MS (Iivanainen, 1981). Thus the etiology of MS is likely multifactorial: The disease may be produced by an early environmental agent in a genetically susceptible individual with abnormal immunologic mechanisms (McDonald, 1986; McKhann, 1982).

Age of Onset

In the United States, approximately 8,800 new cases of MS (4.2 per 100,000) are diagnosed each year, with an average age at first diagnosis of 38 (Baum and Rothschild, 1981). The mean age of symptom onset, however, is from 29 to 33 (Matthews et al., 1985). The 5–9 year discrepancy between symptom onset and diagnosis illustrates the problems inherent in diagnosing MS in the early stages of the disease. Greater than 96 percent of patients are initially diagnosed between the ages of 20 and 59.

Course and Duration

The course of MS is highly variable. In the early stages of the disease, nearly 90 percent of patients, particularly those with onset prior to age 40, experience successive exacerbations and remissions of clinical symptoms (Reder and Antel, 1983). An attack may remit completely or in part, may remain stationary for a prolonged period, or may progress. Approximately 10–20 percent of patients (higher for patients with onset after 40) experience a steady progression of symptoms without episodes of significant improvement (Matthews et al., 1985). The time between attacks varies considerably among patients: While 5 percent of patients may experience exacerbations spaced as many as 20 years apart, nearly one half will sustain a relapse within the first 3 years after onset (Silberberg, 1977). Among the patients with an initial relapsing–remitting course, approximately 25 percent will eventually experience steady symptomatic progression (Confavreux et al., 1980). In general, the shorter the interval between the first two relapses, the poorer the outcome in terms of overall physical disability (Confavreux et al., 1980). The effect of MS on life expectancy varies considerably depending on illness severity. Kurtzke et al. (1970) found that MS patients' survival rate was 73 percent that of healthy individuals 25 years after onset of the disease.

Very little information is available regarding the natural history of dementia in MS (Rao, 1986). Cross-sectional neuropsychological studies have generally not found a relationship between cognitive test performance and length of illness (Ivnik, 1978b; Marsh, 1980; Rao, Hammeke, McQuillen et al., 1984). Results of longitudinal studies (Canter, 1951; Fink and Houser, 1966; Ivnik, 1978a) have produced equivocal results but have been criticized for methodological problems (i.e., small sample size, inadequate controls, and brief retest intervals; Rao, 1986). Clearly, large-scale, prospective neuropsychological investigations are needed.

CLINICAL CHARACTERISTICS

The clinical presentation in MS is highly variable due to the wide distribution and varying extent of demyelinating lesions in the white matter of the cerebrum, brain stem, cerebellum, and spinal cord. Frequent symptoms include: motor weakness and ataxia, spasticity, optic neuritis, diplopia, numbness and paresthesia, pain, bowel and bladder dysfunction, fatigue (which is worsened with warmer weather and after exercise), sexual disturbances, and dysarthria. Much less common are seizures, hemianopia, aphasia, and dysphagia. A more thorough account of the signs and symptoms of MS may be found in Matthews et al. (1985).

DEMENTIA SYNDROME

As is true for other symptoms of MS, cognitive dysfunction is highly variable in MS patients. Controlled neuropsychological studies have identified some degree of cognitive dysfunction in 30–70 percent of patients (Peyser and Poser, 1986; Rao, 1986), with the higher rate of disturbance observed in studies that examined a high proportion of patients with a chronic progressive course (Heaton et al., 1985).

Intelligence

Studies assessing intellectual functions suggest a low frequency of severe dementia. Rao (1986) reviewed eight studies that administered the Wechsler scales to MS patients. Mean Verbal IQ scores were in the average or above average range. These scores were consistently 7–10 points higher than the mean Performance IQs, which may have been adversely affected by primary sensorimotor deficits.

Memory

Memory deficits are commonly observed in MS patients and have been extensively studied. Controlled investigations indicate that the predominant feature of memory loss is the inability to retrieve information spontaneously (both verbal and nonverbal) from long-term storage (Beatty and Gange, 1977; Beatty et al., 1988; Fischer, 1988; Heaton et al., 1985; Jambor, 1969; Rao, Hammeke, McQuillen et al., 1984; Rao, Leo, and St. Aubin-Faubert, in press; Vowels, 1979). Recognition memory is normal or less impaired than retrieval (Caine et al., 1986; Carroll et al., 1984; Rao, Hammeke, McQuillen et al., 1984), suggesting relatively intact encoding and storage mechanisms. In addition, short-term memory appears to be normal when assessed with digit span (Litvan et al., 1988a; Heaton et al., 1985; Jambor, 1969; Rao, Hammeke, McQuillen et al., 1984; Vowels, 1979) and on immediate free recall (i.e., normal recency effect) (Rao, Leo, and St. Aubin-Faubert, in press). However, other methods of assessing short-term memory have yielded mixed findings. For example, on the Brown–Peterson task, which assesses forgetting from short-term storage, some studies indicate that MS patients perform normally (Litvan et al., 1988a; Rao, Leo, and St. Aubin-Faubert, in press), while others have found impairment (Beatty et al., 1988; Grant et al., 1984). Remote memory was evaluated in a recent study by Beatty et al. (1988); chronic progressive MS patients were found to be impaired on the Famous Faces test relative to normal controls.

Abstract–Conceptual Reasoning

MS patients perform poorly on measures of abstract–conceptual reasoning, such as the Category test (Heaton et al., 1985; Peyser et al., 1980; Reitan et al., 1971), Wisconsin Card Sorting Test (Heaton et al., 1985; Rao et al., 1987), Grassi Block Substitution Test (Parsons et al., 1957), Levine Concept Formation task (Rao and Hammeke, 1984), and Weigl Sorting Test (Jambor, 1969). On sorting tasks investigators have frequently noted that MS patients make an inordinate number of perseverative responses.

Rate of Mental Processing

Two recent investigations have examined the rate of information processing in MS patients. Litvan et al. (1988b) administered the Paced Auditory Serial Addition Test to MS patients and normal controls. The former group were less accurate on this task, particularly at the faster of two stimulus presentation rates. We (Rao, St. Aubin-Faubert, and Leo, 1989) recently completed a study comparing MS patients with normal

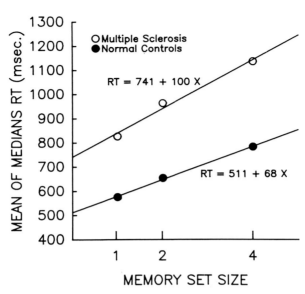

Figure 12-1 Mean of median reaction times for MS and normal control groups as a function of memory set size. (Reproduced with permission from Rao, St. Aubin-Faubert, and Leo, 1989.)

controls on the Sternberg Memory Scanning Paradigm. In this task subjects were asked to memorize one, two, or four single digits. On each trial a probe digit was presented on a screen, and the subject was asked to decide whether the number matched a digit held in memory by pressing one of two response keys. Sternberg (1969) noted a linear relationship between reaction time and the number of digits held in memory. This linear function is characterized by a *y* intercept, which reflects overall reaction time and may be adversely influenced by primary motor dysfunction, and slope, which is a pure measure of mental speed independent of motor impairment. Figure 12-1 indicates that the slope of the MS patients was 1.5 times steeper than that of the control group (100 vs. 68; $p < .03$), suggesting that MS patients exhibit a slowing of mental processing speed.

Language

Linguistic functions have not been extensively studied in MS patients. Clinical case reports (Olmos-Lau et al., 1977) suggest that aphasia with paraphasic disturbance occurs very infrequently in MS and typically results from demyelinating lesions that extend into the gray matter of the dominant hemisphere. Indeed, the low frequency of linguistic distortion in conversational speech may account for the low rate of detection of dementia in MS on bedside mental status evaluations (Peyser et al., 1980).

Controlled studies (Drayer, 1988; Caine et al., 1986; Jambor, 1969; Rao, Leo, and St. Aubin-Faubert, in press; van den Burg et al., 1987) suggest that MS patients are frequently impaired on object naming tasks, such as the Boston Naming Test, and on fluency tasks, such as the Controlled Oral Word Association Test. Tests of repetition speech and oral comprehension are generally performed without difficulty. It is not clear whether the deficits in naming and fluency result from a breakdown of linguistic processes or from defective retrieval of lexical information. Successful performance on the Boston Naming Test requires the patient to recall words of both high and low frequency of usage, whereas tests of object naming on standard aphasia batteries (Goodglass and Kaplan, 1983) only assess responses to high-frequency words. Patients with aphasia are likely to fail items regardless of usage frequency (Goodglass and Kaplan, 1983), while patients with retrieval deficits are more likely to have problems with low-frequency words. While additional work is needed in this area, it is our clinical impression that the "linguistic" deficit in MS results from impaired memory.

Two studies (Jacobson et al., 1983; Rubens et al., 1985) evaluated the effects of demyelination on cross-callosal transfer of verbal information using the dichotic listening paradigm. Both used consonant–vowel syllables and found an exaggeration of the right ear effect in MS patients. These studies suggest that linguistic information initially processed in the right hemisphere does not effectively cross the corpus callosum for subsequent analysis by the language-dominant left hemisphere. It is noteworthy that atrophy of the corpus callosum is commonly reported in autopsy studies of MS patients (Barnard and Triggs, 1974).

Visuospatial Skills

Beatty et al. (1988) administered a simplified version of Money's Road Map Test, a measure of egocentric spatial orientation, to MS patients and normal controls. Mild, but statistically significant, group differences were observed, suggesting deficits in visuospatial reasoning. Caine et al. (1986) found that MS patients were impaired in copying figures but performed normally on measures of clock drawing and written arithmetic computations. Collectively, these studies suggest that visuospatial processes are impaired, albeit mildly, in MS patients.

Affect

Much has been written regarding affect and mood disturbances in patients with MS (for reviews of this literature, see Ron, 1986; Devins and Seland, 1987). Depression and, less commonly, euphoria are the primary psychiatric symptoms observed in MS patients. The high rate of behavioral disturbances in MS relative to other equally disabling conditions strongly suggests a biological basis for the personality changes. A few studies have correlated mood changes with structural abnormalities on brain imaging (Honer et al., 1987; Rabins et al., 1986).

PATHOPHYSIOLOGY

Neuropathology

As noted earlier, autopsy studies have consistently demonstrated that the cerebrum is widely and commonly affected in MS patients (Adams, 1977; Brownell and Hughes, 1962; Powell and Lampert, 1983). Characteristic lesions involve the periventricular white matter, although lesions may also be observed in the gray–white matter junction and occasionally extend into gray matter (Brownell and Hughes, 1962). Ventricular dilatation is also frequently noted in the brains of MS patients. While the exact mechanism causing ventricular enlargement is unknown, it is assumed to occur as a consequence of diffuse periventricular demyelination (Brownell and Hughes, 1962).

The MS plaques are not confined to specific fiber tracts. Furthermore, demyelinated fibers are capable of neuronal transmission, albeit abnormal, since axons and cell bodies remain intact, particularly in the acute and subacute stages of lesion development. These factors distinguish MS from cerebrovascular and neurodegenerative conditions in which neural death occurs in affected fiber tracts. These differences in pathologic mechanisms complicate attempts to relate pathology to specific behavioral disturbances in MS.

Radiology

Recent advances in brain imaging technology make it possible to visualize MS-related pathology during life. Such information may potentially demonstrate important clinico-pathologic relationships, particularly with regard to the study of dementia in MS. Studies attempting to relate behavior and imaging data are reviewed later by imaging modality.

Computed Tomography

The standard enhanced computed tomography (CT) scan has been shown to be relatively insensitive to detecting the pathologic lesions in the cerebrum of MS patients (Haughton et al., 1979). Despite this limitation in detecting MS lesions, CT provides a potentially useful index of ventricular size and cerebral atrophy. Age-inappropriate cerebral atrophy is observed in 40 percent of the CT scans of MS patients (Rao et al., 1985). Cerebral atrophy, therefore, can serve as an indirect marker of cerebral disease activity in MS.

Three studies have correlated cerebral atrophy with cognitive testing. Brooks et al. (1984) administered the Wechsler Adult Intelligence Scale (WAIS), standardized reading tests, and CT scans to 12 MS patients. Cognitive dysfunction was defined as a significant discrepancy between IQ and reading test scores. The former measure served as an indicator of acquired cognitive deterioration, while the latter was used as a predictor of premorbid ability level. Eight patients were rated as having cerebral atrophy on CT scan. Seven of these eight patients exhibited cognitive dysfunction, while none of the four patients without atrophy showed signs of cognitive decline.

Rabins et al. (1986) examined 37 MS patients with CT and the Mini-Mental State Examination (MMSE) cognitive screening examination. In addition, patients were also rated for "euphoric mood state." A ventricular–brain ratio (VBR) was computed by dividing a linear measure of the lateral ventricles at their greatest width by the intracranial width at the same level. Rabins and colleagues found that patients with large ventricles were more likely to be impaired cognitively and to be rated as "euphoric." A significant negative correlation was observed between VBR and MMSE scores ($r = -.33$).

We (Rao et al., 1985) obtained observer ratings and linear measurements of ventricular size from CT scans as well as neuropsychological test information on 47 chronic progressive MS patients. The cognitive measures included: the verbal subtests of the revised WAIS (WAIS-R), the Wechsler Memory Scale, and two experimental measures of verbal and visuospatial learning and memory. CT scans were classified as having either no, mild, or moderate to severe cerebral atrophy. Nineteen patients (40 percent) were judged to have no ventricular enlargement, 19 (40 percent) had mildly enlarged ventricles, and 9 (20 percent) had moderate to severe ventricular dilatation. Statistically significant ($p < .05$) group differences were observed on the WAIS-R Comprehension subtest and on 10 of 13 measures of learning and memory. Figure 12-2 illustrates the learning curves for the three atrophy groups.

We have also measured ventricular size using the linear measurement procedures described by Huckman et al. (1975). These measurements included: (1) the length of the distance between the most lateral portion of each of the frontal horns of the lateral ventricles ("bifrontal" span), (2) the width of the lateral ventricles in the region of the caudate nuclei, that being the width of the two lateral ventricles just anterior to the third ventricle ("bicaudate"), and (3) the maximum width of the third ventricle

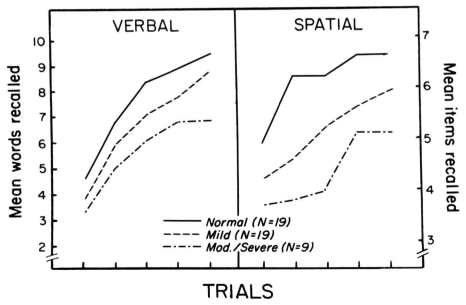

Figure 12-2 Learning curves for free verbal recall test ("verbal") and 7/24 spatial recall test ("spatial") for three subgroups of MS patients having normal ventricular size, mild dilatation, and moderate to severe ventricular enlargement. (Reproduced with permission from Rao et al., 1985.)

("third"). The third ventricle measure correlated significantly, though modestly, with 16 of 19 cognitive measures ($r = -.25$ to $-.41$); the "bifrontal" and "bicaudate" indices, by comparison, were relatively poor predictors of memory–cognitive dysfunction.

The primary conclusion to be drawn from the CT studies is that size of the ventricular spaces is a significant, but weak, indicator of cognitive decline in MS. As noted previously, cerebral atrophy is at best an indirect and late index of cerebral demyelination. The inability of CT to provide meaningful information regarding the severity of cerebral lesions may explain the small correlations that have been obtained.

Magnetic Resonance Imaging

The recent introduction of magnetic resonance imaging (MRI) has dramatically emphasized the significant involvement of the cerebrum in MS patients. The shape, location, and distribution of lesions seen with MRI closely resemble those observed at autopsy (Willoughby and Paty, 1989).

Four recent studies (Franklin et al., 1988; Huber et al., 1987; Medaer et al., 1987; Rao, Leo, Haughton, et al., 1989) have attempted to correlate MRI findings with neuropsychological testing in patients with MS. Franklin et al. (1988) studied 60 chronic progressive MS patients with spin-echo MRI. A neuroradiologist recorded the number, size (using a three-point scale), and location (left vs. right hemisphere) of lesions. They computed weighted lesion scores based on the number and size of lesions; these scores were summed to obtain an overall brain lesion score. This score correlated significantly ($r = .35$) with a summary score derived from a brief (30–45 min) cognitive screening battery.

Huber et al. (1987) examined 30 definite MS patients with a 1.5 T MRI scanner. Four indices were derived from the MRI images: (1) a total lesion score, reflecting the sum of five-point ratings applied on the basis of the size of each lesion, (2) a five-point rating of cerebral atrophy, (3) a five-point rating of corpus callosum atrophy based on midsagittal images, and (4) a five-point rating of periventricular plaque severity. A brief (30 min) battery of neuropsychological tests, including the Mini-Mental State Examination and measures of language, memory, apraxia, visuospatial ability, and depression (Zung Self-Rated Depression Scale), was administered. On the basis of this testing protocol, 9 patients (28 percent) were classified as "demented," 11 (34 percent) were moderately impaired, and 12 (38 percent) were minimally impaired. No significant group differences were observed on three of the four MRI indices: total lesion score, cerebral atrophy, and severity of periventricular involvement. On the corpus callosum atrophy ratings "demented" patients had significantly higher ratings of atrophy than the moderate and minimal cognitive impairment groups. Huber and co-workers concluded that atrophy of the corpus callosum is a meaningful indicator of dementia in MS.

Medaer et al. (1987) administered neuropsychological testing (WAIS, Raven Progressive Matrices, Rey Auditory Verbal Learning Test, and an attentional task) to 33 definite MS patients. Patients were classified into three groups of 11 each on the basis of test performance: normal cognitive functions, "partial" impairment, and "serious" impairment. MRI images were rated on a single five-point scale based on the size and number of lesions and the degree of cerebral atrophy. Mean MRI ratings were significantly higher in the "partial" and "serious" groups relative to the cognitively intact group; no differences were observed between the two cognitively impaired groups on MRI ratings, however.

We (Rao, Leo, Haughton et al., 1989) recently completed a study of 53 definite or probable MS patients. All patients underwent MR imaging on a 1.5 T MRI scanner. Unlike the previous studies that used rating scales, we traced MS lesions and cerebral structures (corpus callosum, third and lateral ventricles, total brain area) on the MRI computer console; the area (in cm^2) subtended by each tracing was then computed. Total lesion area (TLA) was computed by adding the measurements of all lesions. Ventricular–brain ratio was computed by dividing the sum of the ventricular measurements by the sum of the brain area measurements. Size of the corpus callosum (SCC) was recorded for 45 of 53 patients. All patients were administered a 7 hour battery of neuropsychological tests over the course of 2 days. The battery consisted of measures of verbal intelligence, memory, abstract–conceptual reasoning, attention–concentration, language, and visuospatial skills.

The data were analyzed to examine differences between patients with and without cognitive dysfunction on MRI, demographic, and illness variables. Cluster analysis was performed on neuropsychological test data to classify patients into "impaired" ($N = 19$) and "intact" ($N = 34$) groups. The impaired group had significantly greater TLA ($p < .001$) and VBR ($p < .01$), and a smaller SCC ($p < .01$) than the intact group. MRI values for individual subjects in each group are presented in Figure 12-3. Of the three MRI variables TLA had the least amount of group overlap. 10 of 12 (83 percent) patients with a TLA greater than 30 cm^2 were cognitively impaired, while 32 of 41 (78 percent) patients with TLA less than 30 cm^3 were cognitively intact.

No significant differences were observed between the two groups on demographic variables (i.e., age, gender, education, and premorbid occupational status). Patients in the cognitively impaired group, however, were less likely to be employed than patients in the cognitively intact group (16 vs. 44 percent, respectively; $\chi^2 = 4.36$, d.f. $= 1$,

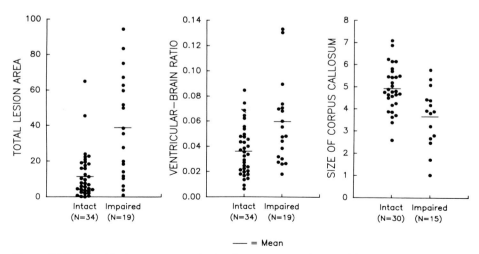

Figure 12-3 Total lesion area, ventricular–brain ratio, and size of the corpus callosum for cognitively intact and impaired MS patients. (Reproduced with permission from Rao, Leo, Haughton, et al., 1989.)

$p < .04$). This finding is particularly noteworthy, since the two groups did not differ in duration of symptoms, disease course, or overall physical disability (Kurtzke Expanded Disability Scale).

To conclude, MRI is a more precise indicator of cognitive dysfunction in MS than CT. While virtually all definite MS patients have abnormal MRI, the overall amount of brain involvement varies considerably between patients. The correlational studies suggest that the overall lesion load is directly proportional to the amount of cognitive dysfunction. Future studies are needed to determine if focal areas of brain involvement are associated with specific patterns of cognitive disruption. A recent MRI study by Honer et al. (1987) suggests that major psychiatric disorders may be associated with focal temporal lobe involvement in MS.

Positron Emission Tomography

Three studies (Brooks et al., 1984; Herscovitch et al., 1984; Sheremata et al., 1984) have examined the possible relationship between degree of cognitive dysfunction and altered cerebral physiology as imaged by positron emission tomography (PET). Brooks et al. (1984) measured regional cerebral oxygen utilization, oxygen extraction, blood flow, and blood volume in 15 MS patients in remission. Patients were administered intelligence and reading tests; 13 patients also underwent CT scanning. Compared with a normal control group ($N = 13$), cerebral oxygen utilization and blood flow were found to be reduced in both the white and cortical gray matter of the MS patients. This effect was most dramatic in those patients with ventricular dilatation as shown on CT scan and in patients with a significant drop in intelligence relative to a prediction of premorbid cognitive ability (i.e., based on reading test scores). They concluded that reduced blood flow in MS is diffuse and caused by a loss of cerebral brain tissue rather than cerebral ischemia.

Sheremata et al. (1984) tested the hypothesis that MS patients were more likely to experience hypometabolism in the frontal lobes on PET imaging. They based their hypothesis on previous neuropsychological studies that have demonstrated a high rate of failure of MS patients on "frontal lobe" cognitive tests (i.e., Wisconsin Card Sorting Test, Verbal Fluency, Category Test). Scanning was performed on three MS patients and three normal controls while they performed a word learning task. Mean metabolic rates were lower in the frontal lobes of the MS patients than controls, but the group difference was even larger for the temporal lobes. Metabolic rates for the parietal and occipital lobes were not presented. Sheremata et al. concluded that, while their original hypothesis was not supported, the overall findings indicated generalized cortical hypometabolism in MS, possibly due to deafferentation.

Herscovitch et al. (1984) used PET to study myelin distribution and regional cerebral blood flow in a 24-year-old clinically definite MS patient, who developed a left hemiparesis and hemisensory deficit during an acute exacerbation. CT demonstrated a hypodense lesion of the right central white matter, which was supported by a diminished radiotracer accumulation in the same region on the myelin image. Regional cerebral blood flow was noted to be decreased in the right frontoparietal cortex superficial to the white matter lesion. A subsequent PET scan noted improvement in cortical blood flow corresponding with resolution of the patient's left-sided deficits. They hypothesized that the reductions in regional cortical blood flow were associated with conduction block in white matter pathways. It should be noted that the patient described by Herscovitch et al. may not be representative of other cognitively impaired MS patients in that focal cortical symptoms (i.e., aphasia, apraxia, lateralized sensorimotor deficits due to cerebral lesions) are relatively rare in MS (Rao, 1986) and likely occur only in association with large, acute lesions extending into gray matter structures.

Electrophysiology

Electroencephalographic recordings show diffuse slowing in approximately two thirds of MS patients (Fuglsang-Frederiksen and Thygesen, 1951; Jasper et al., 1950). Epileptogenic activity, on the other hand, is rare. Clinical case reports note considerable EEG slowing in MS patients with dementia (Bergin, 1957; Koenig, 1968), although systematic studies correlating EEG slowing with cognitive dysfunction have not been reported. In a recent study of 11 MS patients, Honig et al. (1986) found a significant correlation ($r = .81$) between severity of cognitive impairment and P300 latency derived from topographically mapped event-related potentials (Honig et al., 1986).

SUBCORTICAL CONTRIBUTION

It has been previously suggested (Rao, 1986) that the pattern of dementia in MS resembles that seen in subcortical dementia syndromes such as Parkinson's disease, Huntington's disease, and progressive supranuclear palsy (Albert, 1978; Albert et al., 1974; Cummings and Benson, 1984). In addition to neuropathology that is confined primarily to subcortical structures or pathways, patients with subcortical dementia are thought to exhibit a distinct neurobehavioral profile, characterized by memory loss (due to faulty retrieval and forgetfulness), impaired conceptualization and abstraction skills, a slowed rate of information processing, and affective disturbance (depression, euphoria, apathy). In contrast, intellectual and language functions are relatively preserved.

How does the pattern of cognitive dysfunction in MS compare with other dementing conditions? The pattern of neuropsychological deficits found in MS patients (described earlier) recapitulates the profile of dysfunction observed in subcortical dementia. The only study (Caine et al., 1986) that has directly addressed this issue compared the cognitive test performance of MS patients with that of patients in the early stages of Huntington's disease (HD). The two conditions showed substantial similarities in their patterns of impairment. The overall severity of memory impairment, however, was greater in the HD group; the investigators attributed this difference to the specific loss of striatal neurons in HD. Caine et al. also speculated that cognitive impairment in MS results from deficiencies of "modulation" and "tone." According to this view the MS patient uses normal strategies to solve problems but is generally inefficient as a result of mental slowing and a reduced ability to access stored memories.

Taking a more indirect approach, we (Rao, Leo, Bernardin, and Ellington, unpublished) compared the neuropsychological test profiles of 72 representative MS patients with 71 age- and education-matched healthy controls to determine if MS conforms to the clinical "prototype" of a subcortical dementia. Figure 12-4 presents the percentage of MS patients performing below the fifth percentile of the control group on measures

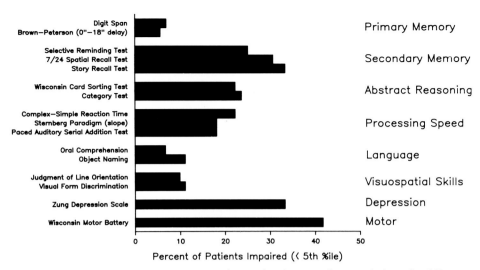

Figure 12-4   Percent of MS patients (total sample of 72) performing below the fifth percentile on neuropsychological testing (left). Cognitive functions assessed by these tests are
also listed (right).

of primary (immediate, short-term) memory, secondary (recent, long-term) memory,
abstract–conceptual reasoning, information processing speed, language, visuospatial
skills, upper-extremity motor speed and coordination, and self-reported depression.

The data in Figure 12-4 suggest that less than 10 percent of MS patients are impaired on measures of primary memory, language, and visuospatial processing. In
contrast, between 20 and 40 percent of MS patients experience deficits on measures
of secondary memory, conceptual reasoning, speed of processing, and primary motor
skills. In addition, patients with MS experience a high rate of self-reported depression.
Thus, on clinical grounds, these data suggest that the pattern of neurobehavioral disturbance in MS resembles the prototype of a subcortical dementia (Cummings and
Benson, 1984).

No study has directly compared MS patients with "cortically" demented patients
(i.e., Alzheimer's disease) on neuropsychological testing. While differences in overall
dementia severity exist between the two conditions, and differences in the age of the
two groups complicate interpretation of cognitive data, such an investigation is needed
to contrast the qualitative patterns in cognitive breakdown.

ACKNOWLEDGMENTS

The research cited in this chapter was supported in part by a Research Career Development
Award (K04 NS01055) and a Research Grant (R01 NS22128) from the National Institute of
Neurological and Communicative Disorders and Stroke. The assistance of Gary J. Leo, Victor
M. Haughton, Sander L. Glatt, Patricia St. Aubin-Faubert, Linda Bernardin, Lee Ellington, and
Thomas A. Hammeke is gratefully acknowledged.

REFERENCES

Adams, C.W.M. Pathology of multiple sclerosis: Progression of the lesion. *Med Bull* 1977; 33:15–9.

Adams, R.O., and Victor, M. *Principles of Neurology, Third edition* McGraw-Hill, New York, 1985.

Albert, M.L. Subcortical dementia. In *Alzheimer's Disease: Senile Dementia and Related Disorders*. Raven Press, New York, 1978, pp. 173–9.

Albert, M.L., Feldman, R.G., and Willis, A.L. The "subcortical dementia" of progressive supranuclear palsy. *J Neurol Neurosurg Psychiatry* 1974; 37:121–30.

Barnard, R.O., and Triggs, M. Corpus callosum in multiple sclerosis. *J Neurol Neurosurg Psychiatry* 1974; 37:1259–64.

Baum, H.M., and Rothschild, B.B. The incidence and prevalence of reported multiple sclerosis. *Ann Neurol* 1981; 10:420–8.

Beatty, P.A., and Gange, J.J. Neuropsychological aspects of multiple sclerosis. *J Nerv Ment Dis* 1977; 164:42–50.

Beatty, W.W., Goodkin, D.E., Monson, N., Beatty, P.A., and Hertsgaard, D. Anterograde and retrograde amnesia in patients with chronic progressive multiple sclerosis. *Arch Neurol* 1988; 45:611–9.

Bergin, J.D. Rapidly progressing dementia in disseminated sclerosis. *J Neurol Neurosurg Psychiatry* 1957; 20:285–92.

Brooks, D.J., Leenders, K.L., Head, G., Marshall, J., Legg, N.J., and Jones, T. Studies on regional cerebral oxygen utilisation and cognitive function in multiple sclerosis. *J Neurol Neurosurg Psychiatry* 1984; 47:1182–91.

Brownell, B., and Hughes, J.F. The distribution of plaques in the cerebrum in multiple sclerosis. *J Neurol Neurosurg Psychiatry* 1962; 25:315–20.

Caine, E.D., Bamford, K.A., Schiffer, R.B., Shoulson, I., and Levy, S. A controlled neuropsychological comparison of Huntington's disease and multiple sclerosis. *Arch Neurol* 1986; 43:249–54.

Canter, A.H. Direct and indirect measures of psychological deficit in multiple sclerosis. *J Gen Psychol* 1951; 44:3–50.

Carroll, M., Gates, R., and Roldan, F. Memory impairment in multiple sclerosis. *Neuropsychologia* 1984; 22:297–302.

Charcot, J.M. *Lectures on the Diseases of the Nervous System*. New Sydenham Society, London, 1877.

Confavreux, C., Aimard, G., and Devic, M. Course and prognosis of multiple sclerosis assessed by the computerized data processing of 349 patients. *Brain* 1980; 103:281–300.

Cummings, J.L., and Benson, D.F. Subcortical dementia: Review of an emerging concept. *Arch Neurol* 1984; 41:874–9.

Devins, G.M., and Seland, T.P. Emotional impact of multiple sclerosis: Recent findings and suggestions for future research. Psychol Bull 1987; 101:363–75.

Drayer, B.P. Imaging of the aging brain. Part II. Pathologic conditions. *Radiology* 1988; 166:797–806.

Ebers, G.C., Bulman, D.E., Sadovnick, A.D., et al. A population-based study of multiple sclerosis in twins. *N Engl J Med* 1986; 315:1638–42.

Fink, S.L., and Houser, H.B. An investigation of physical and intellectual impairment changes in multiple sclerosis. *Arch Phys Med Rehabil* 1966; 47:56–61.

Fischer, J.S. Using the Wechsler Memory Scale–Revised to detect and characterize memory deficits in multiple sclerosis. *Clin Neuropsychol* 1988; 2:149–72.

Franklin, G.M., Heaton, R.K., Nelson, L.M., Filley, C.M., and Seibert, C. Correlation of neuropsychological and MRI findings in chronic/progressive multiple sclerosis. *Neurology* 1988; 38:1826–29.

Fuglsang-Frederiksen, V., and Thygesen, P. The electroencephalogram in multiple sclerosis. *Arch Neurol Psychiatry* 1951; 66:505–17.

Gilbert, J.J., and Sadler, M. Unsuspected multiple sclerosis. *Arch Neurol* 1983; 40:533–6.

Goodglass, H., and Kaplan, E. *The Assessment of Aphasia and Related Disorders, Second edition.* Lea and Febiger, Philadelphia, 1983.

Grant, I., McDonald, W.I., Trimble, M.R., Smith, E., and Reed, R. Deficient learning and memory in early and middle phases of multiple sclerosis. *J Neurol Neurosurg Psychiatry* 1984; 47:250–5.

Haughton, V.M., Ho, K.-C., Williams, A.L., and Eldevik, P. CT detection of demyelinated plaques in multiple sclerosis. *Am J Roentgen* 1979; 132:213–5.

Heaton, R.K., Nelson, L.M., Thompson, D.S., Burks, J.S., and Franklin, G.M. Neuropsychological findings in relapsing-remitting and chronic-progressive multiple sclerosis. *J Consult Clin Psychol* 1985; 53:103–10.

Herscovitch, P., Trotter, J.L., Lemann, W., and Raichle, M.E. Positron emission tomography (PET) in active MS: Demonstration of demyelination and diaschisis. *Neurology* 1984; 34 (Suppl. 1):78.

Honer, W.G., Hurwitz, T., Li, D.K.B., Palmer, M., and Paty, D.W. Temporal lobe involvement in multiple sclerosis patients with psychiatric disorders. *Arch Neurol* 1987; 44:187–90.

Honig, L.S., Ramsay, R.E., Sheremata, W.A., Resillez, M., Wong, P., and Sazant, A. Magnetic resonance imaging (MRI), cognitive impairment, and the P300 event-related potential (ERP) in patients with multiple sclerosis (MS). *Neurology* 1986; 36 (Suppl. 1):157.

Huber, S.J., Paulson, G.W., Shuttleworth, E.C., et al. Magnetic resonance imaging correlates of dementia in multiple sclerosis. *Arch Neurol* 1987; 44:732–6.

Huckman, M.S., Fox, J.H., and Topel, J. The validity of criteria for the evaluation of cerebral atrophy by computed tomography. *Radiology* 1975; 116:85–92.

Iivanainen, M.V. The significance of abnormal immune responses in patients with multiple sclerosis. *J Neuroimmunol* 1981; 1:141–72.

Ivnik, R.J. Neuropsychological stability in multiple sclerosis. *J Consult Clin Psychol* 1978a; 46:913–23.

Ivnik, R.J. Neuropsychological test performance as a function of the duration of MS-related symptomatology. *J Clin Psychiatry* 1978b; 39:304–7.

Jacobson, J.T., Deppe, U., and Murray, T.J. Dichotic paradigms in multiple sclerosis. *Ear Hear* 1983; 4:311–7.

Jambor, K.L. cognitive functioning in multiple sclerosis. *Br J Psychiatry* 1969; 115:765–75.

Jasper, H., Bickford, R., and Magnus, O. The electroencephalogram in multiple sclerosis. *Res Publ Assoc Nerv Ment Dis* 1950; 28:421–7.

Johnson, R.T., Katzman, R., McGeer, E., Price, D., Shooter, E., and Silberberg, D. *Report of the Panel on Inflammatory, Demyelinating and Degenerative Diseases* (Report No. 79-1916). U.S. Department of Health, Washington, DC, 1979.

Kinnunen, E. The incidence of optic neuritis and its prognosis for multiple sclerosis. *Acta Neurol Scand* 1983; 68:371–7.

Koenig, H. Dementia associated with the benign form of multiple sclerosis. *Trans Am Neurol Assoc* 1968; 93:227–8.

Kurtzke, J.F. Neuroepidemiology. *Ann Neurol* 1984; 16:265–77.

Kurtzke, J.F., Beebe, G.W., Nagler, B., Nefzger, M.D., Auth, T.L., and Kurland, L.T. Studies on the natural history of multiple sclerosis. V. Long-term survival in young men. *Arch Neurol* 1970; 22:215–25.

Kurtzke, J.F., Beebe, G.W., and Norman, J.E. Epidemiology of multiple sclerosis in US veterans: III. Migration and the risk of MS. *Neurology* 1985; 35:672–8.

Litvan, I., Grafman, J., Vendrell, P., et al. Multiple memory deficits in patients with multiple sclerosis: Exploring the working memory system. *Arch Neurol* 1988a; 45:607–10.

Litvan, I., Grafman, J., Vendrell, P., and Martinez, J.M. Slowed information processing in multiple sclerosis. *Arch Neurol* 1988b; 45:281–5.

Lyon-Caen, O., Jouvent, R., Hauser, S., et al. Cognitive function in recent-onset demyelinating diseases. *Arch Neurol* 1986; 43:1138–41.

MacKay, R.P., and Hirano, A. Forms of benign multiple sclerosis: Report of two "clinically silent" cases discovered at autopsy. *Arch Neurol* 1967; 17:588–600.

Marsh, G. Disability and intellectual function in multiple sclerosis. *J Nerv Ment Dis* 1980; 168:758–62.

Matthews, W.B., Acheson, E.D., Batchelor, J.R., and Weller, R.O. *McAlpine's Multiple Sclerosis*. Churchill Livingstone, New York, 1985.

McDonald, W.I. The mystery of the origin of multiple sclerosis. *J Neurol Neurosurg Psychiatry* 1986; 49:113–23.

McKhann, G.M. Multiple sclerosis. *Annu Rev Neurosci* 1982; 5:219–39.

Medaer, R., Nelissen, E., Appel, B., Swerts, M., Geutjens, J., and Callaert, H. Magnetic resonance imaging and cognitive functioning in multiple sclerosis. *J Neurol* 1987; 235:86–9.

Olmos-Lau, N., Ginsberg, M.D., and Geller, J.B. Aphasia in multiple sclerosis. *Neurology* 1977; 27:623–6.

Parsons, O.A., Stewart, K.D., and Arenberg, D. Impairment of abstracting ability in multiple sclerosis. *J Nerv Ment Dis* 1957; 125:221–5.

Peyser, J.M., Edwards, K.R., Poser, C.M., and Filskov, S.B. Cognitive function in patients with multiple sclerosis. *Arch Neurol* 1980; 37:577–9.

Peyser, J.M., and Poser, C.M. Neuropsychological correlates of multiple sclerosis. In *Handbook of Clinical Neuropsychology, Vol. 2*. Filskov, S.B., and Boll, T.J. (eds.). Wiley, New York, 1986:364–97.

Poser, C.M. The diagnostic process in multiple sclerosis. In *The Diagnosis of Multiple Sclerosis*. Thieme-Stratton, Inc., New York, 1984, pp. 3–13.

Poser, C.M., Paty, D.W., Scheinberg, L., et al. New diagnostic criteria for multiple sclerosis: Guidelines for research protocols. *Ann Neurol* 1983; 13:227–31.

Powell, H.C., and Lampert, P.W. Pathology of multiple sclerosis. *Neurol Clin* 1983; 1:631–44.

Rabins, P.V., Brooks, B.R., O'Donnell, P., et al. Structural brain correlates of emotional disorder in multiple slcerosis. *Brain* 1986; 109:585–97.

Rao, S.M. Neuropsychology of multiple sclerosis: A critical review. *J Clin Exp Neuropsychol* 1986; 8:503–42.

Rao, S.M., Glatt, S., Hammeke, T.A., et al. Chronic progressive multiple sclerosis: Relationship between cerebral ventricular size and neuropsychological impairment. *Arch Neurol* 1985; 42:678–82.

Rao, S.M., and Hammeke, T.A. Hypothesis testing in patients with chronic progressive multiple sclerosis. *Brain Cogn* 1984; 3:94–104.

Rao, S.M., Hammeke, T.A., McQuillen, M.P., Khatri, B.O., and Lloyd, D. Memory disturbance in chronic progressive multiple sclerosis. *Arch Neurol* 1984; 41:625–31.

Rao, S.M., Hammeke, T.A., and Speech, T.J. Wisconsin Card Sorting Test performance in relapsing-remitting and chronic-progressive multiple sclerosis. *J Consult Clin Psychol* 1987; 55:263–5.

Rao, S.M., Leo, G.J., Haughton, V.M., St. Aubin-Faubert, P., and Bernardin, L. Correlation of magnetic resonance imaging with neuropsychological testing in multiple sclerosis. *Neurology*, 1989; 39:161–6.

Rao, S.M., St. Aubin-Faubert, P., and Leo, G.J. Information processing speed in patients with multiple sclerosis. *J Clin Exp Neuropsychol,* 1989; 4:471–7.

Rao, S.M., Leo, G.J., St. Aubin-Faubert, P. On the nature of memory disturbance in multiple sclerosis. *J Clin Exp Neuropsychol,* in press.

Reder, A.T., and Antel, J.P. Clinical spectrum of multiple sclerosis. *Neurol Clin* 1983; 1:573–99.

Reitan, R.M., Reed, J.C., and Dyken, M. Cognitive, psychomotor, and motor correlates of multiple sclerosis. *J Nerv Ment Dis* 1971; 153:218–24.

Ron, M.A. Multiple sclerosis: Psychiatric and psychometric abnormalities. *J Psychosom Res* 1986; 30:3–11.

Rubens, A.B., Froehling, B., Slater, G., and Anderson, D. Left ear suppression on verbal dichotic tests in patients with multiple sclerosis. *Ann Neurol* 1985; 18:459–63.

Sheremata, W.A., Sevush, S., Knight, D., and Ziajka, P. Altered cerebral metabolism in MS. *Neurology* 1984; 34 (Suppl. 1):118.

Silberberg, D.H. Multiple sclerosis. In *Scientific Approaches to Clinical Neurology, Vol. 1.* Goldensah, E.S., and Appell, S.H. (eds.). Lea and Febiger, Philadelphia, 1977, pp. 299–324.

Sternberg, S. Memory scanning: Mental processes revealed by reaction-time experiments. *Am Scientist* 1969; 57:421–57.

van den Burg, W., van Zomeren, A.H., Minderhoud, J.M., Prange, A.J.A., and Meijer, N.S.A. Cognitive impairment in patients with multiple sclerosis and mild physical disability. *Arch Neurol* 1987; 44:494–501.

Vowels, L.M. Memory impairment in multiple sclerosis. In *Brain Impairment: Proceedings of the 1978 Brain Impairment Workshop.* Molloy, M., Stanley, G.V., and Walsh, K.W. (eds.). University of Melbourne, Melbourne, 1979, pp. 10–22.

Walton, J.N. *Brain's Diseases of the Nervous System, Eighth edition.* Oxford University Press, New York, 1977.

Willoughby, E.W., and Paty, D.W. Brain imaging in multiple sclerosis. In *Neurobehavioral Consequences of Multiple Sclerosis.* Rao, S.M. (ed.). Oxford University Press, New York, 1989.

Young, A.C., Saunders, J., and Ponsford, J.R. Mental change as an early feature of multiple sclerosis. *J Neurol Neurosurg Psychiatry* 1976; 39:1008–13.

13

The AIDS Dementia Complex

BRADFORD A. NAVIA

Since the first cases of the Acquired Immune Deficiency Syndrome (AIDS) were reported in 1981, it was recognized that a large number of AIDS patients developed a variety of disorders of both the peripheral and central nervous system (Snider et al., 1983; Levy et al., 1985). Most common, however, was an unusual encephalopathy that frequently resulted in profound neurologic impairment (Snider et al., 1983; Britton et al., 1984; Navia et al., 1986a; Price et al., 1986). Referred to as a subacute encephalitis or encephalopathy, this disorder was initially believed to result from direct brain infection by cytomegalovirus, a frequent opportunistic pathogen in patients (Snider et al., 1983; Nielson et al., 1984). However, with subsequent clinical–pathologic studies demonstrating that this AIDS encephalopathy was a relatively stereotyped disorder unique to HIV-1 infected patients and the discovery of HIV-1 in brains of AIDS-demented patients initially by Southern blot analysis and subsequently by a variety of other methods, the retroviral etiology of this disorder became established (Shaw et al., 1985; Epstein et al., 1985; Ho et al., 1985; Navia et al., 1986b).

Detailed clinical study clearly indicated that dementia was the most frequent and salient characteristic of this disorder, frequently resulting in global cognitive impairment (Navia et al., 1986a). Further, many of the patients exhibited prominent behavioral or motor disturbances in association with their dementing illness. Thus, in order to differentiate this from other encephalopathic disorders from which it was clearly distinguishable, the terms AIDS dementia complex (ADC) was introduced (Navia et al., 1986a,b). Further study revealed an additional unique feature in that clinically and pathologically ADC appeared to be a predominantly subcortical process (Navia et al., 1986a,b). Many of the clinical features resembled those described in other subcortical dementias, while pathologic, virological, and metabolic studies demonstrated either predominant or primary involvement of subcortical structures with relative preservation of the cerebral cortex both at the regional and cellular level (Albert et al., 1974; Cummings and Benson, 1984; Navia et al., 1986b; Pumarola-Sune et al., 1987; Rottenberg et al., 1987). These results clearly lent additional support to the validity of subcortical dementia as a distinct clinical entity and suggested that ADC may provide an important model to examine further the contribution of subcortical structures to various cognitive and behavioral disorders.

Growing evidence now indicates that ADC is the most frequent neurologic complication of HIV-1 infection, afflicting the majority of AIDS patients at some point in their clinical course (Navia et al., 1986a,b; Price et al., 1988a,b). Indeed, in a few patients it may be the earliest or only clinical manifestation of HIV-1 infection (Navia and Price, 1987). Given its high incidence and its disabling effects on neurologic function, it thus represents a source of great morbidity to the AIDS population. This fact, along with recent findings supporting the etiologic role of HIV-1, has stirred a great deal of clinical and biological interest in this disorder (Price et al., 1988a,c). This chapter proposes to bridge the clinical and biological perspectives on ADC in order to provide a greater understanding of this common problem and a broader basis for future research efforts. It is divided into three major sections: The first reviews clinical, neuropsychological, and pathological features of ADC; the second examines the evidence for its retroviral etiology; and the third discusses major issues of pathogenesis, many of which remain unresolved.

CLINICAL FEATURES

Clinical Studies

The AIDS dementia complex is a distinct clinical syndrome with characteristic disturbances in cognitive, behavioral, and motor function (Navia et al., 1986a) (Table 13-1). Dysfunction in any one of these areas may predominate during the early stages of the disease; for example, progressive lower leg weakness may precede overt intellectual impairment by weeks to months, but clearly the latter is the most frequent presentation, best characterized as slowing with loss of precision in activities that involve either mentation or motor control. Thus, patients who have retained insight into their illness complain of difficulty with concentration and memory. More mental effort is needed to recall once familiar events and information; appointments may be missed, and the patient may resort to using lists. Thinking is slowed; tasks that once were performed readily require more time and become laborious; the loss of concentration may force the patient to reread a paragraph several times in order to grasp content fully. Performing simple calculations, composing a sentence, or typing an overlearned code on the computer becomes difficult and maybe abandoned altogether. This difficulty with attention also causes the patient to lose either track of conversation or his own train of thought. Similarly the patient may feel bewildered or confused when

Table 13-1   AIDS Dementia Complex: Clinical Features

Early Symptoms	
Cognitive	Slowness, impaired attention and concentration, forgetfulness, confusion
Motor	Clumsiness, deterioration in fine motor tasks, tremor, loss of balance, leg weakness
Behavioral	Reduced spontaneity, apathy, social withdrawal
Early Signs	
Mental status	Psychomotor slowing, impaired word reversal, serial subtraction, blunted affect, organic psychosis
Motor	Impaired rapid movements, sustension tremor, hyperreflexia, limb paresis, impaired tandem gait

simultaneously faced with more than one task. This inability to initiate and organize either thoughts or behavior efficiently may result in embarrassing problems at work with eventual loss of professional standing. Verbal and motor responses also become slowed. In many instances the patient is either not aware of or denies the change in his thinking or personality. Friends or colleagues will note loss of spontaneity as the patient becomes disinterested in and withdraws from his usual professional and social activities. The typical picture is, therefore, that of a once vibrant and productive individual who has become dull, apathetic, and subdued.

Such behavioral disturbances are relatively common and, not surprisingly, frequently mistaken for depression (Navia et al., 1986a). Distinguishing features include the general absence of true dysphoria and the lack of response to antidepressant treatment. Differentiating between the two, in reality, is often difficult, but the diagnosis of ADC should be evident with the appearance of additional neurologic signs. Less commonly, the patient may become agitated, hyperactive, and even manic. An organic psychosis is an infrequent but nonetheless well described presentation of ADC (Navia et al., 1986a).

Motor disturbances most often consist of loss of either fine motor coordination or balance. Hand activities become clumsy and slow, particularly handwriting. A fine tremor may appear, contributing further to problems with coordination. Difficulties with gait are manifested typically by either tripping and falling episodes or slowness in movement. Progressive leg weakness, initially unilateral, may be the predominant complaint early in the disease.

The early loss of cognitive function is usually gradual and subtle and thus can either be missed or overlooked, particularly in the context of a systemic illness. Compounding this diagnostic dilemma is the fact that the bedside neurologic examination on initial presentation is either unremarkable or may consist only of slowed verbal or motor responses; difficulty with attention and concentration, a common complaint, may be evident during word reversal or serial subtractions. Memory loss, despite its prevalence, is less often demonstrated at the bedside. In patients with an unusually progressive form of the disorder, affect is typically blunted or flat; insight is poor, and the patient appears strikingly indifferent to his illness and surroundings.

Motor abnormalities include slowing of rapid successive movements of the fingers, a fine tremor of the upper extremities on sustension, and hyperreflexia of the lower extremities; difficulty with either tandem gait or turns may provide the only clue to early ataxia. Tests of ocular mobility may show slowing of smooth pursuit associated with saccadic intrusions.

Onset of dementia is typically insidious, and steady progression occurs over months. Abrupt deterioration in cognitive function occurs in some patients, frequently in the setting of a systemic illness, which when resolved can be associated with some recovery of neurologic function. Less often, onset can be unusually rapid, resulting in global cognitive loss over weeks. Further examination shows that the temporal profile of ADC consists of at least three general patterns that may correspond to different forms of the disorder: insidious onset, steady progression; acute–subacute onset, rapid progression; and insidious onset, minimal or no progression. The relative incidence of these different presentations is not precisely known, although the majority of patients probably fall either in the first or last category. The basis for this difference in clinical expression between the progressive and static forms is also not understood but may be related either to host or virological factors, including the possible existence of neuro-trophic variants (see the following discussion).

With disease progression a more stereotyped clinical picture emerges. Diffuse cognitive impairment, associated with severe impoverishment of speech and progressive motor impairment, leaves the patient with little meaningful contact with his environment. In its most extreme form, the patient is bedridden and mute, shows little spontaneous motor movement, and is incontinent. Tremor or myoclonus of either the focal or multifocal type may also be seen. Less often the patient will appear markedly distractible or agitated and may show disinhibited and socially inappropriate behavior reminiscent of patients with frontal lobe damage. Rarely, an organic psychosis with either hallucinatory or delusional features may predominate. In contrast to other encephalopathies of either infectious or metabolic etiology, consciousness is characteristically preserved unless the patient has developed an interrcurrent systemic illness.

Neuropsychological Studies

A number of neuropsychological studies have been published on the profile of intellectual impairment in ADC (Tross et al., 1988; Sidtis et al., 1987; Grant et al., 1987; Levy et al., 1987; Saykin et al., 1987; Rubinow et al., 1988). These have demonstrated that formal neuropsychological testing can prove to be valuable both in supporting the diagnosis of ADC and in identifying impairment in specific subsets of cognitive function not found by routine bedside testing.

When compared with seronegative controls, patients with early AIDS typically show impairment in sequential problem solving and fine motor speed and control (Table 13-2). With disease progression, the incidence and severity of neuropsychological impairment increases. In late AIDS reduced performance is also found in verbal fluency, verbal and visual memory, and visuospatial performance. Remarkably, despite the severity of cognitive impairment, language function, (e.g., naming and vocabulary) remains relatively preserved. Thus patients with ADC show prominent difficulties in areas that require mental speed, flexibility, spontaneity, fine motor control, and visual motor integration. This profile is consistent with the major clinical features of ADC and provides further support for its prominent subcortical characteristics. As with other subcortical dementias, aphasia, agnosia, or true amnesia are not prominent findings except in some advanced cases. Rather, psychomotor slowing is the salient feature, contributing to many of the areas of neuropsychological impairment. These studies, therefore, provide a set of quantifiable descriptors that should be useful in defining

Table 13-2 The Neuropsychological Profile of Impairment in the AIDS Dementia Complex

Early ADC	Motor control (Finger-tapping and grooved pegboard)[a]
	Sequential problem solving (Trail making A and B)
Late ADC	As above
	Verbal fluency (FAS)
	Visual spatial performance (Block design)
	Visual and verbal memory (Wechsler memory scale)

[a]Specific neuropsychological subtest(s) indicated within parentheses.

further the natural history and clinical course of ADC within the context of either immunosuppression, systemic infection, or antiviral treatment.

The incidence of neuropsychological impairment in HIV-1 seropositive patients remains a controversial yet nonetheless important issue (Grant et al., 1987; Tross et al., 1988). 12 to 44 percent of these patients have been found to show some degree of impairment on formal neuropsychological testing, depending on the study and the criteria used for degree of abnormality. Clearly, additional longitudinal studies are needed to establish unambigous criteria for ADC (Ornitz et al., 1987; Sidtis et al., 1987). Nonetheless, it appears on the basis of these preliminary reports that neuropsychological impairment may be present in a small undefined segment of the HIV seropositive population. The recent isolation of HIV-1 from the cerebrospinal fluid in some of these patients provides further evidence for the early presence HIV-1 in the central nervous system (CNS) (Goudsmit et al., 1986a; McArthur et al., 1988). The incidence and spectrum of the clinical manifestations resulting from early HIV-1 infection of the CNS have not yet been established.

Neurodiagnostic Studies

Neurodiagnostic studies both with computerized tomographic scanning (CT) and magnetic resonance imaging (MRI) have provided some useful though limited information regarding the pathologic and anatomic substrates of ADC (Navia et al., 1986a). The most frequent finding consists of diffuse cerebral atrophy of varying severity, sometimes associated with ventricular dilatation. Although found in the majority of patients at presentation, cerebral atrophy has also been detected months before the onset of clinically overt dementia. Together these findings suggest that histological changes need to be present for some time before dementia becomes clinically evident. It is not surprising then that the majority of presumed nondemented patients were found to have mild pathologic changes at autopsy; some of these patients, however, may have never progressed beyond the subclinical phase of ADC (see the following discussion).

Less frequently, either patchy or diffuse attenuation of the white matter may be observed on CT scans. MRI, however, is much more sensitive in detecting this abnormality, which characteristically appears as a patchy or diffuse increased signal in the white matter on a T2 weighted image (Navia et al., 1986a). Similar changes in signal have also been occasionally noted either in the basal ganglia or thalamus. The pathologic substrate of the white matter findings may be related to the presence of multifocal rarefaction of the white matter and infiltration by macrophages and multinucleated cells, characteristically seen in a subset of patients with the severe form of ADC (see the following discussion). Additionally, these findings correlate with the detection of HIV-1 in the brain by either Southern blot analysis or immunohistochemistry. Thus it is plausible that this MRI abnormality may help identify a subset of AIDS patients more likely to develop the progressive form of ADC and to have HIV-1 in the brain. Further studies are needed to determine the prognostic significance of this finding.

Examination of the cerebrospinal fluid most commonly reveals a mild elevation in protein in about two thirds of patients and a mononuclear pleocytosis in nearly one quarter (Navia et al., 1986a). More specifically, HIV-1 has been isolated from the cerebrospinal fluid (CSF) of patients with various CNS manifestations, including acute

aseptic meningitis, chronic meningitis, and dementia, as well as from HIV-1 seropositive patients without systemic AIDS who were either asymptomatic or found to have
abnormal neuropsychological testing (Ho et al., 1985; Levy et al., 1985; Goudsmit et
al., 1986a; McArthur et al., 1988). Intrathecal synthesis of HIV-1 antibodies has also
been demonstrated, but the diagnostic and prognostic significance of this finding remains to be established (Resnick et al., 1985; Goudsmit et al., 1986b). On the basis
of these studies the following conclusions can be drawn: (1) HIV-1 antigen can be
detected in the CSF in the majority of cases of ADC; (2) failure to isolate HIV-1 in
some cases may reflect the limitation of the culture technique or the poor replication
of certain viral strains in T cells; (3) HIV-1 may be detected in the CSF early in the
course of HIV-1 infection; and (4) the serological profile detected by immunological
methods may differ in the CSF and serum in the same patient. Future prospective
studies correlating the isolation of HIV-1 in the CSF with the appearance of neuropsychological dysfunction should help further define the temporal profile of HIV-1
infection of the CNS and its effects on neurologic function.

The Neuropathology of ADC

The pathologic substrate of ADC was not established until detailed clinical pathologic
study revealed a constellation of characteristic histological abnormalities involving
specific brain regions (Navia et al., 1986b). Grossly mild to moderate cerebral atrophy
is seen in almost all demented patients. On histological examination the brunt of brain
injury is found predominantly in the subcortical structures, notably in the central white
and deep gray matter regions, particularly the basal ganglia and thalamus (Navia et
al., 1986b; Petito et al., 1986). Remarkably, despite profound dementia in many patients, the cortex appears relatively spared (Navia et al., 1986b). The most frequent
histological abnormality found in over 90 percent of autopsied cases, including nondemented patients, consists of a diffuse pallor of the centrum semiovale, usually associated with a reactive astrocytosis (Table 13-3) (Navia et al., 1986b; Petito et al.,
1986). There is a greater predilection for the central and periventricular white matter
than for the subcortical fibers. A predominantly mononuclear inflammatory response
of variable intensity is found in almost all cases, most often in the white and subcortical
gray matter and occasionally in the cortex. In milder forms of ADC, this reaction is
composed of a few brown pigmented macrophages and lymphocytes in a perivascular

Table 13-3 Neuropathology of the AIDS Dementia Complex

Distribution	Central white matter, subcortical gray matter (basal ganglia, thalamus), cerebral cortex relatively preserved except in most advanced cases
Histopathology	
Mild	White matter pallor, perivascular infiltrates: brown pigmented macrophages and lymphocytes
Severe	Diffuse white matter pallor, multifocal rarefaction, reactive astrocytosis, parenchymal and perivascular infiltrates: foamy macrophages, multinucleated cells, neuronal loss in basal ganglia, occasionally in cortex
Additional findings	Demyelination, vacuolation, focal necrosis, microglial modules, prominent focal regional involvement in some

distribution, while in more severe cases the inflammatory response is more prominent, consisting of both parenchymal and perivascular collections of foamy macrophages and multinucleated cells of macrophage origin, in association with discrete multiple foci of rarefaction in the white matter. Neuronal loss with a reactive gliosis can occasionally be found in severe cases, particularly in the caudate and putamen and less often in the frontal and temporal lobes, but generally does not represent a major histological feature of this disorder (Navia et al., 1986b; Petito et al., 1986; de la Monte et al., 1987).

Additional but less frequent findings include focal necrosis, vacuolation of the white matter, and either focal or diffuse demyelination. Occasionally brain pathology may consist predominantly of one of these abnormalities or show prominent focal involvement of either the basal ganglia or brain stem, disproportionate to the severity of white matter involvement. Thus, although ADC pathologically is characterized by a common core of histological findings, variation either in the type or distribution of pathology may be encountered in individual patients.

Microglial nodules consisting of clusters of microglial cells and astrocytes are found in nearly 60% of patients; while cytomegalovirus (CMV) inclusions, typically associated with a microglial nodule encephalitis, are found in 15 to 20% of patients. Although both can occur in patients with multinucleated cells and HIV-1 in brain, neither correlates with either the severity of ADC or its underlying pathology (Navia et al., 1986b). Coinfection with CMV however, may contribute to the degree of clinical dysfunction in some patients (Navia et al., 1986b; Wiley and Nelson, 1988; Vinters et al., 1989).

Clinical–pathological examination shows that the severity of clinical dementia generally correlates with the extent of brain pathology (Table 13-4) (Navia et al., 1986b). With some notable exceptions, progressive severe dementia is associated with diffuse pallor and rarefaction of the white matter with macrophages and multinucleated cells both in the white and deep gray matter regions. In patients with a less pronounced course, abnormalities are few, less diffuse, and, in some, remarkably bland despite

Table 13-4 Clinical, Pathological, and Virological Correlations of the AIDS Dementia Complex

Approximate Percentage of all AIDS Patients	Clincal Severity of ADC[a]	Neuropathologic Severity	Multi-nucleated Cells	Neuroimaging CT/MRI[b]	HIV[c] Detection: Antigen and Southern Blot
25	Severe	Severe	+	Atrophy/increased white matter signal	+
50	Mild to moderate	Mild to moderate	−	Atrophy	−
25	None/ subclinical	Mild	−	Normal/atrophy	−

[a]ADC, AIDS dementia complex.
[b]CT, computed tomography; MRI, magnetic resonance imaging.
[c]HIV, human immunodeficiency virus.

moderate neurologic impairment. Rarefaction is almost never seen, and multinucleated cells are absent. As already mentioned, mild brain pathology consisting most often of white matter pallor is also found in the majority of nondemented patients who may either have had a subclinical or early form of the disorder, possibly overlooked in the context of overwhelming systemic illness. Importantly, this finding provides additional evidence for the high incidence of brain involvement in AIDS patients.

The spinal cord may show similar inflammatory changes, including the presence of multinucleated cells, particularly in severe cases of ADC. However, the most common finding is a vacuolar myelopathy found in approximately 25 percent of all AIDS patients and in nearly 50 percent of those with ADC (Petito et al., 1985). Pathologically, there is vacuolation of the posterior and lateral columns, most commonly seen at the thoracic level. This resembles the subacute combined degeneration of vitamin B12 deficiency; serum B12 levels, however, are normal in these patients. The early histological finding consists of scattered vacuoles resulting from intramyelin swelling and lipid-laden macrophages. In severe cases vacuolation is diffuse and associated with secondary axonal degeneration. Clinically a spastic ataxic paraparesis develops. The severity of this myelopathy generally correlates with that of dementia and forebrain pathology, although it can occur in the absence of major brain abnormalities (Petito et al., 1985; Navia et al., 1986b). This discrepancy further underscores the pathologic heterogeneity of ADC and reinforces the issue of whether the entire spectrum of abnormalities represents variants of a single agent or in fact are related to different etiologies.

Epidemiology and Natural History

The incidence of ADC remains undefined, but, on the basis of retrospective and ongoing prospective studies, it is estimated that between 70 and 90 percent of AIDS patients will develop neuropsychological impairment at some point in their clinical course (Navia et al., 1986a; Price et al., 1988a,b). Nearly two thirds of these patients will have had developed systemic AIDS, as defined by Center for Disease Control (CDC) criteria, before the onset of ADC. Thus, in the majority of patients, ADC appears as a relatively late manifestation in the natural history of HIV-1 infection. It is estimated that, at the time of diagnosis, nearly one third of patients will show overt neurologic impairment and another one quarter will be subclinically affected. Further, it has now been shown that ADC can develop as the initial clinical manifestation of HIV-1 infection and, despite evidence for severe immunosuppression, it may remain its only if not predominant expression (Navia and Price, 1987). It is of interest that dementia in this particular subset of patients is typically progressive and severe, associated at autopsy with widespread changes in the subcortical regions, including the presence of multinucleated cells and HIV-1 (Navia and Price, 1987). One possible explanation is that these patients may be infected with a highly neurotropic variant of HIV-1 compared with patients who initially develop systemic AIDS (see the following discussion).

Recent data indicate that HIV-1 likely enters the central nervous system early in the course of infection (see the following discussion) (Goudsmit et al., 1986a; McArthur et al., 1988; Chiodi et al., 1987). Some patients may develop a self-limiting acute meningitis or encephalitis, but the majority probably remain asymptomatic during this time. It is not clear, however, when after this initial insult patients begin to develop neurologic impairment consistent with ADC. Further studies are, therefore, needed to define the natural history of this disorder within the context of various virological and immunological factors that may contribute to its spread in the human host, including host genetic factors, the role of immunosuppression and background systemic infection, and the existence of HIV-1 variants with differing cell tropism and cytopathology.

ETIOLOGY

It has been sufficiently established that the AIDS dementia complex or at least that form associated with multinucleated cells in the brain results from direct brain infection by HIV-1, the causative agent of AIDS (Shaw et al., 1985; Epstein et al., 1985; Ho et al., 1985). This observation is based on both indirect and direct sources of evidence (Table 13-5). The relatively stereotyped nature of the clinical and pathologic features of the dementia and its unique occurrence in HIV-1 infected patients suggested a retroviral etiology (Navia et al., 1986b). Additional supporting evidence came from various forms of retroviral infection of the CNS in animals. This included the observation that HIV-1 biologically and genetically resembles visna, a nononcogenic retrovirus that causes a chronic neurologic disorder in sheep (Gonda et al., 1985, 1986; Haase, 1986). Shared biological properties include the capacity to cause cell lysis and fusion resulting in synctial or multinucleated cell forms and a strong tropism for cells of the immune system including macrophages. Both viruses show a predilection for the white matter of the CNS, but visna results in a much greater inflammatory response. The general paucity of inflammatory cells in response to HIV-1 infection probably reflects the degree of immunosuppression characteristic of AIDS.

Simian immunodeficiency virus (SIV) is morphologically and antigenically related to HIV-1 and can cause an AIDS-like syndrome when inoculated into macaque monkeys (Daniel et al., 1985; Letvin et al., 1985; Kanki et al., 1985; Ringler et al., 1988). The brains of these infected animals show a multinucleated cell encephalitis characterized by the presence of macrophages and multinucleated cells in the white and gray matter and meninges. With further study these animals may provide a useful model of some of the biological aspects of ADC.

A somewhat more remote retroviral model is provided by the infection of wild mice by the murine leukemia virus (MuLV), which results in spongiform changes of the gray matter of the spinal cord (Gardner, 1988). Pathogenesis is related to the intra-

Table 13-5 Evidence Supporting the Etiology of HIV-1 in the AIDS Dementia Complex

Indirect evidence	Clinical pathological disorder unique to HIV-1 infected patients
	Animal models of CNS retroviral infection (visna, SIV, MuLV)
Direct evidence	Nucleic acid detection
	(Southern blot analysis, in situ hybridization)
	Virions (election microscopy)
	Viral isolation (CSF, brain culture)
	Antigen detection (immunohistochemistry)

cellular and extracellular accumulation of viral products, resulting in neuronal and glial cell injury. Specifically, the paralytic determinant has been localized to the outer membrane envelope glycoprotein (gp70). These observations suggest possible mechanisms that may be relevant to the events leading to cell injury in HIV-1 infection of the brain (see the following discussion).

A direct link between ADC and HIV-1 was first demonstrated by Shaw and colleagues, who detected HIV-1 nucleic acid sequences by Southern blot analysis in brain of AIDS demented patients (Shaw et al., 1985). Three additional and potentially significant observations were made: (1) when compared with peripheral tissues, the brains of some patients contained a greater abundance of HIV-1; (2) unintegrated as well as integrated forms of HIV-1 were found, indicating active viral replication; and (3) different but related forms of HIV-1 were found in the brain among different AIDS patients. The latter observation is consistent with the known polymorphism of the virus, most often observed in the envelope (env) gene, and suggests the possible existence of neurotropic variants (see the following discussion) (Hahn et al., 1985, 1986).

Brain infection by HIV-1 has since been demonstrated by a variety of other methods, including electron microscopy (Epstein et al., 1985), viral isolation from the brain and CSF (Ho et al., 1985; Levy et al., 1985), immunohistochemistry (Wiley et al., 1986; Gabuzda et al., 1986; Pumorola-Sune et al., 1987), in situ hybridization (Shaw et al., 1985; Koenig et al., 1986; Stoler et al., 1986), and intrathecal synthesis of anti-HIV antibodies (Resnick et al., 1985; Goudsmit et al., 1986b). Although these studies have clearly demonstrated the presence of HIV-1 in brains of AIDS demented patients, many issues with respect to pathogenesis remain to be resolved, including which cells harbor the virus in the brain and how the virus disturbs brain function both at the cellular and regional level.

There is an emerging consensus based on studies using either immunohistochemistry or in situ hybridization that the most commonly infected cells in brain consist of macrophages and multinucleated cells derived from viral-induced fusion of macrophages (Wiley et al., 1986; Koenig et al., 1986; Pumorola-Sune et al., 1986; Stoler et al., 1986). In addition, HIV-1 has been identified with less frequency in several different process-bearing cells, including microglia, vascular endothelial cells, astrocytes, and rarely neurons (Wiley et al., 1986; Pumorola-Sune et al., 1986; Vazeux et al., 1987). Similarly, productive infection of brain-derived cells has not been readily demonstrated in vitro; in fact, successful HIV-1 isolation usually requires cocultivation with known permissive cell lines (Chiodi et al., 1987; Cheng-Mayer et al., 1987; Popovic et al., 1988). The small number of infected brain cells with a low yield of viral progeny is more consistent with a latent rather than a productive form of infection and may contribute to persistent infection in brain in a manner analogous to that by visna (Haase, 1986).

The regional distribution of HIV-1 infection in brain generally parallels the neuropathologic findings, with the largest number of infected cells found in the white and deep gray matter structures, particularly the basal ganglia and thalamus; cortical involvement, however, is also sometimes seen.

Analysis of the clinical, pathologic, and virological data allows further classification of the AIDS patients into three general groups depending on the severity of the disease and the presence of HIV-1 in brain as shown in Table 13-4 (Pumarola-Sune et al., 1986; Price et al., 1988c). Nearly 25 percent will develop severe dementia clinically and show multinucleated cells and HIV-1 in the brain. Thus, in the majority of patients, despite moderate to severe dementia in many, brain pathology is remarkably mild, and HIV-1 cannot be detected by the methods described earlier. This observation raises the important question as to whether the entire spectrum of ADC is causally linked to HIV-1 and, if so, what are the host and viral factors contributing to differences in the clinical and pathologic expression of this disorder (see the following discussion).

PATHOGENESIS

Although growing evidence now indicates that HIV-1 is the most likely cause of ADC, many fundamental questions of pathogenesis remain unanswered (Table 13-6). When and how does HIV enter the CNS during the course of systemic infection? Recent data based primarily on reports of CSF abnormalities, including the isolation of HIV-1 either at the time of seroconversion or from asymptomatic seropositive patients, suggest that the CNS may be involved early (Carne et al., 1985; Cooper et al., 1985; Goudsmit et al., 1986a; Ho et al., 1985; Resnick et al., 1985). Meningeal infection may thus represent the initial step in establishing parenchymal disease leading to dementia. It is not known, however, how many or which patients with early meningeal involvement will go on to develop progressive dementia. Future studies are needed to define the relationship between these two events, as well as to identify those factors that determine clinical progression. These include host genetic susceptibility, degree of immunosuppression, and neurotropic variants of HIV-1. The latter may be particularly important in governing the tempo and severity of disease. The source of HIV-1 in the neuroaxis is also not established. Does the virus enter the CNS in free form or

Table 13-6   Major Issues of Pathogenesis in the AIDS Dementia Complex

Viral pathogenesis
    Route of viral entry; timing in relation to systemic infection
    Significance of aseptic meningitis with respect to ADC
    Role of macrophage, Trojan horse hypothesis
    Cell types infected
    Cell surface receptor
    Level of viral expression in different cells
    Heterogeneity in clinical–pathological expression of ADC
    Host genetic factors
    Immunosuppression; systemic infection
    HIV-1 variants; specific neurotropic subtypes
    Genomic sequences responsible for cell tropism and pathogenicity

Mechanisms of brain dysfunction
    Noncytopathic
    Clinical pathologic dissociation
    Metabolic injury
    Specific cells and regions involved
    Role of macrophage
    Host versus viral coded products
    Role of neurotoxins
    Effects of gp120 on neuronal function

is it transported within lymphoid cells such as macrophages that have been infected in the periphery? The latter is consistent with the Trojan horse hypothesis based on observations in visna that the macrophage which harbors the virus provides an essential portal of entry into the CNS (Haase, 1986). It has been recently shown that HIV-1 can latently infect human choroid plexus cells in culture (Harouse et al., 1989). The choroid plexus may, therefore, represent an alternative route of entry and serve as a reservoir for viral seeding of the CNS.

Within the CNS major issues include the spectrum of cells infected by HIV-1 and the nature of the surface receptor. As already discussed, recent data point to the macrophage as the predominant infected cell in the brain, although other cell types, including brain-derived cells, may also be involved but to a much lesser degree. The molecular basis for this difference in susceptibility is unknown but may be related to the presence either of a surface receptor or of cellular factors needed to support viral replication. Expression of the CD4 receptor is essential for HIV-1 entry into lymphocytes (Dagleish et al., 1984; Klatzmann et al., 1984; Maddon et al., 1986). Transfecting the CD4 gene into cell lines can confer HIV-1 infectivity (Maddon et al., 1986). Both a full length and a truncated CD4 messenger RNA have been recently demonstrated in mammalian brain, although the specific regional and cellular localization has not been established (Maddon et al., 1986). Low levels of CD4 messenger RNA have also been reported in astrocyte cultures, which have been shown to be susceptible to a low level of HIV-1 infection. However, what role the CD4 receptor has in mediating the pathogenetic effects of HIV-1 infection in brain still remains undefined (Cheng-Mayer et al., 1987).

Approximately 25 percent of patients develop progressively severe dementia associated with multinucleated cells and HIV-1 in brain. Thus the majority will clinically experience mild to moderate impairment with some or no progression and pathologically show mild abnormalities with no detectable HIV-1. The failure to detect virus in these patients could be explained by a level of expression too low for detection by the usual methods. The finding of nonproductive or latent HIV-1 infection in glial cells in vitro provides some support for this hypothesis (Chiodi et al., 1987; Popovic et al., 1988). Similarly, differences in the onset of dementia with respect to systemic infection also needs to be explained. Specifically, what accounts for the development of dementia as the earliest or only manifestation of HIV-1 infection in 10–15 percent of AIDS patients? Both host genetic factors contributing to susceptibility and differences in viral strains of HIV-1 may be implicated (Eales et al., 1987). Because HIV-1 is highly polymorphic, viral isolates may not only differ among individual patients, but also can be distinguished from each other on the basis of a number of biological properties, including the capacity to infect and replicate in different host cell lines and to cause cell lysis (Cheng-Mayer et al., 1988a,b). Recent reports of different HIV-1 isolates obtained from the neuroaxis of the same patient with differing cell tropism, cytopathology, and patterns of replication in culture provide support for the possible existence of neurotropic variants that may be partly responsible for the clinical and pathologic heterogeneity of ADC (Koyanagi et al., 1987). Additional supporting evidence includes findings that brain isolates may infect macrophages more efficiently than lymph node isolates and that such isolates also show a greater capacity to replicate in macrophages than in T cells and may be noncytocidal to T4 cells (Koyanagi et al., 1987; Cheng-Mayer and Levy, 1988; Anand, 1988). These results suggest that brain isolates from AIDS patients may represent subtypes of HIV-1; whether or not they are specific neurotropic variants, however, remains to be proved. Additional viral isolates need to characterized biologically and molecularly and correlated with various clinical and pathologic features of ADC. Further study of the genomic structure of these different isolates and comparison with other HIV-1 isolates should help determine if there are specific sequences, particularly in the env gene, responsible for differences in neurotropism and cytopathology.

The mechanisms of brain dysfunction in ADC remain similarly elusive, although various hypotheses have been postulated (Navia et al., 1986b; Price et al., 1988a,b). Given that productive HIV-1 infection is essentially restricted to the macrophage and that lysis or loss of specific brain-derived cells (e.g., neurons or atrocytes) is relatively absent in brains of patients with ADC, brain injury may result more from metabolic perturbations than from simple destruction of cells (Navia et al., 1986b; Price et al., 1988a). The observed discrepancy between the degree of clinical impairment and neuropathology noted in many patients, the majority of whom do not show HIV-1 in brain, also points to a primary metabolic basis for ADC. In this particular group nonproductive infection may be sufficient to disturb cellular function by interfering with either host transcriptional or translational events. Indirect evidence for a primary metabolic mechanism is based on studies of infection by murine leukemia virus, which show that the pathogenesis of polioencephalomyelopathy in mice is related to the accumulation of the viral external envelope glycoprotein gp70 (Gardner, 1988). The spongiform degeneration, characteristic of this disorder, may be mediated by binding of this molecule to a cellular receptor, resulting in either competition with a trophic factor or alteration of a specific physiological function.

Because the macrophage represents the most commonly infected cell in the brain, it is likely that it contributes importantly to the pathogenesis of ADC by either rescuing latently infected cells and thereby amplifying the rate of infection or by secreting either viral or cell coded products toxic to the surrounding tissue. It has been postulated that infected monocytes may release monokines e.g. tumor neurosis factor, or profeolyfic enzymes resulting in either cytofoxicity or changes in cellular physiology. Different lines of evidence indicate that the HIV-1 envelope glycoprotein gp120 may have the capacity to interfere with some aspect of either neuronal metabolism or physiology and thereby cause neuronal death (Brenneman et al., 1987; Pert et al., 1988). The problem with a neurotoxic hypothesis is that neuronal loss, although readily demonstrated in tissue culture, is not a major histological feature of ADC until late in its course (Navia et al., 1986b). It is more likely that HIV-1 infection through either direct or indirect mechanisms alters cellular metabolism (glial, neuronal or both) at a level that is noncytocidal but sufficient to disturb cellular and regional function. Clearly, additional studies are needed to define further the mechanisms of brain injury caused by HIV-1 infection.

Direct evidence for metabolic dysfunction in ADC has come recently from studies using position emission tomography and 18-flourodeoxy-glucose (Navia et al., 1987; Rottenberg et al., 1987). Initial studies suggested altered cerebral glucose metabolism in some patients; however, with the use of a novel analytic method termed *scaled subprofile model/factor analysis of variance*, Rottenberg and colleagues identified two distinct metabolic patterns that clearly differentiated ADC patients from normals (Rottenberg et al., 1987). Subcortical hypermetabolism was found in patients with mild or

early ADC and correlated with impairment of fine motor control on neuropsychological testing. With disease progression, a different pattern emerged consisting of cortical
and subcortical hypometabolism. A causal link to HIV-1 infection was shown in two
patients who developed severe ADC as their only clinical manifestation and were
found to have HIV-1 in brain by Southern blot analysis and immunohistochemistry.
Further, despite significant cortical and subcortical hypometabolism in both, the pathology predominantly involved subcortical structures, while the cortex appeared only
mildly affected. Four general conclusions are suggested by the above findings: (1)
subcortical dysfunction likely represents the initial or primary change at the regional
level; (2) disease progression correlates with alterations in subcortical and cortical
metabolism; (3) cortical dysfunction may be prominent in late ADC, although histologically few abnormalities are found; and (4) alterations in subcortical–cortical interactions may differentiate ADC patients from normals and underlie the major clinical
features of ADC.

   Further support for a metabolic basis of the dementia in ADC has come from a
recent study indicating impaired cholinergic transmission in ADC (Navia et al.,
1986c). Regional acetyl choline transferase (ACht) was significantly reduced in the
AIDS group, including nondemented patients compared with controls. This deficiency
generally paralleled the severity of ADC clinically and pathologically and the detection
of HIV-1 in brain. It is noteworthy that many of the patients with the lowest AChT
levels had ADC as the sole manifestation of HIV-1 infection. The basis and specificity
of these findings remain to be established but may be related to interruption of subcortical projections.

AIDS DEMENTIA COMPLEX: A MODEL FOR SUBCORTICAL DEMENTIA

The term *subcortical dementia* was initially introduced by Albert and colleagues in
describing the clinical features of a dementia associated with progressive supranuclear
palsy (Albert et al., 1974). Typically, these patients showed psychomotor retardation,
difficulty in manipulating acquired knowledge, personality change, and memory loss,
which reflected a pathologically slow recall more than a true amnesia. Substantial
controversy, however, has since centered around the validity of subcortical dementia
as a true clinical entity since it has been argued that dementia in these cases may reflect
associated cortical pathology (Whitehouse, 1986). The major clinical features of ADC
as discussed earlier are consistent with those of a subcortical dementia. Typical symptoms of cortical dysfunction such as aphasia, apraxia, or agnosia are absent until late
in the clinical course. These findings are reinforced by neuropsychological studies that
depict a distinct profile of impairment consisting of prominent slowing of cognitive
and motor function, loss of mental flexibility and spontaneity, and difficulty with sequential problem solving, while language function other than verbal fluency remains
relatively well preserved. The pathologic and virological studies demonstrate predominant involvement of subcortical regions. Regional cortical pathology with neuronal
loss characteristic of cortical dementias such Alzheimer's disease is not a prominent
histological finding in ADC. More recently, metabolic studies using position emission
tomography show that early cases of ADC are characterized by primary involvement
of subcortical structures. Although neuropsychological correlation with various met-

abolic indices indicates significant correlation with cortical regions, these are always associated with subcortical dysfunction either in the basal ganglia or thalamus (Rottenberg et al., 1987; Sidtis et al., 1989). Cortical dysfunction in ADC likely represents a secondary event following injury to subcortical regions. The sum of the cortical and subcortical components, however, is highly correlated with disease progression and severity of neuropsychological impairment (Rottenberg et al., 1988; Sidtis et al., 1989).

Disturbances in subcortical–cortical interactions may, therefore, contribute to cognitive, motor and behavioral impairment in ADC, particularly in its later stages. It has been suggested that ADC could be viewed as a disordered neural network encompassing these subcortical and cortical abnormalities (Sidtis et al., 1989). Further study of the behavioral and metabolic characteristics of ADC may therefore suggest mechanisms by which cognition may be impaired in the subcortical dementias. Indeed, such subcortical–cortical interactions may underlie the progression of cognitive dysfunction in these disorders.

ACKNOWLEDGMENT

Support for this chapter was provided by the Robert Wood Johnson Minority Medical Faculty Development Award.

REFERENCES

Albert, M.L., Feldman, R.G., and Willis, A.L. The "subcortical dementia" of progressive supranuclear palsy. *J Neurol Neurosurg Psychiatry* 1974; 41:874–9.

Anand, R. Natural variants of Human Immunodeficiency Virus from patients with neurological disorders do not kill T4 cells. *Ann Neurol* 1988; 23 (Suppl.):566–70.

Brenneman, D.E., et al. External envelope protein gp120 of HIV produces neuronal death in hippocampal cultures. *Soc Neurosci Abst* 1987. Abstract 137.1.

Britton, C.B., and Miller, J.R. Neurologic complications in acquired immunodeficiency syndrome (AIDS). *Neurol Clin* 1984; 2:315–39.

Carne, C.A., et al. Acute encephalopathy coincident with seroconversion for anti-HTLV-III. *Lancet* 1985; 1:1206–8.

Cheng-Mayer, C., and Levy, J.A. Distinct biological and serological properties of human immunodeficiency virus from brain. *Ann Neurol* 1988b; 23(Suppl.):558–61.

Cheng-Mayer, C. et al. Human immunodeficiency virus can productively infect cultured human glial cells. *Proc Natl Acad Sci USA* 1987; 84:3526–30.

Cheng-Mayer, C., et al. Biologic features of HIV-1 that correlate with virulence in the host. *Science* 1988a; 240:80–2.

Chiodi, F., et al. Infection of brain derived cells with the human immunodeficiency virus; *J Virol* 1987; 61:1244–7.

Cooper, D.A., et al. Acute AIDS retrovirus infection: definition of a clinical illness associated with seroconversion. *Lancet* 1985; 1:537–40.

Cummings, J.L., and Benson, D.F. Subcortical dementia–review of an emerging concept. *Arch Neurol* 1984; 41:874–9.

Dagleish, A.G., et al. The CD4 (T4) antigen is an essential component of the receptor for the AIDS retrovirus. *Nature* 1984; 312:763–7.

Daniel, M.D., et al. Isolation of T-cell tropic HILV-III-like retrovirus from Macaques. *Science* 1985; 228:1201–9.

de la Monte, S.M., et al. Subacute encephalomyelitis of AIDS and its relation to HTLVIII infection. *Neurology* 1987; 37:562–9.

Eales, J.J., et al. Association of different allelic forms of group specific component with susceptibility to and clinical manifestation of human immunodeficiency virus infection. *Lancet* 1987; 1:999–1002.

Epstein, L.G., et al. HTLV-III/LAV–like retrovirus particles in the brains of patients with AIDS encephalopathy. *AIDS Res* 1985; 1:447–54.

Gabuzda, D.H. et al. Immunohistochemical identification of HTLV-III antigen in brains of patients with AIDS. *Ann Neurol* 1986; 20:289–95.

Gardner, M.B. Neurotropic retroviruses of wild mice and macaques. *Ann Neurol* 1988; 23 (Suppl.):5201–6.

Gonda, M.A., et al. Sequence homology and morphologic similarity of HTLV-III and visna virus, a pathogenic lentivirus. *Science* 1985; 227:173–7.

Gonda, M.A., et al. HTLV-III shares sequence homology with a family of pathogenic lentiviruses. *Proc Natl Acad Sci USA* 1986; 83:4007–11.

Goudsmit, J., et al. Expression of human immunodeficiency virus antigen (HIV-Ag) in serum and cerebrospinal fluid during acute and chronic infection. *Lancet* 1986a; 2:177–80.

Goudsmit, J., et al. Intrathecal synthesis of antibodies to HTLV-III in patients without AIDS or AIDS-related complex. *Br Med J* 1986b; 292:1231–4.

Grant, I., et al. Evidence for early central nervous system involvement in the acquired immune deficiency syndrome (AIDS) and other human immunodeficiency virus (HIV) infections. *Ann Intern Med* 1987; 107:828–36.

Haase, A.T. Pathogenesis of lentivirus infections. *Nature* 1986; 322:130–6.

Hahn, B.H., et al. Genomic diversity of the acquired immune deficiency syndrome virus HTLV-III: different viruses exhibit greatest divergence in their envelope genes. *Proc Natl Acad Sci USA* 1985; 82:4813–7.

Hahn, B.H., et al. Genetic variation in HTLV-III/LAV over time in patients with AIDS or at risk for AIDS. *Science* 1986; 232:1548–53.

Harouse, J.M., et al. Human choroid plexus cells can be latently infected with human immunodeficiency virus. *Ann Neurol* 1989; 25:406–11.

Ho, D.D., et al. Isolation of HTLV-III from cerebrospinal fluid and neural tissue of patients with neurologic syndromes related to the acquired immunodeficiency syndrome. *N Engl J Med* 1985; 313:1493–7.

Kanki, P.J., et al. Serologic identification and characterization of macaque T-lymphotropic retrovirus closely related to HLTV-III. *Science* 1985; 228:1199–201.

Klatzman, D., et al. T-lymphocytes T4 molecule behaves as the receptor for the human retrovirus LAV. *Nature* 1984; 12:767–68.

Koenig, S., et al. Detection of AIDS virus in macrophages in brain tissue from AIDS patients with encephalopathy. *Science* 1986; 233:1089–93.

Koyanagi, Y., et al. Dual infection of the central nervous system by AIDS viruses with distinct cellular tropism. *Science* 1987; 236:819–22.

Letvin, N.L., et al. Induction of AIDS-like disease in macaque monkeys with T-cell tropic retrovirus STLV-III. *Science* 1985; 230:71–3.

Levy, J.A., et al. Isolation of AIDS-associated retroviruses from cerebrospinal fluid and brain of patients with neurological symptoms. *Lancet* 1985; 2:586–8.

Levy, J.K., et al. Verbal memory disturbance associated with HIV infection. *J Clin Exp Neuropsychol* 1987; 9:45.

Levy, R.M., et al. Neurological manifestations of the acquired immunodeficiency syndrome

(AIDS): experience at VCSF and review of the literature. *J Neurosurg* 1985; 62:475–95.

Maddon, P.J., et al. The T4 gene encodes the AIDS virus receptor and is expressed in the immune system and the brain. *Cell* 1986; 47:333–48.

McArthur, J.C., et al. Cerebrospinal fluid abnormalities in homosexual men with and without neuropsychiatric findings. *Ann Neurol* 1988; 23 (Suppl.):534–7.

Navia, B.A., Jordan, B.D., and Price, R.W. The AIDS dementia complex. I. Clinical features. *Ann Neurol* 1986a; 19:517–24.

Navia, B.A., et al. The AIDS dementia complex. II. Neuropathology. *Ann Neurol* 1986b; 19:525–35.

Navia, B.A., et al. Choline acetyltransferase activity is reduced in the AIDS dementia complex. *Ann Neurol* 1986c (Abstr.); 20:142.

Navia, B.A., and Price, R.W. The acquired immunodeficiency syndrome dementia complex as the presenting or sole manifestation of human immunodeficiency virus infection. *Arch Neurol* 1987; 44:65–9.

Navia, B.A., et al. Metabolic anatomy of the AIDS dementia complex. *J Cereb Blood Flow Metab.* 1987 (Abstr.).

Nielsen, S.L., et al. Subacute encephalitis in acquired immune deficiency syndrome: a post-mortem study. *Am J Clin Pathol* 1984; 82:678–82.

Ornitz, D., et al. Scales for the neurological examination and history in the AIDS dementia complex. Presented at the III International Conference on AIDS, Washington, DC, June 1–5, 1987.

Pert, C.B., et al. AIDS and its dementia as a neuropeptide disorder: role of VIP receptor blockade by human immunodeficiency virus envelope. *Ann Neurol* 1988; 23 (Suppl.):571–3.

Petito, C.K., et al. Vacuolar myelopathy pathologically resembling subacute combined degeneration in patients with acquired immunodeficiency syndrome (AIDS). *N Engl J Med* 1985; 312:874–9.

Petito, C.K., et al. Neuropathology of acquired immunodeficiency syndrome (AIDS): an autopsy review. *J Neuropathol Exp Neurol* 1986; 45:635–46.

Popovic, M., et al. Role of mononuclear phagocytes and accessory cells in human immunodeficiency virus type 1 infection of the brain. *Ann Neurol* 1988; 23 (Suppl.):574–7.

Price, R.W., et al. The AIDS dementia complex: Some current questions. *Ann Neurol* 1988c; 23 (Suppl.):527–33.

Price, R.W., et al. The brain in AIDS: Central Nervous System HIV-1 infection and AIDS dementia complex. *Science* 1988a; 239:586–92.

Price, R.W., et al. The AIDS dementia complex. In *AIDS and the Nervous System*. Rosenblum, M.L., et al. (ed.). Raven Press, New York, 1988b.

Price, R.W., Navia, B.A., and Cho, E.-S. AIDS encephalopathy. *Neurol Clin* 1986; 4:285–301.

Pumarole-Sune, T. et al. HIV antigen in the brains of patients with the AIDS dementia complex. *Ann Neurol* 1987; 21:490–6.

Resnick, L., et al. Intra-blood-brain-barrier synthesis of HTLV-III-specific IgG in patients with neurologic symptoms associated with AIDS or AIDS-related complex. *N Engl J Med* 1985; 313:1498–504.

Ringler, D.T., et al. Simian immunodeficiency virus-induced meningoencepholitis: natural history and retrospective study. *Ann Neurol* 1988; 23 (Suppl.):5101–7.

Rottenberg, D.A., et al. The metabolic pathology of the AIDS dementia complex. *Ann Neurol* 1987; 22:700–6.

Rubinow, D.R., et al. Neuropsychiatric consequences of AIDS. *Ann Neurol* 1988; 23 (Suppl.):524–6.

Saykin, A.J., et al. Cognitive and motor deficits in AIDS-related complex. *J Clin Exp Neuropsychol* 1987; 9:45.

Shaw, G.M., et al. HTLV-III infection in brains of children and adults with AIDS encephalopathy. *Science* 1985; 227:177–82.

Sidtis, J.J., et al. The brief neuropsychological examination for AIDS dementia complex: correlation with functional status scales and other neuropsychological tests. Presented at the III International Conference on AIDS, Washington, DC, June 1–5, 1987.

Sidtis, J., et al. Neuropsychological correlates of subcortical and cortical metabolism in the AIDS dementia complex. Unpublished.

Snider, W.D., et al. Neurological complications of acquired immune deficiency syndrome: analysis of 50 patients. *Ann Neurol* 1983; 14:403–18.

Stoler, M.H., et al. Human T-cell lymphotropic virus type III infection of the central nervous system—a preliminary *in situ* analysis. *JAMA* 1986; 256:2360–4.

Tross, S., et al. Neuropsychological characterization of the AIDS dementia complex: A preliminary report. *AIDS Res* 1988; 2:81–8.

Vazeux, R., et al. AIDS subacute encephalitis; identification of HIV infected cells. *Am J Pathol* 1987; 126:403–10.

Vinters, H.V., et al. Cytomegalovirus in the nervous system of patients with the acquired immune deficiency syndrome. *Brain* 1989; 112:245–68.

Whitehouse, P.J. The concept of subcortical and cortical dementia: another look. *Ann Neurol* 1986; 19:1981–6.

Wiley, C.A., et al. Cellular localization of human immunodeficiency virus infection within the brains of acquired immune deficiency syndrome patients. *Proc Natl Acad Sci USA* 1986; 83:7089–93.

Wiley, C.A. and Nelson, I.A. Role of human immunodeficiency virus and cytomegalovirus in AIDS encephalitis. *Am J Pathol* 1988; 133:73–81.

14

Rare Acquired and Degenerative Subcortical Dementias

DANIEL B. HIER AND JEFFREY L. CUMMINGS

Several unusual acquired disorders such as inflammatory and granulomatous diseases as well as rare degenerative dementias such as Wilson's disease, spinocerebellar degenerations, and Fahr's disease have been reported to produce subcortical dementia syndromes. Too few of these cases have been studied or too little attention paid to the characteristics of the mental status changes to give a comprehensive description of the associated dementia syndromes. Nevertheless, preliminary information is available, and tentative inclusion of these cases in a volume reviewing the syndromes of subcortical dementia is warranted to demonstrate the variety of diseases in which subcortical dementia occurs.

SARCOIDOSIS

Clinical Features

Sarcoidosis is an inflammatory disorder of unknown cause. Histopathologically, the disease is characterized by the formation of multiple noncaseating granulomas. In about 3–10 percent of sarcoidosis cases, the nervous system is involved (Delaney, 1977; James and Williams, 1985). Granulomas may affect the peripheral or cranial nerves, brain, spinal cord, or meninges (Colover, 1948).

The mortality rate of neurosarcoidosis is about 10 percent. The chest is involved in 82 percent of neurosarcoidosis cases and the eye in 58 percent of cases. Patients with sarcoidosis limited to the central nervous system have been reported (James and Williams, 1985).

Presentations of neurosarcoidosis include polyneuropathy, mononeuritis, seizures, hydrocephalus, hypopituitarism, diabetes insipidus, meningitis, encephalopathy, and dementia. Involvement of peripheral and cranial nerves is common; facial nerve palsy has been reported in up to 50 percent of cases (Schonell et al., 1968). Occasionally, sarcoid may present as a mass lesion (Griggs et al., 1973), and sarcoid infiltration of the meninges may produce adhesive arachnoiditis and hydrocephalus. Whelan and Stern (1980) described a sarcoid granuloma presenting as a mass in the posterior fossa with hydrocephalus. Sarcoid may involve the diencephalic areas of the brain, including the hypothalamus, optic chiasm, pituitary gland, and juxtasellar region (Chiang et al., 1984; Weisberg and Jacobs, 1984). With hypothalamic and pituitary involvement, endocrine abnormalities, including amenorrhea, impotence, and pituitary insufficiency, may occur. Hypothalamic dysfunction may result in diabetes insipidus, altered temperature regulation, or lethargy. Visual and hearing loss may occur with granulomatous involvement of the optic and acoustico-vestibular nerves (Babin et al., 1984; Slavin and Glaser, 1983).

The cerebrospinal fluid (CSF) is almost uniformly abnormal in neurosarcoidosis, and a completely normal CSF examination probably excludes the diagnosis (Cordingley, 1981). Common abnormalities include a lymphocytic pleocytosis (reported range 8–1600 per mm^3) and an elevated protein (reported range 46–860 mg/dl). Less commonly the glucose may be decreased.

Neuropathology

The main neuropathologic change in sarcoidosis is infiltration of the brain, spinal cord, and meninges with microscopic granulomata. In patients with basilar meningitis, the meninges are infiltrated with lymphocytes and microscopic granulomata. Hydrocephalus may result from either adhesive arachnoiditis or obstruction of the aqueduct or fourth ventricle. Mass lesions due to giant granulomas in the brain or brain stem are rare. Delaney (1977) found 20 case reports of mass lesions due to sarcoidosis. The third ventricular region (including hypothalamus and pituitary gland) is a common site of cerebral involvement in neurosarcoidosis. These diencephalic lesions are critical to the development of subcortical dementia in neurosarcoidosis.

Dementia Syndrome

A variety of neuropsychiatric impairments may complicate neurosarcoidosis, including delirium, dementia, psychosis, and personality change (Stoudemire et al., 1983). Cordingley et al. (1981) reviewed the literature and found 35 cases of dementia with preserved alterness due to neurosarcoidosis. Men outnumbered women two to one. The median age was 36, with a range of 15–66 years. Findings were variable and included memory loss (all cases), poor concentration (11), hallucinations (4), euphoria, delusions, apathy, depression, aggressiveness, disorientation, and dyscalculia. In 10 of the 35 patients, the sarcoidosis appeared to be limited to the nervous system.

Camp and Frierson (1962) reported autopsy findings in a young man with widespread sarcoidosis affecting the brain, spinal cord, and meninges. Dementia, visual loss, memory impairment, and also diabetes insipidus were noted.

The patient reported by Cordingley et al. (1981) had a dementia syndrome characterized as "a nearly pure memory loss and mild anomia." Dementia in their case was due to a widespread meningitis and ependymitis due to sarcoidosis with associated hydrocephalus. Hydrocephalus appears to be the mechanism of dementia in several of the cases of neurosarcoidosis with intellectual deterioration (Ho et al., 1979). The hydrocephalus may be either the communicating type related to basilar meningitis and adhesive arachnoiditis or a noncommunicating type related to blockage by granuloma of either the aqueduct or fourth ventricle.

Thompson and Checkley (1981) reported a case of neurosarcoidosis with dementia and memory impairment. The Wechsler Adult Intelligence Scale Full Scale IQ in their patient was 78. A marked impairment was noted on the logical memory subtest of the Wechsler Memory Scale. They speculated that the memory loss and dementia in their patient were due to basilar meningitis with limbic system involvement.

Hier et al. (1983) reported an autopsied case of neurosarcoidosis of the fornices and hypothalamus with subcortical dementia (see the following discussion). They speculated that the involvement of subcortical structures critical to memory (especially the fornices and hypothalamus) produced the picture of subcortical dementia.

Case Report

A 40-year-old, right-handed black man was admitted for evaluation of dysarthria, apathy, hearing loss, and amnesia. Past medical history was significant for sickle-cell hemoglobinopathy, malaise, arthralgias, arthralgias, aseptic necrosis of both femoral heads, decreased libido, and panhypopituitarism.

On examination, the patient was apathetic, with little spontaneity of speech or movement. Insight was preserved; memory, calculations, and attention were impaired. Speech was fluent with normal grammatical structure, and repetition of short phrases and naming of objects were intact. Psychometric testing showed relatively intact vocabulary, fund of knowledge, and orientation. Short-term memory, new learning ability, and visuospatial skills were impaired. Lumbar puncture revealed a CSF protein of 282 mg/dl, a CSF glucose of 34 mg/dl, and a cell count of 198 white cells (96 percent lymphocytes). An electroencephalogram showed mild generalized slowing. A computerized tomography (CT) scan of the brain and a cerebral angiogram were normal. A radionuclide brain scan was consistent with a diffuse inflammatory process. His mental function gradually improved, and he was subsequently discharged on thyroid and cortisone replacement therapy. There were subsequent fluctuations in his mental abilities. 3 months later he was readmitted for a massive fat embolism to the lungs due to extensive bone necrosis, and he died.

Psychometric Testing

The patient was examined four times in the 2 months prior to his death. His Wechsler Memory Scale MQ fluctuated between 63 and 105. Performance on the Current Information, Orientation, and Mental Control subtests was relatively normal. Severe deficits were noted on the Digit Span, Logical Memory, Visual Reproduction, and Paired Associates subtests. On the Wechsler Adult Intelligence Scale he performed relatively normally on the Information and Vocabulary subtests but poorly on the Picture Completion and Block Design subtests. The overall pattern was consistent with a subcortical dementia.

Neuropathologic Findings

The brain weighed 1200 g. The meninges were opaque and milky in the interpeduncular fossa and at the base of the brain. Multiple tiny white plaques were seen along the walls of the blood vessels. The infundibulum and the hypothalamus were markedly enlarged, tan, and granular in appearance. Serial coronal sections of the brain revealed

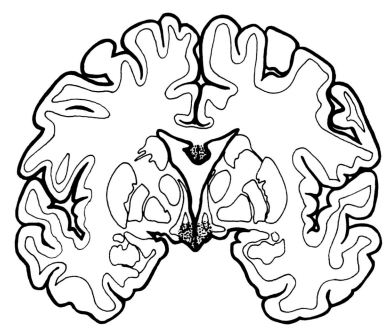

Figure 14-1   Diagram of distribution of sarcoid-related granulomatous changes with lymphocytic proliferation in the hypothalamic region.

an enlarged granular hypothalamus and infundibulum associated with enlargement and granularity of the columns of the fornix. The white matter showed a few petechiae. No other grossly visible granulomata were identified elsewhere in the brain. The ventricles were of normal size. Histologically, the fornix, the hypothalami, and the infundibulum were replaced by noncaseating epithelioid granulomas associated with marked lymphocytic proliferation (Figure 14-1). Cultures and the special stains were negative for bacteria or fungi. Microscopic granulomas were present in the mesial temporal lobes, mamillary bodies, basal ganglia, and occasionally in the outer cortex. In addition, the meninges showed many perivascular granulomas, especially at the base of the brain.

Comment

Pathologically, the sarcoid involved predominantly subcortical structures, including the fornices and hypothalamus. The dementia in this patient had many of the characteristics of subcortical dementia, such as preserved language, impaired memory, preserved insight and orientation, mental slowness, impaired concentration, decreased attention, and apathy.

Treatment

Treatment of neurosarcoidosis remains unsatisfactory, and curative therapy is unavailable. Spontaneous remissions occur in some patients. Regression of mass lesions with corticosteroid therapy has been reported (Griggs et al., 1973). Based on a literature review, Cordingley et al. (1981) reported that 10 of 12 patients with neurosarcoidosis receiving corticosteroids improved at least temporarily. Delaney (1977) reported a favorable response to corticosteroids in 5 of 12 patients with neurosarcoidosis and a transient response in 4 of 12 patients. Neurosurgery is occasionally needed for mass lesions or hydrocephalus that does not respond to corticosteroid therapy. The use of immunosuppressant drugs such as azothioprine and cyclosporine for neurosarcoidosis is under investigation (James and Williams, 1985).

BEHCET'S DISEASE

Clinical Features

The Turkish dermatologist Hulusi Behcet first described Behcet's disease in 1937 as a triad of recurrent oral aphthous ulcers, genital ulcers, and iritis. Other commonly associated features of the disease include arthritis, thrombophlebitis, erythema nodosum, and meningoencephalitis. Jorizzo (1987) suggested that the diagnosis is likely when at least three of six major criteria are present: aphthous stomatitis, aphthous genital ulceration, uveitis, cutaneous pustular vasculitis, synovitis, and meningoencephalitis. The disease is most common in Japan and the eastern Mediterranean region and less common in Europe and the United States.

Neurologic involvement (neuro-Behcet's disease) occurs in approximately 10 percent of patients with Behcet's disease. Kawakita et al. (1967) reviewed 85 previously reported cases of Behcet's disease with neurologic complications and estimated the incidence of neurologic involvement in Behcet's disease as 3–27 percent. In patients with neurologic involvement, the age of onset varies from 20 to 51 years, with a mean age of onset of 33 years. Common neurological findings include headache (52 percent), dysarthria (29 percent), nystagmus (19 percent), ataxia (16 percent), diplopia (19 percent), dysphagia (13 percent), and seizures (13 percent). Approximately 50 percent of patients exhibit impairment of intellectual function, including impaired memory or dementia (Shimizu, 1979).

Neuro-Behcet's disease may present as either a meningoencephalitis, a brain-stem syndrome, or an acute dementia (Pallis and Fudge, 1956). The meningitic presentation may be confused with other rare forms of meningitis, including Harada's disease and Vogt–Koyanagi syndrome. The dementia presentation of neuro-Behcet syndrome may simulate the onset of general paresis, whereas the brain-stem presentation of neuro-Behcet disorder may be confused with multiple sclerosis (Alema and Bignami, 1966). In cases of Behcet's syndrome with neurologic involvement, the spinal fluid is usually abnormal, even when neurologic findings are few (Alema and Bignami, 1966). The most common abnormality is a pleocytosis (4–5,000 cells/mm^3).

Neuropathology

Pathologic involvement of the brain in Behcet's disease is characterized by lymphocytic cuffing of vessels, focal and diffuse gliosis, and areas of necrosis and demyelination (Norman and Campbell, 1966). Topographically involvement is usually confined to the upper brain-stem, hypothalamus, basal ganglia, and internal capsule.

There is some debate as to whether the origin of focal necrosis within the brain is due to inflammation or vascular occlusion (Norman and Campbell, 1966). The cerebral cortex and cerebellum are usually spared (Alema and Bignami, 1966). It is this predilection of Behcet's disease to involve subcortical structures that may lead to the subcortical dementia observed in some affected patients. In addition to these areas of necrosis and demyelination, Behcet's disease often produces an aseptic meningitis that is associated with a lymphocytic infiltration of the meninges and a lymphocytic pleocytosis of the CSF.

Neuroradiology

The most common findings on CT in neuro-Behcet's disease are low-density parenchymal lesions, usually in the brain stem or basal ganglia. These lesions usually show homogeneous enhancement with contrast infusion (Dobkin, 1980; Kozin et al., 1977; Kuroiwa et al., 1986; Weitz et al., 1986; Weilleit et al., 1986). Magnetic resonance imaging (MRI) appears to be a highly sensitive technique for detecting the brain lesions of neuro-Behcet's disease. Generally, high-intensity signals are detected on the $T2$ weighted images. These high-intensity signals may correspond to areas of gliosis, inflammation, or demyelination. Lesions are most likely to be detected in the brain stem, basal ganglia, thalamus, and internal capsule consistent with the hypothesis that neuro-Behcet's disease can be a cause of subcortical dementia.

Dementia Syndrome

Although cognitive impairment is frequent in neuro-Behcet's disease (about 50 percent of cases), the dementia has not been analyzed in detail. Shimizu (1979) reported dementia in 12 of 31 cases of neuro-Behcet's disease. Other symptoms in the 31 patients included memory impairment (49 percent), depression (39 percent), irritability (26 percent), hallucinations (26 percent), euphoria (19 percent), apathy (19 percent), and delusions (16 percent). We have recently seen a patient with neuro-Behcet's disease with prominent involvement of the subcortical structures. Her pattern of cognitive impairment was consistent with a subcortical dementia.

Case Report

A 29-year-old woman presented with a 6-month history of progressive neurologic dysfunction that included blurred vision, diplopia, and headaches. Two months earlier, she had experienced episodes of dysarthria. Subsequently, she noted generalized malaise, occasional light-headedness, and weakness of the left arm and leg. On admission, neurologic examination demonstrated dysarthria, bilateral internuclear ophthalmoplegia, bilateral dysmetria, bilateral dysdiadochokinesia, and a wide-based gait. Ulcerated lesions were noted in the oral mucosa. Cerebrospinal fluid examination showed 121 WBCs/mm³ (74 percent lymphocytes) and protein elevated to 60 mg/dl. Contrast-enhanced CT scans showed an enhancing midbrain lesion. The patient was started on high-dose corticosteroids, and her symptoms resolved. Five months later she was readmitted with recurrent headaches, high fever, and ulcers of the vulvar mucosa. Vulvar biopsy showed nonspecific inflammation. The genital ulcers, in conjunction with her

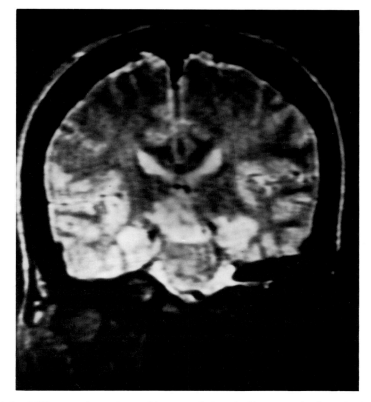

Figure 14-2   MRI scan of a patient with neuro-Behcet's disease and subcortical dementia. Note high signal areas in the midbrain and hypothalamus.

past oral ulcers and recurrent neurologic dysfunction, suggested a diagnosis of Behcet's disease. Three years later, she experienced an exacerbation of her disease characterized by high fever, memory impairment, dementia, and headaches. There were no focal neurologic signs. An MRI scan was obtained with multiple spin-echo sequences using $T1$, $T2$, and proton density weighting in multiple planes. Discrete areas of abnormally high signal intensity, most prominent on $T2$-weighted images, appeared in the midbrain and hypothalamus (Figure 14-2). MRI and clinical findings were consistent with neuro-Behcet's disease with involvement of the midbrain, hypothalamus, and thalamus. The headache and fever resolved with high-dose corticosteroid therapy; however, memory impairment and dementia persisted.

Psychometric testing

The patient had a Verbal IQ of 68, a Performance IQ of 60, and a Full Scale IQ of 62. Scores on the Digit Span, Orientation, and Personal Information subtests of the Wechsler Memory Scale were normal. The Visual Reproduction and Logical Memory subtests showed a marked impairment in new learning ability and also in recent memory, as noted on the Rey Auditory Verbal Learning Test. Speech was fluent but dysarthric, and the score fell within the normal range on the Token Test. Overall test performance was characterized by slow and inefficient cognitive processing, poor problem solving and reasoning skill, impaired visuospatial skills, and markedly impaired new learning ability. Language skills, including comprehension and repetition, were largely preserved, although anomia was noted on visual confrontation naming.

Comment

Behcet's disease has a special predilection for involvement of subcortical structures including the hypothalamus, thalamus, and basal ganglia. By MRI and CT criteria this patient had lesions largely confined to these subcortical structures, and intellectual impairment was consistent with a pattern of subcortical dementia (defective memory and reasoning in the setting of relatively preserved insight, orientation, and language).

Treatment

Therapy for this condition remains controversial. Most cases of neuro-Behcet's disease are treated first with corticosteroids, and neurologic symptoms and signs generally regress rapidly on high-dose oral therapy. Systemic corticosteroids are usually effective in suppressing acute exacerbations, but their effect on long-term outcome is less certain. Recurrences may be frequent when corticosteroids are discontinued.

Long-term therapy of neuro-Behcet's disease is problematic, since the hazards of chronic corticosteroid therapy are well established. Some authorities recommend immunosuppressive therapy with either cyclophosphamide, azothioprine, chlorambucil, or cyclosporine. However, the effectiveness and safety of these more aggressive therapies are unproved (Jorizzo, 1987).

WILSON'S DISEASE

Wilson's disease is an autosomal recessive genetic condition in which an absence of the copper-carrying protein ceruloplasmin leads to excessive copper deposition in body tissues, particularly the liver, cornea, and basal ganglia (Scheinberg and Sternlieb, 1984). It has a prevalence of roughly 1 in 200,000 members of the population.

The disease was first described by Samuel Alexander Kinnier Wilson in 1912 in Great Britain and has since been observed in virtually every country of the world. Wilson used the name *progressive lenticular degeneration* for the condition, emphasizing the neurologic aspects of the disorder, although he also observed the accompanying cirrhosis of the liver. Involvement of other organ systems was described over the following several decades, and a biochemical assay capable of identifying the diminished level of serum ceroplasmin was developed in 1952 (Scheinberg and Sternlieb, 1984).

Clinical Features

Wilson's disease typically becomes evident between the ages of 12 and 32 years and is equally common in males and females. The most common presentation of Wilson's disease is with signs of neurologic dysfunction, including temor, poor coordination, dystonia, rigidity, micrographia, or gait abnormalities (Cartwright, 1978; Starosta-Rubenstein et al., 1987). Signs of impairment of bulbar function are common and may be evident as dysarthria, dysphagia, or hypophonia. As the disease progresses, bulbar signs, dystonia, tremor, and evidence of cerebellar involvement are the principal clinical manifestations.

In addition to the neurologic findings, Wilson's disease may produce chronic hepatitis or hemolytic anemia. Proximal renal tubular reabsorption is abnormal in most cases, leading to aminoaciduria, peptiduria, glucosuria, urisocuria, and phosphaturia. The loss of phosphate in the urine eventually leads to phosphatemia and bone disease with osteoporosis and pseudofractures (Cartwright, 1978). Kayser–Fleischer rings, consisting of brown or green discolorations near the limbus of the cornea, are present in nearly all patients with neurologic manifestations of Wilson's disease and a substantial proportion of those with other presentations.

CT scans in Wilson's disease demonstrate ventricular enlargement and cerebral cortical atrophy in a majority of cases. In addition, approximately one half of the patients have brain-stem atrophy and hypodense areas in the region of the basal ganglia, particularly the putamen. Nearly all patients with neurologic dysfunction have basal ganglia abnormalities as seen on CT scans (Williams and Walshe, 1981). MRI is more sensitive than CT to the brain abnormalities; $T2$-weighted images demonstrate bilaterally symmetric areas of increased signal in the lenticular nuclei, caudate nuclei, thalami, dentate nuclei, and brain stem (Aisen et al., 1985).

The diagnosis of Wilson's disease in a patient presenting with neurologic dysfunction depends on slit-lamp examination and assessment of copper metabolism. Slit-lamp studies reveal Kayser–Fleischer rings in the great majority of cases, and laboratory studies will demonstrate a serum ceruloplasmin level of less than 20 mg/dl, a 24-hour copper excretion of more than 100 mg, or a very low rate of incorporation of radio-copper into ceruloplasmin. In some cases liver biopsy may be necessary and will reveal a hepatic copper concentration of greater than 250 mcg per g of dry weight (Scheinberg and Sternlieb, 1984).

Dementia Syndrome

Wilson noted the presence of mental status changes in the patients he studied and could be credited with the first description of subcortical dementia. Although descriptions of dementia in Parkinson's disease and Huntington's disease preceded the discovery of Wilson's disease, in neither case was the disease known to be associated with pathology of the basal ganglia. Wilson was the first to ascribe the presence of a movement disorder to basal ganglia dysfunction. He also noted that the patients were facile, docile, and childish and exhibited mental status changes that could be readily distinguished from senile dementia, dementia paralytica, and dementia praecox. He observed that the mental condition resembled that of Huntington's disease. He doubted that the word *dementia* was appropriate, since the patients lacked apraxia and agnosia and suggested the phrase "narrowing of the mental horizons" to describe their intellectual decline.

There have been few studies of the mental status changes of Wilson's disease. Dening (1985) noted that the observed behavioral changes could usefully be divided into four types: affective, behavioral–personality, schizophrenia-like, and cognitive. The categories are not mutually exclusive and commonly co-occur. The mood changes may be depressive or mixed manic–depressive in quality. The behavioral features commonly manifested include aggressive, childish, and self-destructive or antisocial acts and schizoid, hysterical, or sociopathic personality traits. Psychosis is the least common of the major neuropsychiatric manifestations but probably occurs more frequently than expected in the general population.

Intellectual deterioration in Wilson's disease is mild in degree, and the pattern of deficits resembles that seen in other subcortical dementias. Knehr and Bearn (1956) were among the first to administer formal neuropsychological tests to patients with Wilson's disease. They studied seven patients and found that vocabulary skills were preserved but abstraction abilities as assessed with the Progressive Matrices Tests were impaired. Goldstein et al. (1968) examined 22 patients with Wilson's disease before and after treatment. They noted improvement after therapy in the Wechsler Adult Intelligence Scale subtests involving Information, Comprehension, Similarities, and Block Design. Similarly, scores on the Wechsler Memory Scale also improved. Davis and Goldstein (1974) found significant differences between pretreatment Wilson's disease patients and normal controls on the Verbal IQ, Trails A and B, and several tests dependent on precision of motor performance. Recently, Medalia and co-workers (1988) used a more extensive neuropsychological test battery and compared 19 patients with neurologically symptomatic Wilson's disease, 12 patients with asymptomatic disease, and 15 normal controls. Differences between the three groups (with the symptomatic patients being most impaired) were documented for the Performance IQ, Full Scale IQ, Wechsler Memory Scale, Mattis Dementia Rating Scale, Trails A, and Trails B. There were no differences for Verbal IQ, Boston Naming Test, Animal Naming, or Wisconsin Card Sorting Test. Together these few studies indicate that the patients have memory, cognitive, and behavioral abnormalities consistent with subcortical dementia. Their language skills are largely spared, as noted in most subcortical dementia syndromes.

Neuropathology

The external appearance of the brain is usually normal, although in some cases gross atrophy and loss of hemispheric white matter is apparent. Cavitary necrosis of the putamena is obvious on coronal sections. The external capsule and claustrum are also involved, and the caudate and the globus pallidus show limited changes. Atrophy of the brain stem and dentate nuclei of the cerebellum may be severe. Microscopically, the changes range from severe cavitation and liquification to mild astrogliosis. In involved areas there is marked proliferation of protoplasmic astrocytes, and Opalski cells are seen in the margins of affected regions (Scheinberg and Sternlieb, 1984).

Treatment

The principal agent used in the treatment of Wilson's disease is penicillamine. Patients receive 1 g/day in divided doses between meals and continue therapy for life (Scheinberg and Sternlieb, 1984). Pyridoxine (25 mg daily) must be coadministered to combat the antipyridozine effects of penicillamine. Ancillary treatment measures include decreasing copper intake by limitation of copper-containing foods in the diet (liver, chocolate, cocoa, nuts, mushrooms, molasses, dried peas, broccoli, shellfish) and prevention of copper absorption in the gastrointestinal tract by administration of potassium sulfide (20 mg twice daily after meals) (Barbeau, 1981). Neurologic symptoms improve with long-term therapy and, as noted above, the dementia syndrome also responds to treatment (Goldstein et al., 1968).

Comment

The dementia syndrome of Wilson's disease is among the preventable and treatable subcortical dementia syndromes. In addition, it was the earliest dementia syndrome recognized in a disorder known to be related to pathologic changes in the basal ganglia. The severity of the dementia is relatively limited, as expected in a disease having its primary effect on the putamen. The principal connections to the putamen arise from the motor cortex, whereas prefrontal fibers mediating cognitive abilities project primarily to the caudate nuclei (Kish et al., 1988). The neuropsychological characteristics of the dementia are similar to those of other subcortical dementias described in this volume. The mood alterations and personality changes accompanying the dementia of Wilson's disease are also common in other subcortical dementia syndromes.

ATAXIC SYNDROMES AND SPINOCEREBELLAR DEGENERATION

The ataxic syndromes and spinocerebellar degeneration are a heterogeneous group of disorders that continue to defy coherent classification. An expanding number can be ascribed to definable biochemical deficits, and the inheritance patterns are being delineated with increasing precision. Progressive and intermittent ataxic disorders are encompassed within the group, and there are both childhood- and adult-onset forms. The mental status changes accompanying the syndromes have been either completely ignored or inadequately characterized. In this brief section, the clinical and pathologic aspects of progressive adult-onset spinocerebellar degeneration with documented intellectual alterations will be summarized.

Clinical Features

A classification of progressive adult-onset ataxias is presented in Table 14-1. This classification is adapted from Currier (1984) and emphasizes the neuropathologic heterogeneity of the ataxias. It also incorporates a separation between common and rare types of ataxia and between those with and without extra-cerebellar and extra–central nervous system features. In all cases, the syndrome is gradually progressive and is dominated by signs of cerebellar dysfunction, including ataxic gait, intention tremor, dysdiadochokinesia, past-pointing, loss of rebound checking abilities, titubation, and dysarthria. Primary forms of ataxia produced by degenerative or inherited biochemical disturbances must be distinguished from acquired ataxic syndromes secondary to toxins (e.g., mercury, phenytoin, alcohol), remote effects of carcinoma, multiple sclerosis, trauma, hypothyroidism, and malabsorption syndromes with vitamin E deficiency.

Evaluation of patients with primary spinocerebellar degeneration reveals evidence of cerebellar degeneration on CT or MRI scans (Figure 14-3). EEG studies may dem-

Table 14-1   Classification of Progressive Adult-Onset Ataxias[a]

Primary
  Common forms
    Autosomal dominant
      Adult onset (20–50 years old)
        "Pure" cerebellar type
          With decreased reflexes
          With extrapyramidal signs
          With spastic ataxia
      Old-age onset (> 50 years old)
    Recessive inheritance
      Adult onset (20–50 years old)
        With increased reflexes
        With decreased reflexes
      Old-age onset (> 50 years old)
        GDH[b] deficiency
  Rare forms (dominant, x-linked, or recessive inheritance)
    Neuropathologic variants
      Spinocerebellar degeneration
      Posterior column involvement
      Cerebello-olivary degeneration
      Anterior horn cell and peripheral nerve involvement
      Cerebral cortical involvement
      Others
    With sense organ abnormality
        Ocular: retina, optic never, extraocular muscles
        Ear: deafness

Secondary
  Remote effects or systemic carcinoma
  Multiple sclerosis
  Hypothyroidism
  Trauma
  Toxic
  Malabsorption with vitamin E deficiency

[a]Based on Classification of Currier, 1984.
[b]GDH, glutamate dehydrogenase.

onstrate nonspecific slowing in the theta range. Fluorodeoxyglucose positron emission tomography (PET) studies of patients with olivopontocerebellar degeneration reveal diminished metabolic activity in the cerebellar hemispheres, cerebellar vermis, and brain stem (Gilman et al., 1988).

Treatment for the degenerative ataxic syndromes is not yet available.

Neuropathology

The diversity of locations of degenerative changes in the brains of patients with progressive ataxic syndromes mirrors the clinical heterogeneity of the disorders. In most of the diseases, there is marked involvement of the cerebellum with loss of Purkinje cells, atrophy of the inferior olivary and pontine nuclei, and pallor of the cerebellar white matter. Torpedoes (expanded Purkinje cell axons) may be visible in the granular layer of the cerebellum. In addition, the spinal cord frequently shows degenerative

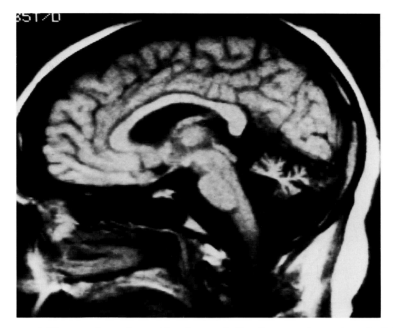

Figure 14-3   MRI scan of a patient with spinocerebellar degeneration, subcortical dementia, and psychosis, demonstrating marked cerebellar atrophy.

changes in the posterior corticospinal and spinocerebellar tract. Pathologic changes beyond the cerebellum and spinal cord are also common; there may be involvement of the substantia nigra, globus pallidus, putamen, thalamus, subthalamic nuclei, red nuclei, brain-stem nuclei, and even the cerebral cortex.

At the light-microscopic level there are no distinctive histopathologic features. There is marked cell loss in the involved areas without an accompanying inflammatory response. Gliosis is evident in affected structures, and Bergmann glia are increased in the cerebellum. Biochemical studies of patients with olivopontocerebellar degeneration reveal a marked loss of acetylcholinesterase, a marker enzyme for the neurotransmitter acetylcholine (Koeppen and Barron, 1984). Choline acetyltransferase, another cholinergic marker, has been shown to be markedly reduced in the cerebral cortex of patients with dominantly inherited olivopontocerebellar atrophy (Kish et al., 1987). Glutamate dehydrogenase deficiency has also been identified in some patients with progressive ataxia (Duvoisin et al., 1983).

Dementia Syndrome

As previously noted, there have been few studies systematically assessing the mental status of patients with ataxic syndromes using instruments sensitive to a broad range of neuropsychological deficits and assessing the individuals periodically throughout the course of their illness. Existing studies suggest that many of the ataxic disorders are unaccompanied by intellectual deterioration until the terminal phases of the illness, when it might be ascribed to systemic disturbances rather than intrinsic brain dysfunction. As expected, dementia is more often recorded in patients with evidence of more widespread central nervous system involvement (cerebellar signs as well as extrapyramidal and pyramidal tract disorders) than in patients manifesting spinal and cerebellar syndromes exclusively. In one of the few studies to include information relevant to the frequency of dementia in patients with spinocerebellar degeneration, Skre (1974) reported that dementia was the most common behavioral disorder to occur; it was observed in 36.4 percent of patients with autosomal dominant spinocerebellar degeneration, 58.3 percent of patients with the autosomal recessive cerebellar disease, and 81.8 percent of the autosomal recessive spinocerebellar type.

The pattern of the mental status deficits in affected patients remains obscure, but preliminary evidence suggests that the patients manifest abnormalities consistent with the subcortical dementia syndrome. Memory disturbances are the most frequently observed abnormalities, and attentional deficits are common. Apathy and psychomotor retardation are also described. Language abnormalities are not prominent, although auditory comprehension may be compromised late in the course of the disease (Cummings and Benson, 1983). Depression and a schizophrenia-like psychosis have been observed in a minority of patients.

FAHR'S DISEASE (IDIOPATHIC BASAL GANGLIA CALCIFICATION)

Fahr's disease refers to idiopathic calcification of the basal ganglia. It is a rare inherited (usually autosomal dominant) disorder that produces an extrapyramidal movement disorder, subcortical dementia, neuropsychiatric disturbances, and calcific deposits in the basal ganglia, thalamus, cerebellar nuclei, and hemispheric white matter. Tests of calcium and phosphorous metabolism reveal no abnormalities.

Clinical Features

Calcification of the basal ganglia is often detectable on skull x-rays and CT scans prior to the appearance of neurologic or behavioral abnormalities. The onset of symptoms tends to follow a biomodal pattern, with some patients presenting in early adulthood with a schizophrenia-like psychosis or mood disorder and others remaining asymptomatic until the sixth decade, when they manifest an extrapyramidal syndrome, subcortical dementia, and mood disturbances (Cummings et al., 1983). Either gender may be affected, and the syndrome is identical in the two sexes.

A variety of types of extrapyramidal movement disorders have been described in Fahr's disease. Parkinsonism may be the most common manifestation, but choreathetosis, cerebellar ataxia, dystonia, and paroxysmal chorea and dystonia have been described (Boller et al., 1977; Caraceni et al., 1974; Larsen et al., 1985; Micheli et al., 1986; Moskowitz et al., 1971; Sandyk, 1983). There is no effective treatment for the disorder, and no therapy that will prevent the appearance of symptoms in presymptomatic patients with visible calcifications.

The diagnosis of Fahr's disease is appropriate when dense bilateral calcification of the basal ganglia extending well beyond the globus pallidus is identified on CT (Figure

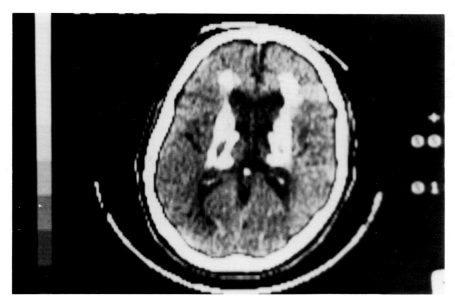

Figure 14-4 CT scan of a patient with Fahr's disease, demonstrating calcification of the basal ganglia and periventricular white matter.

14-4) or MRI scans and other causes of such calcification (hypoparathyroidism, pseudohypoparathyroidism, hyperparathyroidism, mitrochondrial encephalopathy, trauma, infection) have been excluded.

Dementia Syndrome

Fahr's disease is a rare disorder, and there have been few studies of the accompanying mental status changes. Trautner and colleagues (1988) demonstrated that organic mood disturbances, primarily of the depressed type, are common, and Cummings et al. (1983) showed that schizophrenia-like disorders with delusions and hallucinations are frequent among younger patients.

Dementia occurs in most patients with Fahr's disease and may be an early manifestation in some cases. Apathy, memory disturbances, and impaired judgment are the most prominent features; language function is spared. The profile of the dementia is consistent with that of subcortical dementia (Adachi et al., 1968; Boller et al., 1977; Cummings et al., 1983; Pilleri, 1966; Trautner et al., 1988).

Neuropathology

At autopsy, mineral deposits are found in the globus pallidus, putamen, thalamus, corona radiata, cerebellar dentate nuclei, and cerebellar white matter. Histologically, the calcific deposits form around a central nidus of mucopolysaccharides and related substances. The ferro-calcific deposition occurs primarily in the walls of the arterioles and capillaries (Adachi et al., 1968; Friede et al., 1961; Kalamboukis and Molling, 1962; Kasanin and Crank, 1935; Neumann, 1963; Strassman, 1949).

Comment

There are many unanswered questions regarding the mental status changes of Fahr's disease. First, since calcification is evident before the disease becomes clinically symptomatic, what determines the relationship between calcific deposition and clinical evidence of basal ganglia dysfunction? Second, why do some patients develop psychoses early in life, whereas others are without symptoms until an extrapyramidal syndrome and dementia emerge? Third, what is the cause of calcification, and why are the deep nuclei the most vulnerable areas to deposition?

Despite these unresolved issues, it is evident that Fahr's disease represents another rare cause of subcortical dementia. The focus of the pathologic changes is in the subcortical nuclei, particularly the basal ganglia, and the profile of neuropsychological alterations is like that of other subcortical diseases. The disease also emphasizes the important relationship between basal ganglia dysfunction, mood disorders, and psychosis.

ACKNOWLEDGMENT

This project was supported by the Veterans Administration.

REFERENCES

Adachi, M., Wellman, K.F., and Volk, B.W. Histochemical studies on the pathogenesis of idiopathic non-arteriosclerotic cerebral calcification. *J Neuropathol Exp Neurol* 1968; 27:483–99.

Aisen, A.M., Martel, W., Gabrielson, T.O., Glazer, G.M., Brewer, G., Young, A.B., and Hill, G. Wilson disease of the brain: MR imaging. *Radiology* 1985; 157:137–41.

Alema, G., and Bignami, A. Involvement of the nervous system in Behcet's disease. In *Behcet's Disease*. Monacelli, M., and Navarro, P., (eds.). Karger, Basel, 1966, pp. 52–66.

Babin, R.W., Liu, C., and Aschenbrener, C. Histopathology of neurosensory deafness in sarcoidosis. *Ann Otol Rhinol Laryngol* 1984; 93:389–93.

Barbeau, A. Treatment of Wilson's disease. In *Disorders of Movement*. Barbeau, A. (ed.). J.B. Lippincott, Philadelphia, 1981, pp. 209–20.

Boller, F., Boller, M., and Gilbert, J. Familial idiopathic cerebral calcifications. *J Neurol Neurosurg Psychiatry* 1977; 40:280–5.

Camp, W.A., and Frierson, J.G. Sarcoidosis of the central nervous system. *Arch Neurol* 1962; 7:432–41.

Caraceni, T., Broggi, G., and Avazini, G. Familial basal ganglia calcification exhibiting "dystonia musculorum deformans" features. *Eur Neurol* 1974; 12:351–9.

Cartwright, G.E. Diagnosis of treatable Wilson's disease. *N Engl J Med* 1978; 298:1347–50.

Chiang, R., Marshall, M.C., Rosman, P.M., et al. Empty sella turcica in intracranial sarcoidosis. *Arch Neurol* 1984; 41:662–5.

Colover, J. Sarcoidosis with involvement of the nervous system. *Brain* 1948; 71:451–75.

Cordingley, G., Navarro, C., Brust, J.C.M., and Healton, E.B. Sarcoidosis presenting as senile dementia. *Neurology* 1981; 11:1148–51.

Cummings, J.L., and Benson, D.F. *Dementia: A Clinical Approach.* Butterworths, Boston, 1983.

Cummings, J.L., Gosenfeld, L.F., Houlihan, J.P., and McCaffrey, T. Neuropsychiatric disturbances associated with idiopathic calcification of the basal ganglia. *Biol Psychiatry* 1983; 18:591–601.

Currier, R.D. A reclassification for ataxia. In *The Olivopontocerebellar Atrophies.* Duvoisin, R.D., and Plaitakis, A. (eds.). Raven Press, New York, 1984, pp. 1–4.

Davis, L.J., Jr., and Goldstein, N.P. Psychologic investigation of Wilson's disease. *Mayo Clin Proc* 1974; 49:409–11.

Delaney, P. Neurological manifestations in sarcoidosis: Review of the literature, with a report of 23 cases. *Ann Intern Med* 1977; 897:336–45.

Dening, T.R. Psychiatric aspects of Wilson's disease. *Br J Psychiatry* 1985; 147:677–82.

Dobkin, B.H. Computerized tomographic findings in neuro-Behcet's. *Arch Neurol* 1980; 37:58–9.

Duvoisin, R.C., Chokroverty,, S., Lepore, F., and Nicklas, W. Glutamate dehydrogenase deficiency in patients with olivopontoverebellar atrophy. *Neurology* 1983; 33:1322–6.

Friede, R.L., Magee, K.R., and Mack, E.W. Idiopathic nonarteriosclerotic calcification of cerebral vessels. *Arch Neurol* 1961; 5:279–86.

Gilman, S., Markel, D.S., Koeppe, R.A., Junck, L., Kluin, K.J., Gebarski, S.S., and Hichwa, R.D. Cerebellar and brainstem hypometabolism in olivopontocerebellar atrophy detected with positron emission tomography. *Arch Neurol* 1988; 23:223–30.

Goldstein, N.P., Ewert, J.C., Randall, R.V., and Gross, J.B. Psychiatric aspects of Wilson's disease (hepatolenticular degeneration): Results of psychometric tests during long-term therapy. *Am J Psychiatry* 1968; 124:1555–61.

Griggs, R.C., Markesbury, W.R., and Condemi, J.J. Cerebral mass due to sarcoidosis: Regression during corticosteriod therapy. *Neurology* 1973; 23:981–9.

Hier, D.B., Thomas, C.T., and Shindler, A.G. A case of subcortical dementia due to sarcoidosis of the hypothalamus and fornices. *Brain Cogn* 1983; 2:189–98.

Ho, S., Berenberg, R.A., Kim, K.S., and Dal Canto, M.C. Sarcoid encephalopathy with diffuse inflammation and focal hydrocephalus shown by sequential CT. *Neurology* 1979; 29:1161–5.

James, D.G., and Williams, W.J. *Sarcoidosis and Other Granulomatomous Disorders.* W.B. Saunders, Philadelphia, 1985.

Jorizzo, J.L. Behcet's disease. *Neurol Clin* 1987; 5:427–40.

Kalamboukis, Z., and Molling, P. Symmetrical calcification of the brain in the predominance in the basal ganglia and cerebellum. *J Neuropathol Exp Neurol* 1962; 21:364–71.

Kasanin, J., and Crank, R.P. A case of extensive calcification in the brain. *Arch Neurol Psychiatry* 1935; 34:164–78.

Kawakita, H., Nishimura, M., Satoh,, Y., and Shabat, N. Neurological aspects of Behcet's disease: A case report and clinico-pathological review of literature in Japan. *J Neurol Sci* 1967; 5:417–39.

Kish, S.J., Currier, R.D., Schut, L., Perry, T.L., and Morito, C.L. Brain choline acetyltransferase reduction in dominantly inherited olivopontocerebellar atrophy. *Ann Neurol* 1987; 22:272–5.

Kish, S.J., Shannak, K., and Hornykiewicz, O. Uneven pattern of dopamine loss in the striatum of patients with idiopathic Parkinson's disease. *N Engl J Med* 1988; 318:876–80.

Knehr, C.A., and Bearn, A.G. Psychological impairment in Wilson's disease. *J Nerv Ment Dis* 1956; 124:251–5.

Koeppen, A.H., and Barron, K.D. The neuropathology of olivopontocerebellar atrophy. In *Olivopontocerebellar Atrophies*. Duvoisin, R.C., and Plaitakis, A. (eds.). Raven Press, New York, 1984, pp. 13–38.

Kozin, F., Haughton, V., and Bernhard, G.C. Neuro-Behcet disease: Two cases and neuroradiologic findings. *Neurology* 1977; 27:1148–52.

Kuroiwa, H., Tongi, H., Kanayama, H., Fujimori, M., and Aoki, H. Neuro-Behcet's disease with alternating hemiparesis. *Neuroradiology* 1986; 28:284.

Larsen, T.A., Dunn, H.G., Jan, J.E., and Calne, D.B. Dystonia and calcification of the basal ganglia. *Neurology* 1985; 35:533–7.

Medalia, A., Isaacs-Glaberman, K., and Scheinberg, I.H. Neuropsychological impairment in Wilson's disease. *Arch Neurol* 1988; 45:502–4.

Micheli, F., Pardal, M.M.F., Parera, C., and Giannaula, R. Sporadic paroxysmal dystonic choreoathetosis associated with basal ganglia calcifications. *Ann Neurol* 1986; 20:750.

Moskowitz, M.A., Winickoff, R.N., and Heinz, E.R. Familial calcification of the basal ganglions. *N Engl J Med* 1971; 285:72–7.

Neumann, M.A. Iron and calcium dysmetabolism in the brain. *J Neuropathol Exp Neurol* 1963; 22:148–63.

Norman, R.M., and Campbell, A.M.G. The neuropathology of Behcet's disease. In *Behcet's Disease*. Monacelli, M., and Nazzaro, P. (eds.). Karger, Basel, 1966, pp. 67–78.

Pallis, C.A., and Fudge, B.J. The neurological complications of Behcet's syndrome. *Arch Neurol Psychiatry* 1956; 75:1–14.

Pilleri, G. A case of morbus Fahr (nmonarteriosclerotic, idiopathic intracerebral calcification of the blood vessels) in three generations. *Psychiatr Neurol* 1966; 152:43–58.

Sandyk, R. Parkinsonism, gait apraxia and dementia associated with intracranial calcifications. *S Afr Med J* 1983; 63:738–9.

Scheinberg, I.H., and Sternlieb, I. *Wilson's Disease*. W.B. Saunders, Philadelphia, 1984.

Schonell, M.E., Gillespie, W.J., and Maloney, A.F.J. Cerebral sarcoidosis. *Br J Dis Chest* 1968; 62:195–9.

Shimizu, T. Clinicopathological studies on Behcet's disease. In *Behcet's Disease*. Dilsen, N., Konice, M., and Ovul, C. (eds.). Excerpta Medica, Amsterdam, 1979, pp. 9–37.

Skre, H. Spino-cerebellar ataxia in Western Norway. *Clin Genet* 1974; 6:265–8.

Slavin, M.L., and Glaser, J.S. Optic neuropathy and cerebral sarcoidosis. *J Clin Neuro Opthalmol* 1983; 3:259–62.

Starosta-Rubenstein, S., Young, A.B., Kluin, K., Hill, G., Aisen, A.M., Gabrielsen, T., and Brewer, G.J. Clinical assessment of 31 patients with Wilson's disease. *Arch Neurol* 1987; 44:365–70.

Stoudemire, A., Linfors, E., and Houpt, J.L. Central nervous system sarcoidosis. *Gen Hosp Psychiatry* 1983; 5:129–32.

Strassman, G. Iron and calcium deposits in the brain; their pathological significance. *J Neuropathol Exp Neurol* 1949; 8:428–35.

Thompson, C., and Checkley, S. Short term memory deficit in a patient with cerebral sarcoidosis. *Br J Psychiatry* 1981; 139:160–1.

Trautner, R.J., Cummings, J.L., Read, S.L., and Benson, D.F. Idiopathic basal ganglia calcification and organic mood disorder. *Am J Psychiatry* 1988; 145:350–3.

Weilleit, J., Schmutzhard, E., Aichner, F., Mayr, U., Weber, F., and Gerstenbrand, F. CT and MR imaging in neuro-Behcet disease. *J Comput Assist Tomogr* 1986; 10:313–5.

Weisberg, L.A., and Jacobs, L. Clinical and computed tomography findings in intracranial sarcoidosis involving the juxtasellar region. *Comput Radiol* 1984; 8:107–11.

Weitz, Z., Machtey, I., Rothman, G.M., Davidovich, S., and Shifter, T. Computed axial tomography of brain in neuro-ocular Behcet's syndrome. *J Rheumatol* 1986; 45:310–1.

Whelan, M.A., and Stern, J. Sarcoidosis presenting as a posterior fossa mass. *Surg Neurol* 1980; 15:455–7.

Williams, F.J.B., and Walshe, J.M. Wilson's disease. An analysis of the cranial computerized tomographic appearances found in 60 patients and the changes in response to treatment with chelating agents. *Brain* 1981; 104:735–52.

Wilson, S.A.K. Progressive lenticular degeneration: A familial nervous disease associated with cirrhosis of the liver. *Brain* 1912; 34:295–507.

15

Depression

DEBORAH A. KING AND ERIC D. CAINE

For much of the twentieth century, traditional attempts to understand the nature of depressive disorders have addressed the most obvious behavioral manifestation of the illness: depressed mood. Nonemotional, intellectual aspects of the illness have rarely been the focal point of psychiatric or psychological investigations. These traditional mind- or emotion-oriented psychological models have not had the potential for defining or studying the neurobiologic underpinnings of depression. In contrast, neuropsychiatric methods combine the study of behavior and brain. For example, investigation of cognitive functioning as a behavioral manifestation of depressive disorder allows one to explore behavior–brain relationships and provides the opportunity to develop inferences about the potential neuroanatomic substrates of the illness.

In this chapter we shall review selected findings derived from several diverse neuropsychiatric research methods used to study unipolar major depression, a clinical syndrome that affects an estimated 3–7 percent of Americans in the course of a lifetime (Robins et al., 1984). The primary symptoms of the disorder fall within three broad behavioral categories: (1) dysphoric mood, (2) neurovegetative changes, such as disturbed sleep, appetite, and sexual drive, and (3) difficulties in thinking (American Psychiatric Association, 1987).

A variety of broadly defined neuropsychiatric methodologies have been used to investigate behavior–brain relationships in depression. A neuropsychological method attempts to infer the nature of central nervous system impairment from the pattern of observed cognitive deficits. Similarly, an electrophysiological approach attempts to identify the nature of central nervous system disruption by studying patterns of electrical activity generated by the brain. Recently, more direct neuroanatomic, morphologic, and metabolically sensitive methods (e.g., computed tomography, positron emission tomography) have been used to study abnormalities in brain structure or function. Finally, studies of patients with cerebrovascular accidents (strokes) provide an alternate method for examining the neurobiology of mood disorders. Rather than using mood as an independent variable and exploring brain function as the dependent variable, these investigations relate the locus of lesion as an independent variable to specific syndromes as dependent variables.

Each of these neuropsychiatric methods can be viewed as a specialized lens providing a unique, but somewhat distorted, view of depressive disorders. Different conclusions may be drawn about the nature of illness, depending on which lens is used to study particular subjects. For example, a technique designed to find focal, structural abnormalities (e.g., computed tomography) will lead to different conclusions when compared with a technique used to study more diffusely controlled processes (e.g., electroencephalography). Similarly, studies of depressed patients whose symptom picture fulfills specific diagnostic criteria will likely yield distinct results from investigations of nonpatient or student subjects with induced negative mood states or high scores on self-assessment inventories.

The practice of applying neuropsychiatric techniques to the study of psychopathology is relatively new. Many unanswered questions remain. Nonetheless, we will present in this chapter current knowledge about the nature of brain dysfunction that underlies the polymorphic syndrome we call "depression."

NEUROPSYCHOLOGICAL STUDIES

Early anecdotal reports suggested that severely depressed patients often presented with memory disturbance and apparent intellectual decline (Kiloh, 1961). Further clinical observation revealed the depressive's marked variability in performance on tasks of similar difficulty and frequent use of "I don't know" responses (Wells, 1979). The results of psychological studies of depressives yielded a variety of findings, making it difficult to isolate an agreed-upon pattern of deficit that characterized depression (Miller, 1975). In recent years, however, there have been at least three major trends in the neuropsychological literature that have proved productive for investigating the brain basis of depression.

Comparative Approaches

One neuropsychological approach compares a known or specific neurobehavioral disease with a less-well-defined psychopathologic disorder (Caine and Joynt, 1986). Rather than simply inferring the locus of brain dysfunction from the pattern of test results, this approach seeks to use established neurologic diseases as "anchor points" from which to make inferences about the nature of brain–behavior relationships in depression. Like all neuropsychiatric methods, this approach is subject to its own unique limitations. For example, similar patterns of cognitive deficit may result from different types of underlying neuropathy; that is, there are relatively few final common behavioral pathways for manifesting central nervous system dysfunction. Thus, whenever possible, it is important to combine neuropsychological test findings with other, more direct pathophysiological methods such as imaging techniques.

Consistent with this comparative neuropsychological approach, Cummings and Benson (1984) summarized the distinction between "higher cortical" dementias characterized by aphasia, amnesia, and agnosia (e.g., Alzheimer's disease, AD); and subcortical diseases characterized by forgetfulness, mental slowing, aberrant problem-solving strategies, and impaired spontaneous use of stored information (e.g., Huntington's and Parkinson's disease). Caine (1981) surveyed depressed inpatients and found a pattern of impairment suggestive of a subcortical syndrome, including inattention, slowed mental processing, and decreased verbal elaboration. He concluded that this admittedly loosely defined series of depressives suffered from impairment of those structures that modulate or control higher cortical centers. However, these early descriptive findings could not be viewed as definitive because of the lack of appropriate control groups.

In a recent controlled study Caine and colleagues (unpublished) formally tested the notion that depressives suffer from a "subcortical" pattern of impairment by comparing the neuropsychological profiles of unipolar depressed inpatients with the profiles of matched normal volunteers and patients with a known subcortical disease (i.e., Huntington's disease, HD).

The depressives were significantly impaired compared with normal controls on the following tests: spontaneous, timed generation of words beginning with the letter f and categorical word lists (e.g., animals); verbal memory tasks, including immediate recall of a 10-word list, delayed list recall, immediate recall of a story, and multiple-choice story recognition; and immediate and delayed recall of geometric shapes. There were no significant differences between depressives and normals on primary language tasks, delayed recognition of the word list, visuospatial tasks, or ideomotor praxis. In addition, there were no significant differences between depressives and HD patients on any of these tasks.

The depressives' deficit in spontaneous word generation, in the context of other intact language functions, was consistent with the prediction that they would have particular difficulty with verbal elaboration, but not with primary linguistic functions, such as confrontation naming. It was our observation that depressed subjects found word generation demanding in terms of attention and concentration. Weingartner et al. (1984) failed to find deficits on similar word-production tasks in Parkinson's disease (PD) patients who were impaired on other "effortful" tasks (e.g., free recall of words; see Hasher and Zacks, 1979, on "automatic" versus "effortful" processing). Thus, timed retrieval from the store of overlearned, semantic information may be preserved in one subcortical disorder (PD) but not in another (HD). However, distinctions between so-called automatic and effortful processing need to be more rigorously defined and demonstrated, especially within the domain of semantic memory, before the meaning of this apparent difference between disorders can be fully understood.

The pattern of memory failure demonstrated by the depressives during word list learning (i.e., impaired recall in the context of intact recognition) suggested particular difficulty retrieving learned information from episodic, or context-specific, memory. This finding was consistent with other reports of intact recognition or improved memory performance when cues were provided to aid retrieval (Dunbar and Lishman, 1984; Miller and Lewis, 1977; Weingartner et al., 1981). However, the fact that depressives were impaired on story recognition points out the importance of considering the nature of the recognition task. Our story recognition task employed a multiple-choice format that required the subject to choose each response from a set of four alternatives. This procedure demanded greater resistance to distraction or interference, in comparison to a word list recognition task that simply required the subject to distinguish 10 "old" words from 10 similar "new" ones. Thus it may be that depressives are more impaired on recognition tests that tax attentional and decision-making capacity, either at the time of initial encoding or ultimate retrieval. There are other reports suggesting that recognition is impaired in depression (Watts et al., 1987; Wolfe et al., 1987). Given the discrepant findings in this area, more studies are needed that control for difficulty, mode of presentation (auditory vs. visual), response bias factors, and severity of depressive illness.

Differences between recall and recognition can result from encoding and retrieval deficits. Weingartner and colleagues (1981) conducted an elegant series of studies demonstrating that depressives fail to use semantic learning strategies spontaneously, although they benefit from semantic cues and strategies when these are inherent to the task. This same group of investigators found that severity of depression was strongly associated with impaired memory and motor performance (Cohen et al., 1982). They hypothesized a "generalized deficit in the central motivational state" of depressives and suggested that these patients are impaired on all complex, effortful memory tasks. Similarly, our qualitative analysis of word list learning revealed that depressives failed to use a normal learning strategy, serial position, efficiently (Glanzer, 1966). Their performance was qualitatively similar to that of patients with early HD, and quite distinct from that of AD patients.

In summary, the pattern of deficits observed in the depressed group involved impaired verbal elaboration, difficulty accessing learned information, and inefficient use of a normal learning strategy. HD patients evidenced a similar pattern of deficits, suggesting a common disruption of "psychomotor" or "modulatory functions," rather than primary linguistic, gnostic, or practic deficits (Bamford and Caine, 1986). This pattern of deficits is similar to that found in other studies of patients with known subcortical pathology (Albert et al., 1974; Cummings, 1986).

In order to understand patterns of neuropsychological performance in elderly depressives and to explore the construct of "pseudodementia" further, we conducted a study that compared the neuropsychological test performance of rigorously diagnosed elderly unipolar depressed inpatients with AD patients and normal controls (King et al., unpublished). The pattern of cognitive performance of elderly depressives was clearly different from that of AD patients on most measures. However, there was considerable heterogeneity within the depressed group such that one subgroup of patients evidenced the same pattern of modulatory impairment revealed in our earlier study, whereas a second subgroup was older and manifested clearly deficient performance on language, visuospatial, and memory tasks. These more severely impaired depressives had a greater frequency of parenchymal abnormalities on computer tomography (CT) or magnetic resonance imaging (MRI) scans (e.g., periventricular lucencies, isolated small white matter lesions); however, there was no specifically localized pattern of abnormality.

These impaired elderly depressives may suffer from some form of progressive, age-related neuropathology that was not evident from clinical history, presentation, or physical examination. It remains to be seen if theirs is a more "malignant" disorder. Perhaps some elderly depressives experience a combination of structural, higher cortical pathology and either structural or physiological disruption of subcortical functions.

Experimental Studies of Information Processing

Cognitive psychological methods have been used to assess the relative contributions of cognitive and motor components to overall psychomotor slowing in major depression. Some of these investigations have directly compared depression and subcortical disease. These investigations have assessed overall reaction time in relation to varied cognitive and/or motor demands. For example, a memory scanning procedure developed by Sternberg (1975) systematically varies the amount of information to be processed, while motor demands remain constant. Depressed patients have been found to exhibit prolonged overall reaction time on this task in comparison to normals, but normal response latency as a function of increasing cognitive demand (Glass et al., 1981; Hart and Kwentus, 1987). In contrast, patients with known subcortical diseases (i.e., Parkinson's disease and Friedreich's ataxia) have demonstrated both cognitive and motor slowing on this type of task (Wilson et al., 1980; Hart and Kwentus, 1987).

Results from a carefully designed study that systematically varied both motor and cognitive task demands suggested that subtypes of major depression may affect the nature of psychomotor slowing. Cornell and colleagues (1984) found that both melancholic and nonmelancholic depressives were slowed in comparison to normals on reaction time tasks with increasing motor demands, but only melancholic depressives were impaired on reaction time tasks with relatively greater cognitive demands.

Thus it appears that motor slowing on complex reaction time tasks is common in most patients with major depression and in some specific subcortical disorders. The cognitive slowing demonstrated by patients with subcortical dysfunction may be characteristic only of melancholic depressives, although this remains to be tested in direct comparative studies.

Test-Based Localizing Approaches

A third neuropsychological approach is to infer the locus of neuropathology from the pattern of cognitive test findings. Reports of depressives' selective deficits on visuospatial and motor tasks putatively associated with the nondominant cerebral hemisphere exemplify this methodology (Abrams and Taylor, 1987; Goldstein et al., 1977; Gray et al., 1987; Kronfol et al., 1978). These data are consistent with other studies suggesting lateralized cerebral deficits in depression (see Silberman and Weingartner, 1986, for a review). However, much of this work must be interpreted cautiously due to methodological shortcomings, such as lack of normal controls (Goldstein et al., 1977; Kronfol et al., 1978) or failure to include controls matched for educational level (Abrams and Taylor, 1987; Gray et al., 1987). Additionally, it is important to note that some investigators failed to find evidence of nondominant hemisphere deficits in depressives (Taylor et al., 1979). Others have reported evidence of significant verbally mediated learning and memory deficits (McAllister, 1981; Watts, et al., 1987; Wolfe, et al., 1987). Thus there appears to be disruption of functions associated with both cerebral hemispheres in depression.

A more fundamental reason for exercising caution in interpreting these studies arises from concerns regarding test-based inferences about cerebral localization, as well as our overall understanding of "where" discrete cognitive processes are controlled. Many putatively "localizing" neuropsychological procedures were derived from studies of patients with focal lesions, such as stroke or missile wounds. They reflect a view of brain–behavior relationships largely based upon vascular anatomy, or the confounded nature of high-impact traumatic injuries. Whether this understanding of cerebral localization adequately applies to less focal neurochemical systems diseases remains to be determined. Attempts to "find the lesion" that are solely based upon lesion-characteristic test deficits may lead to invalid or incomplete conclusions. For example, we now know that some neurotransmitter systems implicated in arousal, mood, and cognition are distributed asymmetrically in subcortical brain regions prior to reaching the cortex (Tucker and Williamson, 1984). Apparently lateralized differences in higher hemispherically controlled cognitive functions may be due to primary disruption of subcortical structures.

ELECTROPHYSIOLOGICAL STUDIES

Another means of studying behavior–brain relationships in depression is to look at the electroencephalogram (EEG) for asymmetries in hemispheric activation associated with negative emotional states. In most studies the major dependent variable is power in the alpha band (8–13 Hz; Davidson, 1988). Asymmetries in activation between cerebral hemispheres are examined by comparing alpha-band power recorded from homologous electrode sites. This technique has been applied to normal subjects in whom negative moods are induced, as well as to "depressed" college students identified by self-report inventories. Studies of normals revealed significantly greater left-frontal alpha during positive affect and relatively greater right-frontal alpha during negative affect (Davidson et al., 1979; Tucker, 1981). More recent work revealed that individual differences in resting frontal asymmetry predicted the intensity of subjective response to emotional films (Davidson, 1988). While it has been suggested that the presence of greater relative right-frontal activation may reflect a vulnerability for the experience of negative emotion, this remains to be tested in more natural settings. Furthermore, one cannot make inferences about a major depressive syndrome from studies of transient, induced mood states.

Consistent with the results of mood induction studies, Schaffer et al. (1983) found that college students with high scores on the Beck Depression Inventory had less resting left-frontal activation than low scoring subjects. Examination of depressives' frontal and parietal patterns of activation during the viewing of affective facial stimuli revealed opposite patterns of EEG asymmetry in frontal and parietal regions, while normals showed similar patterns of activation in these regions (Davidson et al., 1985). These investigators speculate that depressives' relative right-sided frontal activation may be associated with right-parietal inhibition and that posterior right-sided inhibition may be the cause of depressives' performance deficits observed by some investigators on cognitive tasks mediated by the right hemisphere (Davidson, 1988).

While these results provide valuable leads regarding the nature of brain function in some depressed states, they cannot be used to draw conclusions about major depressive syndromes. Subclinically depressed college student subjects selected solely on the basis of Beck Depression Inventory scores are clearly a different population from clinically depressed patients selected according to standardized diagnostic criteria. Furthermore, selection of subjects on the basis of one self-report inventory does not allow one to rule out other forms of psychopathology in the depressed group. More studies are needed that focus on rigorously diagnosed depressives, as compared to normals and other psychopathologic groups. Furthermore, it is unsatisfactory to generalize from patterns of activation demonstrated by one population of subjects (i.e., subclinically depressed college students) in one study to neuropsychological deficits demonstrated by another population (i.e., patients with a major depressive syndrome) in other studies. The speculation that right-frontal activation and right-parietal inhibition are associated with impairment on visuospatial cognitive tasks needs to be tested by comparing EEG and neuropsychological measures obtained from the same subjects.

Consistent with EEG studies, several other lines of evidence reveal altered hemispheric relationships in depressives. These include studies of the differential effects of left- versus right-sided electroconvulsive therapy (ECT), skin conductance studies, studies of the effects of unilateral amobarbital injections on mood, dichotic listening experiments, and investigations of visual field advantages for verbal or nonverbal–emotional material (see Silberman and Weingartner, 1986, for a review). Unlike the EEG studies, many of these investigations were conducted with carefully diagnosed depressed patients. For example, Silberman et al. (1983) found a tendency towards reversal of the normal left hemisphere advantage for processing verbal material in depressives. Jaeger et al. (1987) found that depressed patients had significantly less right-hemispheric advantage for processing chimeric faces than normals. Taken together, these results suggest an alteration of hemispheric relationships in major depressive disorder. However, even these findings must be considered tentative, as some patients in both studies were already being treated with antidepressant medications.

EEG studies suffer from similar conceptual limitations as the "lesion-characteristic" neuropsychological approach, which attempts to make inferences about localization without reference to neurologically defined control groups. First, the generators or sources of EEG activity are not known; apparent changes in hemispheric relationships could be due to disruption of asymmetrically organized subcortical structures that control arousal and autonomic activity. Second, EEG slowing at a particular site on the scalp could be caused by damage or altered brain chemistry at that site or in an adjacent area that normally provides inhibitory input to the site (perhaps in the opposite hemisphere). Until there is a better understanding of the physiological underpinnings of electrophysiological activation, confident inferences about localization are not possible.

COMPUTED TOMOGRAPHY AND POSITRON EMISSION TOMOGRAPHY

The development of specialized methods to evaluate structural brain features (e.g., computed tomography, CT) or ongoing brain metabolism (e.g., positron emission tomography, PET) has allowed more direct evaluation of behavior–brain relationships than inferential techniques, such as cognitive testing and EEG. Studies of diagnostically heterogeneous groups of clinically depressed patients generally have revealed subgroups of patients with enlarged ventricles (Dolan et al., 1985; Jacoby and Levy, 1980; Schlegel and Kretzschmar, 1987a; Shima et al., 1984; Targum et al., 1983), although some investigators failed to find such differences (Rossi et al., 1987). There is a diversity of findings regarding the characteristics of depressives with enlarged ventricles. Age, age of onset, delusions, and melancholia have all been associated with ventricular enlargement in depressives, although older age (Dolan et al., 1985; Jacoby and Levy, 1980) and older age of onset (Jacoby and Levy, 1980; Shima et al., 1984) appear to be the most consistently reported associated variables. There is also evidence of sulcal widening associated with enlarged ventricles in depressives (Dolan et al., 1986) and of abnormal brain density in elderly depressives (Jacoby et al., 1983), although the latter point has been disputed (Schlegel and Kretschmar, 1987b).

There is a variety of potential methodological reasons for the inconsistencies of the CT findings, including different mixtures of bipolar, unipolar, and dysthymic patients in the depressed groups; the use of different types of nondepressed controls (e.g., healthy nonpatients vs. neurologic patients); and the use of different methods of measurement (e.g., absolute values vs. ratios, linear vs. area or volume measures). The findings are difficult to interpret because the etiology and pathogenesis of the abnormalities are not known. Furthermore, the finding of a structural brain abnormality such as ventricular enlargement is nonspecific and not unique to depression; there is considerable evidence of ventricular enlargement in schizophrenics (cf. Weinberger et al., 1979). Methods of brain assessment that are sensitive to specific changes in brain activity may be better suited to the study of depressive disorders.

The use of PET to study glucose metabolism in the brain has opened a new avenue for the study of brain–behavior relationships. This method offers a more direct means of studying brain function than EEG or neuropsychological testing. Unlike computed tomography, which is limited to the study of structural abnormalities, PET allows the observation of regional metabolic activity in the resting state or during task performance. Baxter et al. (1985) found a significantly lower rate of metabolic activity in the caudate nucleus of carefully diagnosed, unipolar depressed patients who were free of all psychoactive medications. The same study found a subgroup of depressives with a strikingly lower metabolic rate in the left-frontal cortex compared with the right. This finding is consistent with a report of decreased blood flow in the left hemisphere of depressives (Mathew, et al. 1980). Another study of carefully diagnosed, antidepressant-free unipolar depressives undergoing brief electrical stimulation to the arm reported decreased metabolism in the basal ganglia, along with higher frontal-to-occipital ratios of metabolic activity (Buchsbaum et al., 1986). However, this study included only four unipolar subjects.

Taken together, these preliminary studies strongly implicate the basal ganglia as a primary site of metabolic abnormality in depressed patients. This contrasts with findings in schizophrenics that point to specifically diminished frontal glucose metabolism (Cohen et al., 1987).

DEPRESSION AND STROKE

There is an extensive literature that confirms Kraepelin's early observation that depressive disorder could result from focal brain lesions. These investigations reverse the method undertaken by the neuropsychological and electrophysiologic studies. Rather than starting with depressed mood as the independent variable, this approach begins with carefully defined focal cerebral lesions and subsequently describes their effects on mood. The work of Robinson and colleagues has been exemplary. They (Robinson et al., 1984) conducted a series of studies demonstrating that left-anterior cortical or subcortical vascular lesions were associated with depression, while right-anterior lesions were associated with inappropriate cheerfulness or apathy. Most recently, this group of investigators reported that significant depression was also associated with purely subcortical lesions (Starkstein 1987). They found that patients with left-sided damage to the basal ganglia had a significantly higher frequency and greater severity of depression than patients with either right- or left-sided thalamic lesions.

Furthermore, these results could not be explained by differences in the degree of physical, cognitive, or social impairment.

Patients with right-hemispheric cortical and subcortical damage also experience generally lowered mood, but it appears that they have few specific depressive complaints and are characterized by a tendency towards inertia and lack of initiative (Finset, 1988). These findings are consistent with the results of a variety of studies with divergent methodologies that report right-hemispheric control for the processing of emotional information and for modulating cortical arousal levels (Silberman and Weingartner, 1986). It appears that patients with focal right-sided damage to cortical and/ or subcortical areas may lose the ability or the energy to perceive and express emotions accurately.

In summary, studies of patients with focal brain lesions suggest that both cortical and subcortical regions are involved in the production of depressed mood states. Lesions in left-anterior cortical and left subcortical regions result in the experience of a dysphoric mood that resembles unipolar depressed states. These patients manifest the full range of syndromically defined depressive symptoms. Damage to right-hemispheric structures often results in hypo- or hyperarousal, which is frequently encountered in affective disorders. These patients may also manifest alterations in the expression and perception of emotion, but typically they fail to conform to specific diagnostic criteria. Thus it appears that left-hemisphere pathology is primarily implicated in disturbed *mood*, while the right-hemisphere dysfunction is more often associated with disturbed *affect*.

SUMMARY AND CONCLUSIONS

What conclusions can be drawn from these diverse neuropsychiatric perspectives? Neuropsychological findings suggest an underlying deficit in the efficiency or modulation of cognitive processing in depressives that is akin to the pattern of deficits found in Huntington's disease. These results are consistent with the findings of selective deficits on effortful cognitive tasks reported by Weingartner and colleagues. However, our data suggest that the situation becomes more complex when elderly depressives are studied. Depression in late life (i.e., age 70 and older) may be a more neuropsychologically and pathophysiologically heterogeneous phenomenon.

Evidence derived from various approaches, including neuropsychological and electrophysiologic studies, indicates that depression is associated with altered hemispheric relations. Most lesion-characteristic neuropsychological and EEG studies are subject to methodological and conceptual shortcomings that prevent confident conclusions about hemispheric localization. Studies of stroke patients report depressive syndromes after left-frontal and left-basal-ganglion lesions, but one may interpret these data in several ways. A typical interpretation is that a left-hemisphere lesion allows the right hemisphere to function "unopposed," thus causing "bad thoughts and feelings." Alternatively, it could be that a left-sided lesion may release aberrant responses from remaining ipsilateral structures, causing the left hemisphere to generate depressive psychopathology. Finally, deficient innervation from beneath the cortex could also result in seemingly lateralized hemispheric deficits.

None of these competing explanations can be conclusively discounted at this time. However, we are drawn to the consistency in findings of controlled neuropsychological studies of patients with subcortical lesions from stroke and PET studies. Each of these diverse methodologies implicate the basal ganglia in the development of clinical depressive syndromes.

Evidence from a diverse array of experimental studies suggests that the basal ganglia are involved in a variety of cognitive and motor functions, including attention, motivation, memory, and general planning and modulation of responding (see Bamford and Caine, 1986, for a review). There is evidence that the cortex receives sensory information from a multisynaptic neuronal ascending system that runs through the neostriatum and thalamus, and that the basal ganglia influence cognitive processing via a loop from the frontal cortex to the neostriatum to the thalamus to the frontal cortex. Furthermore, the striatum has been conceptualized as a center for integration and focusing, while the pallidum has been implicated in the initiation and activation of responding. Thus disruption of basal ganglion function could be expected to result in a fundamental psychomotor breakdown, that is, a primary disturbance in the initiation and modulation of motor and cognitive responses as found in major depression.

Recent animal studies have revealed that lesions in the ventral striatum produced asymmetric behavioral effects (Kubos et al., 1987; Starkstein et al., in press). It has been suggested that asymmetries in the distribution of biogenic amines within the basal ganglia may account for lateralized effects on mood and behavior associated with basal ganglion lesions (Starkstein et al., 1988). This proposal remains to be tested further.

In conclusion, we propose that unipolar major depression is a neuropsychiatrically complex phenomenon that reflects the dynamic interplay of subcortical and higher cortical structures. There is considerable preliminary evidence that neurobiological systems originating in subcortical regions are associated with depressed mood and with a "psychomotor or modulatory dementia," characterized by impaired verbal elaboration, difficulty accessing learned information, and inefficient use of normal learning strategies. At the same time, these same subcortical structures ultimately project to the cortex and may generate apparent "higher cortical" deficits or an altered relationship between the hemispheres.

Through the use of neuropsychiatric research methods, we are now beginning to recognize neuroanatomic substrates for the dementia of depression. The intellectual deficits of depressed patients had been viewed by some as epiphenomena to their mood disturbance. However, studying such discrete behaviors, rather than difficult-to-define emotional constructs, has allowed for clinical–pathologic correlation. Indeed, the dementing disorder of depression is not "pseudo" at all!

REFERENCES

Abrams, R., and Taylor, M.A. Cognitive dysfunction in melancholia. *Psychol Med* 1987; 17:359–62.

Albert, M.L., Feldman, R.G., and Willis, A.L. The subcortical dementia of progressive supranuclear palsy. *J Neurol Neurosurg Psychiatry* 1974; 37:121–30.

American Psychiatric Association. *Diagnostic and Statistical Manual of Mental Disorders, Third Edition, Revised.* American Psychiatric Association, Washington, 1987.

Bamford, K.A., and Caine, E.D. The neuropsychology of Huntington's disease: Problems of clinical–pathological correlation in a progressive brain illness. In *Advanced in Clinical Neuropsychology, Vol. 3.* Goldstein, E., and Tarter, R.E. (eds.). Plenum Press, New York, 1986, pp. 181–212.

Baxter, L.R., Phelps, M.E., Mazziotta, J.C., Schwartz, J.M., Gerner, R.H., Selin, C.E., and Sumida, R.N. Cerebral metabolic rates for glucose in mood disorders. *Arch Gen Psychiatry* 1985; 42:441–7.

Buchsbaum, M.S., Wu, J., DeLisi, L.E., Holcomb, H., Kessler, R., Johnson, J., King, A.C., Hazlett, E., Langston, K., and Post, R.M. Frontal cortex and basal ganglia metabolic rates assessed by position emission tomography with [18F]-2-deoxyglucose in affective illness. *J Affective Disord* 1986; 10:137–52.

Caine, E.D. Pseudodementia: Current concepts and future directions. *Arch Gen Psychiatry* 1981; 38:1359–64.

Caine, E.D., Bamford, K.A., King, D.A., Booth, H.A., Cox, C., and Yerevanian, B. The neuropsychology of depression: A controlled and comparative study. (Manuscript in preparation.)

Caine, E.D., and Joynt, R.J. Neuropsychiatry . . . again. *Arch Neurol* 1986; 43:325–7.

Cohen, R.M., Weingartner, H., Smallberg, S.A., Pickar, D., and Murphy, D.L. Effort and cognition in depression. *Arch Gen Psychiatry* 1982; 39:593–8.

Cohen, R.M., Semple, W.E., Gross, M., Nordahl, T.E., Delisi, L.E., Holcomb, H.H., King, A.C., Morihisa, J.M., and Pickar, D. Dysfunction in a prefrontal substrate of sustained attention in schizophrenia. *Life Sci* 1987; 40:2031–9.

Cornell, D.G., Suarez, R., and Berent, S. Psychomotor retardation in melancholic and non-melancholic depression: Cognitive and motor components. *J Abnorm Psychol* 1984; 93:150–7.

Cummings, J.L. Subcortical dementia: Neuropsychology, neuropsychiatry, and pathophysiology. *Br J Psychiatry* 1986; 149:682–97.

Cummings, J.L., and Benson, F. Subcortical dementia: Review of an emerging concept. *Arch Neurol* 1984; 41:874–9.

Davidson, R.J. Cerebral asymmetry, affective style, and psychopathology. In *Cerebral Hemisphere Function in Depression.* Kinsbourne, M. (ed.). American Psychiatric Press, Washington, 1988, pp. 2–22.

Davidson, R.J., Schaffer, C.E., and Saron, C. Effects of lateralized presentations of faces on self-reports of emotion and EEG asymmetry in depressed and nondepressed subjects. *Psychophysiology* 1985; 22:353–64.

Davidson, R.J.,, Schwartz, G.E., Saron, C., Bennett, J., and Goleman, D.J. Frontal versus parietal EEG asymmetry during positive and negative effect. *Psychophysiology* 1979; 16:202–3.

Dolan, R.J., Calloway, S.P., and Mann, A.H. Cerebral ventricular size in depressed subjects. *Psychol Med* 1985; 15:873–8.

Dolan, R.J., Calloway, S.P., Thacker, P.F., and Mann, A.H. The cerebral cortical appearance in depressed subjects. *Psychol Med* 1986; 16:775–9.

Dunbar, G.-C., and Lishman, W.A. Depression, recognition-memory, and hedonic tone: A signal detection analysis. *Br J Psychiatry* 1984; 144:376–82.

Finset, A. Depressed mood and reduced emotionality after right-hemisphere brain damage. In *Cerebral Hemisphere Function in Depression.* Kinsbourne, M. (ed.). American Psychiatric Press, Washington, 1988, pp. 50–64.

Glanzer, M., and Curity, A.R. Two storage mechanisms in free recall. *J Verb Learn Verb Behav* 1966; 5:351–60.

Alison.

you might have already see
the chapter in this book

pls the programme. I promised.

O...

Glass, R.M., Uhlenhuth, E.H., Hartel, F.W., Matuzas, W., and Fischman, M.W. Cognitive dysfunction and imipramine in outpatient depressives. *Arch Gen Psychiatry* 1981; 38:1048–51.

Goldstein, S.G., Filskov, S.B., Weaver, L.A., and Ives, J.O. Neuropsychological effects of electroconvulsive therapy. *J Clin Psychol* 1977; 33:798–806.

Gray, J.W., Dean, R.S., Rattan, G., and Cramer, K.M. Neuropsychological aspects of primary affective depression. *Int J Neurosci* 1987; 32:911–8.

Hart, R.P., and Kwentus, J.A. Psychomotor slowing and subcortical-type dysfunction in depression. *J Neurol Neurosurg Psychiatry* 1987; 50:1263–6.

Hasher, L., and Zacks, R.T. Automatic and effortful processes in memory. *J Exp Psychol [Gen]* 1979; 108:356–88.

Jaeger, J., Borod, J.C., and Peselow, E. Depressed patients have atypical biases in the perception of emotional chimeric faces. *J Abnorm Psychol* 1987; 96:321–4.

Jacoby, R.J., and Levy, R. computed tomography in the elderly: Affective disorder. *Br J Psychiatry* 1980; 136:270–5.

Jacoby, R.J., Dolan, R.J., Levy, R., and Baldy, R. Quantitative computed tomography in elderly depressed patients. *Br J Psychiatry* 1983; 143:124–7.

Kiloh, L.G. Pseudodementia. *Acta Psychiatr Scand* 1961; 37:336–51.

King, D.A., Caine, E.D., and Conwell, Y. The neuropsychology of depression in the elderly: A controlled study of depression, Alzheimer's disease, and healthy elderly. (Manuscript in preparation.)

Kronfol, Z., Hamsher, K., Digre, K., and Waziri, R. Depression and hemispheric functions: Changes associated with unilateral ECT. *Br J Psychiatry* 1978; 132:560–7.

Kubos, K.L., Moran, T.H., and Robinson, R.G. Differential and asymmetrical behavioral effects of electrolytic or 6-hydroxydopamine lesions in the nucleus accumbens. *Brain Res* 1987; 401:147–51.

Mathew, R.J., Meyer, J.S., Francis, D.J., Semchuk, K.M., Mortel, K., Claghorn, J.L. Cerebral blood flow in depression. *Am J Psychiatry* 1980; 137:1449–50.

McAllister, T.W. Cognitive functioning in the affective disorders. *Comp Psychiatry* 1981; 22:572–86.

Miller, W.R. Psychological deficit in depression. *Psychol Bull* 1975; 82:238–60.

Miller, E., and Lewis, P. Recognition memory in elderly patients with depression and dementia: A signal detection analysis. *J Abnorm Psychol* 1977; 86:84–6.

Robins, L.N., Helzer, J.E., Weisman, M.M., Orvaschel, H., Gruenberg, E., Burke, J.D., and Regier, D.A. Lifetime prevalence of specific psychiatric disorders in three sites. *Arch Gen Psychiatry* 1984; 41:959–67.

Robinson, R.G., Kubos, K.L., Storr, L.B., Rao, K., and Price, T.R. Mood disorder in stroke patients. *Brain* 1984; 107:81–3.

Rossi, A., Stratta, P., Petruzzi, C., Donati, M.D., Nistico, R., and Casacchia, M. A computerized tomographic study in DSM-III affective disorders. *J Affective Disord* 1987; 12:259–62.

Schaffer, C.E., Davidson, R.J., and Saron, C. Frontal and parietal EEG asymmetries in depressed and nondepressed subjects. *Biol Psychiatry* 1983; 18:753–62.

Schlegel, S., and Kretzschmar, K. Computed tomography in affective disorders. Part I. Ventricular and sulcal measurements. *Biol Psychiatry* 1987a; 22:4–14.

Schlegel, S., and Kretzschmar, K. Computed tomography in affective disorders. Part II. Brain density. *Biol Psychiatry* 1987b; 22:15–23.

Shima, S., Shikano, T., Kitamura, T., Masuda, Y., Tsukomo, T., Kanba, S., and Asai, M. Depression and ventricular enlargement. *Acta Psychiatr Scand* 1984; 70:275–7.

Silberman, E.K., and Weingartner, H. Hemispheric lateralization of functions related to emotion. *Brain Cogn* 1986; 5:322–63.

Silberman, E.K., Weingartner, H., Stillman, R., Chen, H.J., and Post, R.M. Altered lateralization of cognitive processes in depressed women. *Am J Psychiatry* 1983; 140:1340–4.

Starkstein, S.E., and Robinson, R.G. Lateralized emotional response following stroke. In *Cerebral Hemisphere Function in Depression.* Kinsbourne, M. (ed.). American Psychiatric Press, Washington, 1988, pp. 23–47.

Starkstein, S.E., Robinson, R.G., and Price, T.R. Comparison of cortical and subcortical lesions in the production of post-stroke mood disorders. *Brain* 1987; 110:1045–59.

Starkstein, S.E., Moran, T.H., and Bowersox, J.A. Behavioral abnormalities induced by frontal cortical and nucleus accumbens lesions. *Brain Res* (in press).

Sternberg, S. Memory scanning: New findings and current controversies. *Q J Exp Psychol* 1985; 27:1–32.

Targum, S.D., Rosen, L.N., Delisi, L.E., Weinberger, D.R., and Citrin, C.M. Cerebral ventricular size in major depressive disorder: Association with delusional symptoms. *Biol Psychiatry* 1983; 18:329–36.

Taylor, M.A., Greenspan, B., and Abrams, R. Lateralized neuropsychological dysfunction in affective disorder and schizophrenia. *Am J Psychiatry* 1979; 136:1031–4.

Tucker, D.M. Lateralized brain function, emotion and conceptualization. *Psychol Bull* 1981; 89:19–46.

Tucker, D.M., and Williamson, P.A. Asymmetric neural control systems in human self-regulation. *Psychol Rev* 1984; 91:185–215.

Watts, F.N., Morris, L., and MacLeod, A.K. Recognition memory in depression. *J Abnorm Psychol* 1987; 96:273–5.

Weinberger, D.R., Torrey, E.F., Neophytides, A., and Wyatt, R.J. Lateral ventricular enlargement in chronic schizophrenia. *Arch Gen Psychiatry* 1979; 36:735–9.

Weingartner, H., Burns, S., Diebel, R., and LeWitt, P.A. Cognitive impairment in Parkinson's disease: distinguishing between effort-demanding and automatic cognitive processes. *Psychiatr Res* 1984; 11:223–35.

Weingartner, H., Cohen, R.M., Murphy, D.L., Martello, J., and Gerdt, C. Cognitive processes in depression. *Arch Gen Psychiatry* 1981; 38:42–7.

Weingartner, H., and Silberman, E.K. Models of cognitive impairment: cognitive changes in depression. *Psychopharm Bull* 1982; 18:27–42.

Wells, C.E. Pseudodementia. *Am J Psychiatry* 1979; 136:895–900.

Wilson, R.S., Kaszniak, A.W., Klawans, H.L., and Garron, D.C. High speed memory scanning in Parkinsonism. *Cortex* 1980; 16:67–72.

Wolfe, J., Granholm, E., Butters, N., Saunders, E., and Janowsky, D. Verbal memory deficits associated with major affective disorders: A comparison of unipolar and bipolar patients. *J Affective Disord* 1987; 13:83–92.

16

Subcortical Features of Normal Aging

WILFRED G. VAN GORP AND MICHAEL MAHLER

Significant changes in brain structure and function occur during the normal aging process, resulting in selective cognitive changes during advanced age. Surprisingly, there have been few attempts to integrate data from within the neurosciences, such as neurobiology and neuropsychology, into a coherent view of both the structural and functional changes associated with normal aging. This chapter represents such an attempt.

Several issues of definition and methodology must first be addressed, including definitions of *aging* and *normal elderly*. Comfort (1979) defined senescence as "the group of effects that lead to a decreasing expectation of life with increasing age." This definition is simple and conforms to Gompertz's classic observation (1825) of the exponential relationship between mortality and chronological age. This definition does not require a unitary, intrinsic biological process of aging but implies that multiple effects may contribute to an overall loss of functional competence for survival. These effects may be primary, or endogenous to an aging organism, or they may be secondary, or exogenous, such as infection, trauma, toxins, environmental, or societal changes. Birren and colleagues (Birren and Renner, 1977; Birren and Cunningham, 1985, p.5) define aging as "the regular changes that occur in mature genetically representative organisms living under representative environmental conditions." This definition demands specification of the population under study, since aging may proceed differentially according to genetic and environmental influences. Also, this definition acknowledges the possibility that aging is not necessarily a *deterioration* of biological, psychological, or social function.

The term *normal elderly* also has multiple definitions. A high proportion of the elderly have one or more chronic illnesses and take several prescription medicines. Thus, *normal elderly* may encompass a heterogeneous group in which the effects of illness and medications on neurologic and neuropsychological function complicate intrinsic age-related processes. On the other hand, many researchers exclude older adults with obvious medical problems from study populations to evaluate the effects of age independent of age-related medical illnesses. This exclusion results in a group of ideally fit and active older individuals, supernormals, who demonstrate the best function attainable but who may not represent the majority of their peers. In general, researchers who have studied optimally healthy elderly have found fewer or less dramatic age-related changes than those who have examined less healthy subjects with less independent function (LaRue and Jarvik, 1982; Botwinick and Birren, 1963; Correll, Rokosz, and Blanchard, 1966; Willis et al., 1988; Obler and Albert, 1985; Steuer and Jarvik, 1981; Botwinick and Storandt, 1974; Rinn, 1988).

Differences between cross-sectional and longitudinal designs also result in difficulties in comparing various studies of cognitive change during older adulthood (Schaie and Hertzog, 1985; Nesselroade and Labouvie, 1985; Browning and Spilich, 1981). Many investigators use cross-sectional designs to decrease the time and expense of studies. However, generational differences in the quality and quantity of education, culture, health, nutrition, and other factors may exaggerate the age-related changes that might be seen without these cohort differences.

For this reason, some researchers have embarked upon ambitious longitudinal studies, following a group of adults for several years or even decades. Despite the many advantages of this approach, subject attrition during the course of the study may influence the results. For instance, a precipitous decline in cognitive function in a subset of older adults shortly before death, called *terminal drop*, may result in the appearance of a steeper decline with age among the entire group (Jarvik and Blum, 1971; Riegel and Riegel, 1972). Alternatively, selective attrition of the more disabled individuals leads to an augmentation in group means, producing a survivor effect.

Few studies of normal aging have examined a large number of neuropsychological functions simultaneously. Thus, researchers have traditionally derived conclusions about broad neuropsychological changes in aging by compiling studies examining primarily one cognitive domain, such as memory or language. Finally, few studies have correlated neuropsychological function directly with changes in the brains of normal aged individuals.

BRAIN CHANGES WITH NORMAL AGING

Gross Morphology

Several researchers have studied brain weight in the elderly. Tomlinson, Blessed, and Roth (1968) examined the brains of 28 nondemented subjects aged 65–92. They found a slight, though statistically significant, decrease from young adult norms in the male brains, but no significant decrease for the females. The brain weights of the older half of the study group did not differ from those of the younger half, implying that any changes in brain weight occurred before age 65. In contrast, Dekaban and Sadowsky (1978) reported a 7–8 percent loss of brain weight in elderly humans compared with peak young adult brain weights. Haug (1984), after correcting for long-term secular changes in body dimensions and brain weights, concluded that average brain weights are stable until age 60. Thereafter, brain weight decreases about 0.4 percent per year to age 75.

Changes in brain weight parallel changes in brain volume. Investigators using different techniques estimate a 10 percent decrease in the ratio of brain volume to cranial vault occurs between ages 55 and 90 (Davis and Wright, 1977; Yamamura et al., 1980). Cortical atrophy is slight in nondemented individuals (Tomlinson, Blessed, and Roth, 1968), and when present it appears to affect mainly the frontal and parietal parasagittal gyri (Katzman and Terry, 1983).

A significant portion of older brains show decreased cerebral volume associated with increased ventricular size, suggesting selective tissue loss in subcortical structures (Tomlinson, Blessed, and Roth, 1968). In one series (Tomlinson, Blessed, and Roth, 1968), 7 of the 28 brains examined had completely normal ventricles, 10 had slight ventricular dilatation (between 20 and 30 ml), and 11 had moderate ventricular enlargement (between 30 and 62 ml, mean 39 ml). Basal ganglia softening was the pathology most commonly associated with ventricular dilatation. Other studies demonstrated no change in ventricle dimensions until age 60 (Last and Tompsett, 1953), but beyond 60 ventricular size increases (Morel and Wildi, 1952). Planimetry on x-ray computerized tomography (CT) scans of older adults showed increased ventricular size (Barron et al., 1976; Jacobs et al., 1978; Jacoby et al., 1980), with the ventricles enlarging from 3–4 percent of brain volume in young adults (age 20–49) to 14–17 percent in old adults (age 80–89).

Cerebrovascular Changes

The brains of seemingly normal older people frequently contain ischemic lesions. In the Tomlinson, Blessed, and Roth study (1968), most of the 28 brains had lesions ranging from 0 to 91 ml, mean 13.2 ml. One or more minute foci of ischemia, not visible to the naked eye, occurred in 7 individuals who had been asymptomatic. In 13 others, grossly visible areas of softening occurred, especially in the basal ganglia. These larger lesions had caused motor signs and symptoms, but not dementia, during life.

Newer imaging techniques also demonstrate ischemic lesions in the brains of older adults. Between 10 and 20 percent have areas of low attenuation in the white matter on CT, consistent with ischemic lesions (George et al., 1986; London et al., 1986; Inzitari et al., 1987; Rezek et al., 1987). On magnetic resonance imaging (MRI) similar evidence of ischemia appears as areas of high signal intensity on T_2-weighted sequences (Salgado et al., 1986), predominantly in the deep white matter. These are found in the MRI scans of most elderly patients, including normals (Zimmerman et al., 1986; Brant-Zawadzki et al., 1985), and correlate with risk factors for cerebrovascular disease (Gerard and Weisberg, 1986; Sarpel et al., 1987). The foci of hyperintensity correspond to incomplete white matter infarctions or other pathologic changes in white matter (Kirkpatrick and Hayman, 1987; Englund et al., 1987).

Several pathologic processes may contribute to these ischemic changes in older brains. In the elderly, atherosclerosis regularly affects the major blood vessels, including the cerebral arteries. Also, there is a high prevalence of hypertension, which frequently leads to hyalinosis and occlusion of smaller-caliber arterioles. Finally, amyloid infiltrates occur increasingly with age in pial and penetrating vessels (Kemper, 1984). This amyloid angiopathy is most extensive in the occipital and temporal lobes, and it is more severe in patients with Alzheimer's disease.

Histologic Changes

Classic studies by Brody (1955) on the histology of brain over the life span demonstrated marked decrease in neuronal populations. Cell loss in elderly brains (70–95 years old) compared to young brains (16–21) ranged from 30 to 50 percent, depending

Table 16-1   Estimates of Neuron Loss in Brains of Elderly Subjects[a]

Brain Region	Percent Decrease
Pre-central gyrus	30–40
Post-central gyrus	0–7
Superior temporal gyrus	45–55
Putamen	27–30
Substantia nigra	33
Locus ceruleus	33–37

[a]Figures adapted from Katzman and Terry, 1983.

upon the specific brain region examined (see Table 16-1). The superior frontal, pre-central, and superior temporal gyri show significant neuronal loss, especially in cortical layers II and IV (Creasey and Rapoport, 1985). In contrast, the post-central gyrus of the parietal lobe undergoes little, if any, loss of cells. The picture that emerges is one of neuronal loss in selected regions (Creasey and Rapoport, 1985) rather than decreases in cell counts throughout the cortex.

Selected subcortical regions also show dramatic decreases in neuronal populations. Both large and small neuron populations in the putamen decline approximately 30 percent with age (Bugiani et al., 1978). Purkinje cell numbers in the cerebellum decline by 25 percent by old age (Corsellis, 1976). McGeer (1978) reported a loss of one third of the dopaminergic neurons of the substantia nigra between early and late adulthood. Similar results are noted in the locus ceruleus, which has norepinephrine-containing cells (Vijayashankar and Brody, 1979). While some authors find no age-related changes in the cholinergic cells of the nucleus basalis of Meynert (Whitehouse et al., 1983), others report substantial cell loss in this structure (McGeer et al., 1984; Mann et al., 1984). Thus major neurotransmitter systems are affected by cell loss in aging.

More recently, Haug (1984) challenged previous findings on the extent of cell loss, arguing that failure to account for differential age effects on tissue shrinkage during fixation may have resulted in an overestimate of cell loss associated with age. He concluded that there is no net cellular loss since an actual increase in neuronal density balanced a decrease in total size of the aging frontal cortex. However, individual cells in portions of the frontal lobe did decrease in volume.

The loss of neurons constitutes but one of the common histologic features of the aging brain. The presence of lipofuscin pigments, granulovacuolar degeneration, senile plaque formation, and neurofibrillary tangles are also typical in normal elderly. Lipofuscin, a brownish cytoplasmic deposit, accumulates in many cell types throughout the body and probably results from lysosomes containing hydrolytic enzymes and Golgi membranes (Bondareff, 1985). The deposition of lipofuscin in neurons increases linearly with age, although its effect is unclear (Beregi, 1982).

Granulovacuolar degeneration (GVD), a process unique to humans (Kemper, 1984), consists of cytoplasmic vesicles with dark granular cores that seem to be related to autophagic vacuoles. Tomlinson et al. (1968) found GVD present to some degree in 14 out of 28 normal older brains. GVD in normal brains is located only in the hippocampus (Tomlinson et al., 1968; Kemper, 1984), and GVD in other locations is usually pathologic. GVD affecting more than 10 percent of hippocampal cells is usually indicative of Alzheimer's disease (Tomlinson and Kitchener, 1972).

Senile plaques are extracellular aggregates seen largely in the cortical neuropil, hippocampus, and amygdala (Kemper, 1984; Tomlinson et al., 1968). They are seen only in human brains. Three subtypes of plaques occur, perhaps representing different stages in the development of plaques. The smallest ones are about 10 microns in diameter and consist of granular deposits of amyloid displacing adjacent fibers. Classical plaques are large, up to 100 micrometers, and contain an amyloid core surrounded by reactive astroglia, macrophages, and degenerating axons and dendrites. Primitive plaques resemble the classic ones but without the dense amyloid core. Investigations of the protein components of senile plaques demonstrate the presence of amyloid peptides and neurofilamentous peptides (Davies, 1988). The peptides within plaques in normal-aged brains show dissimilarities compared with Alzheimer's disease plaques (Davies, 1988).

Although large numbers of senile plaques occur in Alzheimer's disease, they are also present in other conditions and in the brains of normal elderly (Tomlinson et al., 1968; Kemper, 1984). Tomlinson et al. (1968) found no plaques in 6 of their 28 normal elderly brains, fewer than 1 plaque per low power field in 5 specimens, between 1 and 5 plaques per field in 9 brains, and 6 to 13 in 8 specimens. When small numbers of plaques occurred the distribution was limited to the hippocampus, and there was a tendency towards an increased number of plaques with age. Therefore, age-adjusted quantitative analysis may be necessary to differentiate plaques resulting from normal aging and those associated with disease.

Neurofibrillary tangles are also unique to human brains. These intraneuronal fibrils consist of argentophilic, paired helical filaments. Tangles seem related to normal neurofilament proteins, but the nature of their biochemical abnormality remains obscure (Kemper, 1984). Antibodies that label neurofibrillary tangles cross react with the amyloid peptides of senile plaques; however, there is no cross reaction with any protein that is found in normal brain (Davies, 1988).

Tomlinson et al. (1968) observed neurofibrillary tangles in over one half of the normal brians in their sample, especially in the hippocampus and adjacent entorhinal cortex. The percentage of brains showing this change increases with age from the fourth to the ninth decade, when almost all brains contain some tangles (Kemper, 1984). Neurofibrillary tangles may also affect the locus ceruleus. In normal brains tangles are rare in the neocortex, but this distribution is common in Alzheimer's disease. Neurofibrillary tangles are also present in dementia pugilistica, postencephalitic parkinsonism, and other neurologic degenerations (Kemper, 1984).

Scheibel (1981) studied Golgi preparations of brain tissue from aged individuals. This technique allows visualization of neuronal cell structure, especially the dendritic array, in great detail. The pyramidal neurons in cortical layers 3 and 5 of the prefrontal, temporal, and parieto-occipital association areas show clear-cut changes in dendrite structure. Dendritic spines decrease in number along the shafts, and the basilar shafts shrivel. These "dendrite-sick neurons" (Scheibel, 1981, p. 35) then become swollen, and eventually pyknotic. Scheibel postulates that this process is relatively selective for dendrites that are the terminal synapses from intracortical projections, perhaps explaining some of the cognitive changes that accompany advanced age.

However, these changes are not restricted to the association cortex. The giant py-ramidal cells of Betz, motor neurons, are particularly vulnerable to these aging changes; there is a loss of three fourths the normal complement of this cell type by the seventh decade (Scheibel, 1979). The spiny cells that make up 85 percent of neurons in the caudate nucleus are also affected, with a 50–75 percent decrease in dendrites as well as changes in dendrite morphology. These changes in the morphology and number of dendritic synapses in forebrain motor system pathways may affect the initiation and integration of motor activities, leading to observable declines in motor performance in the elderly.

The histologic changes described above occur even in the brains of clinically nor-mal people. Scheibel (1981) proposes the term *gerohistology* for alterations in neuronal soma and dendrite structure that may be normal developmental change in late adult-hood. Just as massive cell loss is normal and essential to nervous system development during gestation, cellular changes within allowable limits in older brains might not necessarily be pathologic. Scheibel (1981) emphasizes the loss of dendrites and syn-apses in cortical and subcortical regions of the forebrain, but he notes that other neu-ronal dendrite systems show plasticity and growth in aging animals. "Just as we as-sume that the former group of changes bring with them decreased neural processing capacity, so we would like to assume that the latter changes make up for such decre-ments by enhancing capacities for information processing" (Scheibel, 1981, p. 39).

Neurochemical and Metabolic Changes

In a concise review of the neurochemical changes of aging, Selkoe and Kosik (1984) list the many components of the brain that vary with age. Quantitative studies of nu-cleic acids show no change in DNA content. Whole-brain RNA levels remain stable, but RNA content in at least some brain areas decreases with age. Both DNA and RNA undergo structural and functional changes that could lead to increased errors in tran-scription. Protein synthesis decreases significantly during brain maturation, and this decline is slower later in life. Other changes in brain proteins include decreases in activity in some of the enzymes of intermediary metabolism. Brain lipid content also decreases in the course of aging, including loss of myelin.

Age affects several neurotransmitter systems as well (McGeer, 1978; Selkoe and Kosik, 1984). Studies of dopamine synthesis reveal marked declines in tyrosine hy-droxylase in the caudate and putamen in childhood and young adulthood, with much smaller changes after age 60 (McGeer, 1978). Choline acetyltransferase and other markers of acetylcholine activity are clearly reduced in the cortex in Alzheimer's dis-ease, but there is no consensus among investigators on whether cholinergic activity decreases in normal elderly (Bartus et al., 1982). Synthetic enzymes for gamma-ami-nobutyric acid (GABA) also decrease with age, but again the decline is more rapid in younger than in older groups (McGeer, 1978).

Brain metabolism has been measured by several techniques. Early studies using direct samples of carotid artery and jugular vein blood have given way to positron emission tomography (PET) to measure cerebral blood flow (CBF) and cerebral met-abolic rate of oxygen (CMR02) and glucose (CMRG1c). Kuhl et al. (1984) found decreases in the mean local CMRG1c in normal subjects between ages 18 and 78, with more rapid age-related decline in the superior frontal cortex and posterior inferior frontal cortex. This finding was challenged by other investigators (de Leon et al., 1984; Duara et al., 1984), who found no correlation between age and local or whole-brain mean CMRG1c. These variations may result from differences in technique or health status of subjects between studies (Creasey and Rapoport, 1985).

Summary

These findings reveal the alterations in gross morphology, histology, neurochemistry, and metabolism found in the aging brain. There is a small decrease in total brain weight, with an enlargement of the ventricles as the most obvious manifestation of gross atrophy. Ischemic changes are observed even in asymptomatic individuals, especially in deep white matter and the basal ganglia. On a microscopic level neuronal loss occurs selectively in brain regions such as pre-central frontal gyrus, putamen, substantia nigra, and locus ceruleus. Other histologic changes include lipofuscin accumulation, granulovacuolar change, senile plaque formation, and the presence of neurofibrillary tangles. Degeneration of dendrites occurs, most notably in the prefrontal cortex and other association cortex, Betz cells in motor cortex, and the caudate nucleus. Decreased activity of the enzymes of neurotransmitter synthesis affects dopaminergic and other catecholaminergic neurons, although the bulk of this decrement occurs in early adulthood. Cerebral metabolism may decrease with aging, with more of a decline within the frontal lobes. However, some authors report no age-related change in cerebral metabolic activity.

NEUROPSYCHOLOGICAL CHARACTERISTICS OF NORMAL AGING

General Intelligence and Global Cognitive Function

Most studies of the neuropsychological processes associated with normal aging have examined one functional domain in isolation, limiting the understanding of how several information processing functions interact and change with time. One exception to this is a study by Benton, Eslinger, and Damasio (1981), who administered a comprehensive neuropsychological test battery to a cross-sectional group of older adults over age 65 and found little evidence of generalized cognitive decline before the age of 80 years. The most significant declines occurred in tests of short-term visual memory, serial digit learning, and facial recognition. Bak and Greene (1980) found that a group aged 67–86 performed worse then one aged 50–62 on 10 out of the 18 neuropsychological measures studied. Van Gorp et al. (in press) also found significantly worse performance in old-old subjects (over 70 years) compared with the young-old group (under 70 years) on nonverbal and timed cognitive measures.

Considerable research has been conducted on differences in general intelligence between young and old individuals. Standard intelligence tests use age-adjusted, deviation IQ scores, assigning a score of 100 as the mean for each age group. To examine performance of subjects *independent* of their age, Rinn (1988) plotted normative data for all age groups studied from the Wechsler series test manuals, using criteria for assigning IQs to persons in their 20s and 30s to persons of all ages. As Figure 16-1 indicates, verbal intellectual abilities show far less age-related change than do nonver-

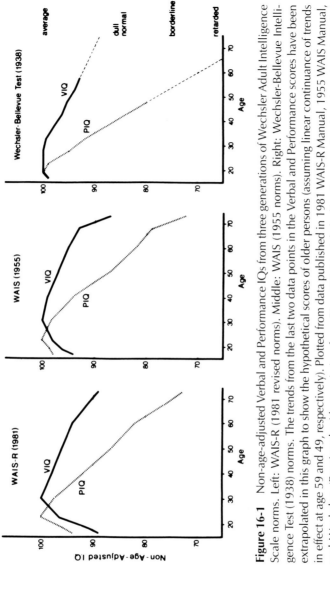

Figure 16-1 Non-age-adjusted Verbal and Performance IQs from three generations of Wechsler Adult Intelligence Scale norms. Left: WAIS-R (1981 revised norms). Middle: WAIS (1955 norms). Right: Wechsler-Bellevue Intelligence Test (1938) norms. The trends from the last two data points in the Verbal and Performance scores have been extrapolated in this graph to show the hypothetical scores of older persons (assuming linear continuance of trends in effect at age 59 and 49, respectively). Plotted from data published in 1981 WAIS-R Manual, 1955 WAIS Manual, and Wechsler. (Reprinted with permission from Rinn, W. Mental decline in normal aging: A review. *J Geriat. Psychiatry Neurol.* 1988, 1:144–58., by PSG Publishing Company, Inc., Littleton, Massachusetts.)

Table 16-2 Common Factor Structure, Varimax Rotation with Kaiser's Normalization for Neuropsychological Battery (N = 156)

Variable	I	II	III
1. Logical prose—delay	0.888	0.000	0.000
2. Logical prose—immediate	0.887	0.000	0.000
3. RAVLT/Trial 5	0.626	0.000	0.307
4. Sum of verbal tests (WAIS-R)	0.521	0.000	0.472
5. Visual reproduction—delay	0.000	0.753	0.334
6. Rey Osterrieth delay	0.000	0.740	0.000
7. Rey Osterrieth copy	0.290	0.714	0.000
8. Visual reproductions—immediate	0.000	0.683	0.374
9. Trails B	0.000	0.000	0.743
10. Trails A	0.000	0.000	0.700
11. Sum of WIA-R performance subtests	0.000	0.422	0.648
12. Boston naming test	0.298	0.000	0.626

bal abilities; the latter show a clear decline beyond age 60. In fact, Rinn notes that for the Wechsler Adult Intelligence Scale–Revised (WAIS-R), only 4 percent of individuals aged 20–24 performed as poorly as the average individual in the 70–74-year-old group.

The differential sensitivity of the timed, nonverbal skills measured by the performance subtests of the WAIS-R illustrated in Figure 16-1 has been called "the classic aging pattern" (Albert and Kaplan, 1980). As mentioned above, this pattern is especially prominent for those in the old-old group, over age 70 (Benton et al., 1981; Van Gorp, Satz, and Mitrushina, in press; Bak and Greene, 1980; Whelihan and Lesher, 1985).

Van Gorp et al. (in press) administered a neuropsychological battery to 156 normal elderly individuals and, based on a factor analysis of their performance, determined that three primary factors accounted for 62 percent of the overall variance (Table 16-2). Factor I consisted mostly of verbal cognitive and memory tests; Factor II consisted mostly of nonverbal cognitive and memory tests; and Factor III consisted mostly of timed cognitive and motor tasks. Figure 16-2 shows the correlation of each factor score with age. Tasks involving speed of processing, Factor III, correlated most with advancing age, while nontimed, verbal tasks demonstrated the least change with age.

The best known conceptualization of the intellectual changes associated with normal aging comes from the two-factor model of intelligence proposed by Cattell (1963) and elaborated by Horn and Donaldson (Horn, 1970; Horn and Donaldson, 1980). In this model, *crystallized intelligence* refers to long-held verbal abilities and well-learned knowledge. *Fluid intelligence* refers to novel, often time-dependent abilities that lack familiarity. Crystallized intelligence is relatively age insensitive; in contrast, fluid intelligence declines more precipitously with age.

Attention and Arousal

Attention is defined as the capacity for selective perception (Lezak, 1983) and is most simply assessed with the Digit Span test of immediate recall, or primary memory. Data from the Digit Span subtest of the WAIS-R and other indices of attention show that

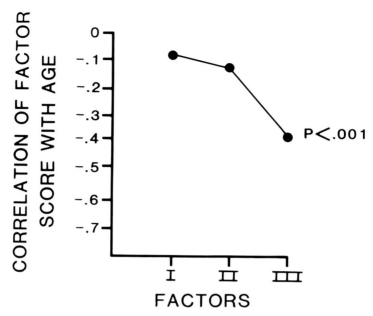

Figure 16-2   The correlation of each total factor score with age.

this function is relatively insensitive to changes in age (Craik, 1977; Fozard, 1980; Kinsbourne, 1980; Poon, 1985). In fact, the Digit Span subtest from the Wechsler intelligence tests requires little age correction for individuals over age 60.

Closely related to attention is the overall level of arousal or alertness of the individual. Woodruff's (1985) comprehensive review of the literature on arousal, sleep, and aging presents electrophysiological evidence for underarousal in the elderly. Because the elderly have fragmented sleep patterns, Woodruff suggests there is dysfunction in the brain-stem reticular activating system, a part of the brain involved in arousal and attention. He concludes that this results in a lowered state of alertness during the day for older people. Although this effect on arousal could account for some of the motor and cognitive slowing in the elderly, it does not produce major differences in digit span or attention.

Language

Language functions show general stability in older adulthood. In the study described above examining neuropsychological performance factors in a cross-section of normal older adults, Van Gorp et al. (in press) found that the Verbal Cognitive/Memory Factor did not decline significantly with age. This concurs with the stability with age of verbal intelligence as assessed by the WAIS-R.

However, tests of general verbal intelligence may yield different results from careful assessments of language capabilities in older adults. Confrontation naming is the best studied linguistic function in normal elderly. Montgomery (1982) and Van Gorp et al. (1986) found no significant differences in confrontation naming between geriatric subjects under 70 and those over 70, although the variability and range of scores were greater in the older group. Obler, Albert and Goodglass (1981) did not find a change with age in semantic substitutions, even though the incidence of circumlocutions increased.

Verbal fluency, the capacity to generate words in a specified semantic category within a time limit, has also been studied. In a cross-sectional sample of older adults, Benton et al. (1981) found that verbal fluency remained intact until age 80. However, this contradicts other researchers (Furry and Baltes, 1973; Schaie and Strother, 1968; Veroff, 1980). Rosen (1980) found that normal elderly did better with an animal category list than a letter category. Hence, it appears that most semantic and language functions studied remain relatively stable during older adulthood, except for a timed task requiring the generation of words from a semantic category. It is unclear to what extent diminished speed accounts for the age-related decline in word list generation.

Learning and Memory

Extensive studies of learning and memory function show that age affects some aspects of memory in most elderly, and in some these changes are dramatic. The term *age-associated memory impairment* (Crook et al., 1986) describes greater than expected forgetfulness in an otherwise apparently normal elderly person.

Delayed recall of both verbal and nonverbal information is sensitive to the effects of aging (see Craik, 1977, and Poon, 1985, for comprehensive reviews). A consistent finding is a differential decline in nonverbal recall as compared with verbal recall (Benton et al., 1981; Bak and Greene, 1980, 1981; McCarty, Siegler, and Logue, 1982; Arenberg, 1982; Eslinger, Pepin, and Benton, 1988). Haaland et al. (1983) confirmed this differential decline in 175 optimally functioning older adults but also found no age-related effects on the percentage recalled on delay (the ratio of immediate to delayed recall) for either verbal or nonverbal information. Clarkson-Smith and Halpern (1983) found that meaningful verbal labels for nonverbal stimuli aided recall for older subjects.

Less structured material requiring spontaneous organization, such as paired associate paradigms or list learning tasks, also appears particularly sensitive to age effects (Poon et al., 1980; Poon, 1985). As has been found in other domains, health status may be an important variable since optimally functioning, healthy subjects retain a greater percentage of material than do those who are less healthy.

Speed of Information Processing

Speed of information processing is one of the most studied functions in the neuropsychology of aging (Salthouse, 1980, 1985; Jacewicz and Hartley, 1987; Strayer, Wickens, and Braune, 1987). Birren (1974) compared the slowness of performance in older adulthood to "electrical brown out." Speed of performance declines especially on motor tasks, particularly by the sixth decade (Jacewicz and Hartley, 1987). In their factor analysis, Van Gorp and colleagues (in press) found that all timed tests loaded solely on Factor III, Speed of Performance, the factor most affected by age (Figure 16-2). This age-related decline was evident on tasks involving both motor and complex cognitive operations. Strayer, Wickens, and Braune (1987) studied the performance of normal elderly on a Sternberg memory search paradigm (which examines cognitive processing capacity independent of motor speed) to determine the components responsible for the decrease in speed of information processing. They concluded the primary contributions to slowing are perceptual–motor slowing and a deliberate cautiousness (requiring greater accuracy at the expense of speed of response), not a decline in central processing speed or capacity with age.

Concept Formation and Novel Problem Solving

In a comprehensive review of the literature on concept formation and problem solving in the elderly, Reese and Rodeheaver (1985, p. 495) concluded:

> In general, old and young adults perform differently on problem-solving tasks. On concept identification tasks, the elderly use less efficient strategies, are less successful at attaining solutions, commit more errors, and are less likely to change strategies when their responses are incorrect. On classification and categorization tasks, old adults use more primitive strategies.

Samuels and Podbros (1988) administered a hypothesis formation task to young, middle aged, and elderly subjects in two conditions, with and without memory aids. They found that the elderly were deficient on these tasks under both conditions, and the older subjects perseverated on their favored hypotheses.

Willis et al. (in press) found no deficits on the Halstead Categories Test in exceptionally healthy older adults, suggesting that this deficiency does not occur among optimally healthy older adults. However, Ernst (1987) did not find any relationship between health status and performance on problem-solving tasks such as the Trail Making Test or Halstead Booklet Categories Test.

A number of researchers have documented age-sensitive performance on tests traditionally thought to be sensitive to frontal lobe disturbance. Veroff (1980) found a significant correlation between age and the percentage of perseveration and segmentation features on the Visual Reproduction subtest from the Wechsler Memory Scale and concluded that there was a significant increase in frontal signs in older adults. Whelihan and Lesher administered tests of frontal lobe function (Stroop Color Naming Test, WAIS-R Similarities, Verbal Fluency, and others) as well as nonfrontal measures to cognitively intact subjects from a geriatric clinic. All six frontal lobe measures showed significant differences between the young-old and the old-old, whereas only 5 of the 19 nonfrontal measures were significantly different between the groups.

Summary

This review of the neuropsychology of aging literature suggests that psychomotor slowing, lowered arousal, diminished performance on nonverbal tasks, forgetfulness for nonverbal information, and poor performance on tasks of cognitive flexibility, set shifting, classification, and categorization are the neuropsychological changes associated with normal aging. In contrast, naming, attention (primary memory), and predominantly verbal neuropsychological tasks all appear relatively insensitive to changes with age.

CONCLUSIONS: NEUROPSYCHOLOGICAL MODELS

Two neuropsychological models have been proposed to explain the pattern of changes associated with normal aging. One model proposes that right-hemisphere dysfunction accounts for these changes while the other emphasizes alterations of frontal–subcortical function.

Klisz (1978) reanalyzed data from a study by Reed and Reitan (1963) and found that tests traditionally thought to be mediated by the right hemisphere best discriminated a middle-aged versus older group. Schaie and Schaie (1977) also noted that the performance of older adults on the WAIS was similar to patients with right-hemisphere dysfunction. The "classic aging pattern" of Albert and Kaplan (1980), decreased Performance IQ and relatively stable Verbal IQ with age, lends credence to a right-hemisphere hypothesis of cognitive deterioration on aging.

Several authors disagree with this, however. Shelton, Parsons, and Leber (1982) administered verbal and nonverbal cognitive tests equated for difficulty to middle-aged and older adult males matched for education. In this study the authors did not find a disproportionate decline on the performance of nonverbal relative to verbal tasks, arguing against the hypothesis. Mittenberg et al. (1988) compared a group of older adults and matched younger controls with selected tests believed to be mediated by specific brain regions on the basis of double dissociation findings in lesion studies. They did not find evidence of greater right-hemisphere vulnerability to aging, but did find that tests mediated by each hemisphere were equally sensitive to aging.

There is little support for the notion of differential right-hemisphere effects in the data on the gross morphologic, histologic, or metabolic changes of the older brain. The only evidence that favors an asymmetric aging process is that electroencephalogram (EEG) slowing is more prominent in the left temporal lobe than in the right in normal elderly (Harner, 1975).

The pattern of differential neuropsychological performance on verbal and nonverbal tasks may have several explanations. As noted above, when the verbal and nonverbal tasks were matched for difficulty, no differences in performance were found. Nonverbal, performance-oriented tests are novel, time-dependent tasks, and the dichotomy of crystallized and fluid intelligence predicts that these functions, representing fluid intelligence, show a greater decline with age. Finally, Van Gorp et al. (in press) demonstrated that a speed of processing factor was most affected by advanced age, and timed, nonverbal tests loaded heavily on this factor. The "classic aging pattern" may reflect differences in tests, with the effect of time-dependent, novel tasks more significant than differences in the hemispheres.

An alternative to the right-hemisphere hypothesis was proposed by Hicks and Birren (1970). They concluded that the basal ganglia, with connections to frontal cortical structures, may be particularly affected by the aging process, since these structures are involved in the speed of initiating and executing movement, a function specifically affected in the elderly. Pointing to the many connections between the frontal lobes and subcortical structures described by Nauta (1971), Albert and Kaplan (1980) also favored a frontal—subcortical model to explain the neuropsychological changes associated with normal aging. Albert and Kaplan (1980) and Verhoff (1980) noted a remarkable similarity between the qualitative performance of normal elderly adults and patients with frontal lobe disease. Mittenberg et al. (1988) suggested that the greatest correlations between age and neuropsychological tests occurred on measures indicative of frontal lobe dysfunction.

Van Gorp, Mitsushina, Cummings, Satz and Modessitt, et al. (1989) compared the neuropsychological performance of a group of normal elderly adults (mean age 70 years) with a young dementia group (mean age 37) with subcortical dementia (acquired immune deficiency syndrome [AIDS] dementia complex) and an older group with cortical dementia of the Alzheimer type (DAT). Despite dramatic age differences between the normal elderly and the AIDS dementia patients, there was a remarkable similarity in the raw test scores of these two groups. Both groups had difficulties on timed motor tests, learning and recall tests, tests sensitive to proactive interference, and nonverbal tests of secondary memory despite the expected superiority of younger individuals on these tasks. In contrast, patients with Alzheimer's disease were notably worse on nearly all neuropsychological measures with an inability to learn new information and language dysfunction characterized by a severe anomia. These findings suggest the neuropsychological alterations produced by normal aging and the subcortical changes of AIDS encephalopathy are remarkably similar and different from the cortical dysfunction of DAT. These data are consistent with the hypothesis that alterations in the frontal–subcortical system are responsible for the behavioral and cognitive changes noted in the course of normal aging.

Taken together, the neuropsychological and neurobiological literature of normal aging support a frontal–subcortical model to account for the cognitive changes of advanced age. Many normal older adults have ischemic changes in the deep white matter and basal ganglia of the brain, and ventricular enlargement results from this subcortical tissue loss. Neuronal cell loss is most prominent in frontal areas of the cerebral cortex and in the basal ganglia. Further, the most severe deterioration of dendrites observed by Scheibel (1981) occurred in the frontal motor cortex, prefrontal association cortex (and parieto-temporal association cortex), and the caudate nucleus. Dopaminergic neurons and neurotransmitter function are reduced in subcortical–frontal systems. Finally, cerebral metabolism is either invariant with age or shows age-related changes that are most prominent in the frontal area.

One caution to the frontal–subcortical hypothesis is the proposal of Goldberg (1986) that any diffuse brain damage will first disrupt frontal executive functions. Thus, generalized cellular or biochemical alterations in the aging brain could also produce the pattern of neuropsychological changes described above. The neurobiological data, however, suggest that frontal–subcortical systems are indeed the most vulnerable to aging and are most responsible for the vast array of age-related effects.

Further research is needed to explore fully the relationship between behavior and brain changes in the elderly. For instance, longitudinal data on cognition and adaptive function before death must be correlated with detailed necropsy analyses in the same subjects. Studies examining the effect of health status on cognitive function are also needed. Finally, cognitive approaches that do not depend upon speed of performance need to be developed to study executive functions specifically in the elderly.

REFERENCES

Albert, M.S., and Kaplan, E. Organic implications of neuropsychological deficits in the elderly. In *New Directions in Memory and Aging: Proceedings of the George A. Talland Memorial Conference.* Poon, L.W., Fozard, J.L., Cermak, L.S., Arenberg, D., and Thompson, L.W. (eds.). Lawrence Erlbaum Associates, Hollsdale, New Jersey, 1980, pp. 403–32.

Arenberg, D. Estimates of age changes on the Benton Visual Retention Test. *J Gerontol* 1982; 37:87–90.

Bak, J.S., and Greene, R.L. Changes in neuropsychological functioning in an aging population. *J Consult Clin Psychol* 1980; 48:359–99.

Bak, J.S., and Greene, R.L. A review of the performance of aged adults on various Wechsler Memory Scale subtests. *J Clin Psychol* 1981; 37:186–8.

Barron, S.A., Jacobs, L., and Kinkel, W.R. Changes in size of the lateral ventricles during aging determined by computerized tomography. *Neurology* 1976; 26:1101–3.

Bartus, R.T., Dean, R.L., Beer, B., and Lippa, A.S. The cholinergic hypothesis of geriatric memory dysfunction. *Science* 1982; 217:408–17.

Benton, A.L., Eslinger, P.J., and Damasio, A.R. Normative observations on neuropsychological test performance in old age. *J Clin Neuropsychol* 1981; 3:33–42.

Beregi, E. The significance of lipofuscin in the aging process, especially in the neurons. In *Neural Aging and its Implications in Human Neurological Pathology.* Terry, R.D., Bolis, C.L., and Toffano, G. (eds). *Aging, Vol. 18.* Raven, Press, New York, 1982, pp. 15–21.

Birren, J.E. Translations in gerontology—From lab to life: Psychophysiology and the speed of response. *Am Psychol* 1974; 29:808–15.

Birren, J.E., and Cunningham, W. Research on the psychology of aging: Principles, concept, and theory. In *Handbook of the Psychology of Aging, Second edition.* Birren, J.E., and Schaie, K.W. (eds.). Van Nostrand Reinhold, New York, 1985, pp. 3–34.

Birren, J.E., and Renner, V.J. In *Handbook of the Psychology of Aging.* Birren, J.E., and Schaie, K.W. (eds.) Van Nostrand Reinhold, New York, 1977, pp. 3–38.

Bondareff, W. The neural basis of aging. In *Handbook of the Psychology of Aging, Second edition.* Birren, J.E., and Schaie, K.W. (eds.). Van Nostrand Reinhold, New York, 1985, pp. 95–112.

Botwinick, J., and Birren, J.E. Cognitive processes: Mental abilities and psychomotor responses in healthy aged men. In *Human Aging: A Biological and Behavioral Study.* Birren, J.E., Butler, R.N., Greenhouse, S.W., Sokoloff, L., and Yarrow, M. (eds.). U. S. Government Printing Office, Washington, D.C., 1963, pp. 95–108.

Botwinick, J., and Storandt, M. Cardiovascular status, depressive affect, and other factors in reaction time. *J Gerontol* 1974; 29:543–8.

Brant-Zawadzki, M., Fein, G., Van Dyke, C., Kiernan, R., Davenport, L., and de Groot, J. MR Imaging of the aging brain: Patchy white matter lesions and dementia. *Am J Neuroradiol* 1985; 6:675–82.

Brody, H. Organization of the cerebral cortex. III. A study of aging in the human cerebral cortex. *J Comp Neurol* 1955; 102:511–66.

Browning, G.B., and Spilich, G.J. Some important methodological issues in the study of aging and cognition. *Exp Aging Res* 1981; 7:175–86.

Bugiani, O., Salvarani, S., Perdelli, F. et al. Nerve cell loss with aging in the putamen. *Eur Neurol* 1978; 17:286–91.

Cattell, R.B. Theory of fluid and crystallized intelligence: A critical experiment. *J Educ Psychol* 163; 54:1–22.

Clarkson-Smith, L., and Halpern, D.F. Can age-related deficits in spatial memory be attenuated through the use of verbal coding? *Exp Aging Res* 1983; 9:179–84.

Comfort, A. *The Biology of Senescence, Third edition.* Elsevier, New York, 1979.

Correll, R.E.,, Rokosz, S., and Blanchard, B.M. Some correlations of WAIS performance in the elderly. *J Gerontol* 1966; 21:544–9.

Corsellis, J.A.N. Some observations on the Purkinje cell population and on brain volume in human aging. In *Neurobiology of Aging.* Terry, R.D., and Gershon, S. (eds.). *Aging, Vol. 3.* Raven Press, New York, 1976, p. 205.

Craik, F.I.M. Age differences in human memory. In *Handbook of The Psychology of Aging.* Birren, J.E., and Schaie, K.W. (eds.). Van Nostrand Reinhold, New York, 1977, pp. 384–420.

Creasey, H., and Rapoport, S.I. The aging human brain. *Ann Neurol* 1985; 17:2–10.

Crook, T., Bartus, R.T., Ferris, S.H., Whitehouse, P., Cohen, G.D., and Gershon, S. Age associated memory impairment: Proposed diagnostic criteria and measures of clinical change—Report of a National Institute of Mental Health work group. *Dev Neuropsychol* 1986; 2:261–76.

Davies, P. Neurochemical studies: An update on Alzheimer's disease. *J Clin Psychiatry* 1988; 49 (Suppl.):23–8.

Davis, P.J.M., and Wright, E.A. A new method for measuring cranial cavity volume and its application to the assessment of cerebral atrophy at autopsy. *Neuropathol Appl Neurobiol* 1977; 3:341–58.

Dekaban, A.S., and Sadowsky, D. Changes in brain weights during the span of human life: Relation of brain weights to body heights and body weights. *Ann Neurol* 1978; 4:345–56.

de Leon, M.J., George, A.E., Ferris, S.H., Christman, D.R., Fowler, J.S., Gentes, C.I., Brodie, J., Reisberg, B., and Wolf, A.P. Positron emission tomography and computed tomography assessments of the aging human brain. *J Comput Assist Tomogr* 1984; 8:88–94.

Duara, R., Grady, C., Haxby, J., Ingvar, D., Sokoloff, L., Margolin, R.A., Manning, R.G., Cutler, N.R., and Rapoport, S.I. Human brain glucose utilization and cognitive function in relation to age. *Ann Neurol* 1984; 16:702–13.

Englund, E., Brun, A., and Persson, B. correlations between histopathologic white matter changes and proton MR relacation times in dementia. *Alzheimer Dis Rel Disord* 1987; 1:156–70.

Ernst, J. Neuropsychological problem-solving skills in the elderly. *Psychol Aging* 1987; 2:363–5.

Eslinger, P.J., Pepin, L., and Benton, A.L. Different patterns of visual memory errors occur with aging and dementia. *J Clin Exp Neuropsychol* 1988; 10:60–1 (Abstr.).

Fozard, J.L. The time for remembering. In *New Directions in Memory and Aging: Proceedings of the George A. Talland Memorial Conference,* Poon, L.W., Fozard, J.L., Cermak, L.S., Arenberg, D., and Thompson, L.W. (eds.). Lawrence Erlbaum Assoc., Hillsdale, NJ, 1980.

Furry, C.A., and Baltes, P.B. The effect of age differences in ability—extraneous performance variables on the assessment of intelligence in children, adults and the elderly. *J Gerontol* 1973; 28:73–80.

George, A.E., de Leon, M.J., Gentes, C.I. et al. Leukoencephalopathy in normal and pathologic aging: 1. CT of brain lucencies. *Am J Neuroradiol* 1986; 7:561–6.

Gerard, G., and Weisberg, L.A. MRI periventricular lesions in adults. *Neurology* 1986; 36:998–1001.

Goldberg, E. Varieties of perseveration: A comparison of two taxonomies. *J Clin Exp Neuropsychol* 1986; 8:701–5.

Gompertz, B. On the nature of the function expressive of the law of human mortality, and a new mode of determining the value of life contingencies. *Philosophical Trans R Soc London*, 513, June 9, 1825.

Haaland, K.Y., Linn, R., Hunt, W.C., and Goodwin, J.S. A normative study of Russell's variant of the Wechsler Memory Scale in a healthy elderly population. *J Consult Clin Psychol* 1983; 51:878–81.

Harner, R.N. EEG evaluation of the patient with dementia. In *Psychiatric Aspects of Neurologic Disease, Vol. 1*. Benson, D.F., and Blumer, D. (eds.). Grune and Stratton, New York, 1975, p. 64.

Haug, H. Macroscopic and microscopic morphometry of the human brain and cortex: A survey in light of new results. In *Brain Pathology, Vol. 1*. Pilleri, G., and Tagliavini, F., (eds.). Brain Pathology Institute, Bern, Switzerland, 1984, 123:49.

Hicks, L.H., and Birren, J.E. Aging, brain damage, and psychomotor slowing. *Psychol Bull* 1970; 74:377–96.

Horn, J. Organization of data on life-span development of human abilities. In *Life-Span Developmental Psychology: Research and Theory*. Goulet, L.R., and Baltes, P.B. (eds.). Academic Press, New York, 1970, pp. 424–66.

Horn, J.L., and Donaldson, G. Cognitive development in adulthood. In *Constancy and Change in Human Development*. Brim, O.G., and Kagan, J. (eds.). Harvard University Press, Cambridge, Massachusetts, 1980, pp. 445–529.

Inzitari, D., Diaz, F., Fox, A., Hachinski, V.C., Seingart, A., Lau, C., Donald, A., Wade, J., Mulic, H., and Merskey, H. Vascular risk factors and leuko-araiosis. *Arch Neurol* 1987; 44:42–7.

Jacewicz, M.M., and Hartley, A.A. Age differences in the speed of cognitive operations: Resolution of inconsistent findings. *J Gerontol* 1987; 42:86–8.

Jacobs, L., Kinkel, W.R., Painter, F. et al. Computerized tomography in dementia with special references to changes in size of normal ventricles during aging and normal pressure hydrocephalus. In *Alzheimer's Disease: Senile Dementia and Related Disorders*. Katzman, R., and Terry, R.D., and Bick, K.L. (eds.). *Aging, Vol. 7*. Raven Press, New York, 1978, p. 21.

Jacoby, R.J., Levy, R., and Dawson, J.M. Computed tomography in the elderly: I. The normal population. *Br J Psychiatry* 1980; 136:256–69.

Jarvik, L.F., and Blum, J.E. Cognitive declines as predictors of mortality in discordant twin pairs: A twenty-year longitudinal study of aging. In *Prediction of Life Span*. Palmore, E.B. and Jeffers, F.C. (eds.). Heath, Lexington, Massachusetts, 1971, pp. 199–211.

Katzman, R., and Terry, R. Normal aging of the nervous system. In *The Neurology of Aging*. Katzman, R., and Terry, R.D. (eds.). F.A. Davis, Philadelphia, 1983, pp. 15–50.

Kemper, T. Neuroanatomical and neuropathological changes in normal aging and dementia. In *Clinical Neurology of Aging*. Albert, M.L. (ed.). Oxford University Press, New York, 1984, pp. 9–52.

Kinsbourne, M. Attentional dysfunctions and the elderly: Theoretical models and research perspectives. In *New Directions in Memory and Aging: Proceedings of the George A. Talland Memorial Conference*. Poon, L.W., Fozard, J.L., Cermak, L.S., Arenberg, D., and Thompson, L.W. (eds.). Lawrence Erlbaum Associates, Hillsdale, New Jersey, 1980, pp. 113–29.

Kirkpatrick, J.B.,and Hayman, L.A. White-matter lesions in MR imaging of clinically healthy brains of elderly subjects: Possible pathologic basis. *Radiology* 1987; 162:509–11.

Klisz, D. Neuropsychological evaluation in older persons. In *The Clinical Psychology of Aging*. Storandt, M., Stiegler, I.C., and Elias, M.F. (eds.). Plenum Press, New York, 1978, pp. 71–95.

Kuhl, D.E., Metter, E.J., Reige, W.H., and Hawkins, R.A. The effects of normal aging on patterns of local cerebral glucose utilization. *Ann Neurol* 1984; 15 (Suppl.):S133–7.

LaRue, A., and Jarvik, L.F. Old age and biobehavioral changes. In *Handbook of Developmental Psychology*. Wolman, B.B. (ed.). Prentice Hall, Englewood Cliffs, New Jersey, 1982, pp. 791–806.

Last, R.J., and Tompsett, D.H. Casts of the cerebral ventricles. *Br J Surg* 1953; 40:525.

Lezak, M. *Neuropsychological Assessment, Second edition*. Oxford University Press, New York, 1983.

London, E., de Leon, M.J., George, A.E., Englund, E., Ferris, S., Gentes, C., and Reisberg, B. Periventricular lucencies in the CT scans of aged and demented patients. *Biol Psychiatry* 1986; 21:960–2.

Mann, D.M.A., Yates, P.O., and Marcyniuk, B. A comparison of changes in the nucleus basalis and locus coeruleus in Alzheimer's disease. *J Neurol Neurosurg Psychiatry* 1984; 47:201–3.

McCarty, S.M., Siegler, I.C., and Logue, P.E. Cross-sectional and longitudinal patterns of three Wechsler Memory Scale subtests. *J Gerontol* 1982; 37:169–75.

McGeer, E.G. Aging and neurotransmitter metabolism in the human brain. In *Alzheimer's Disease: Senile Dementia and Related Disorders*. Katzman, R., Terry, R.D., and Bick, K.L. (eds.). *Aging, Vol. 7*. Raven Press, New York, 1978, pp. 427–40.

McGeer, P.L., McGeer, E.G., Suzuki, J., Dolman, C.E., and Nagai, T. Aging, Alzheimer's disease, and the cholinergic system of the basal forebrain. *Neurology* 1984; 34:741–5.

Mittenberg, W., Seidenberg, M., O'Leary, D.S., and DiGuilio, D.V. Changes in cerebral functioning associated with normal aging. Paper presented at the 16th annual meeting of the International Neuropsychological Society, New Orleans, Louisiana, 1988.

Montgomery, K. A normative study of neuropsychological test performance of a normal elderly sample. Unpublished doctoral dissertation, University of Victoria, Victoria, Canada, 1982.

Morel, F., and Wildi, E. General and cellular pathochemistry of senile and presenile alterations of the brain. In *Proceedings of the 1st International Congress of Neuropathology*. Rosenberg, R., and Squier, T. (eds.). Torina, Rome, 1952, pp. 347–74.

Nauta, W.J.H. The problem of the frontal lobe: A reinterpretation. *J Psychiatr Res* 1971; 8:176–87.

Nesselroade, J.R., and Labouvie, E.W. Experimental design in research on aging. In *Handbook of the Psychology of Aging, Second edition*. Birren, J., and Schaie, K.W. (eds.). Van Nostrand Reinhold, New York, 1985, pp. 35–60.

Obler, L., Albert, M.L., and Goodglass, H. The word finding difficulties of aging and dementia. Presented at the annual meeting of the Gerontological Society of America, Toronto, Canada, 1981.

Obler, L., and Albert, M.L. Language skills across adulthood. In *Handbook of the Psychology of Aging, Second edition*. Birren, J., and Schaie, K.W., (eds.). Van Hostrand Reinhold, New York, 1985, pp. 463–73.

Poon, L.W. Differences in human memory with aging: Nature, causes, and clinical implications. In *Handbook of the Psychology of Aging, Second edition*. Birren, J., and Schaie, K.W. (eds.). Van Nostrand Reinhold, New York, 1985, p. 427–62.

Poon,, L.W., Walsh-Sweeney, L., and Fozard, J.L. Memory skill training for the elderly: Salient issues on the use of imagery mnemonics. In *New Directions in Memory and Aging: Proceedings of the George A. Talland Memorial Conference*. Poon, L.W., Fozard, J.L., Cermak, L.S., Arenberg, D., and Thompson, L.W. (eds.). Lawrence Erlbaum Associates, Hillsdale, New Jersey, 1980, pp. 461–84.

Reed, H.B.C., Jr., and Reitan, R.M. Changes in psychological test performance associated with the normal aging process. *J Gerontol* 1963; 18:271–4.

Reese, H.W., and Rodeheaver, D. Problem solving and complex decision making. In *Handbook of the Psychology of Aging, Second edition.* Birren, J., and Schaie, K.W. (eds.). Van Nostrand Reinhold, New York, 1985, pp. 474–99.

Rezek, D.L., Morris, J.C., Fulling, K.H., and Gado, M.H. Periventricular white matter lucencies in senile dementia of the Alzheimer type and in normal aging. *Neurology* 1987; 37:1365–8.

Riegel, K.F., and Riegel, R.M. Development, drop, death. *Dev Psychol* 1972; 6:309–16.

Rinn, W.E. Mental decline in normal aging: A review. *J Geriatr Psychiatry Neurol* 1988; 1:144–58.

Rosen, W.G. Verbal fluency in aging and dementia. *J Clin Neuropsychol* 1980; 2:135–46.

Salgado, E.D., Weinstein, M., Furlan, A.J., Modic, M.T., Beck, G.J., Estes, M., Awad, I., and Little, J.R. Proton magnetic resonance imaging in ischemic cerebrovascular disease. *Ann Neurol* 1986; 20:502–7.

Salthouse, T. Age and memory: Strategies for localizing the loss. In *New Directions in Memory and Aging: Proceedings of the George A. Talland Memorial Conference.* Poon, L.W., Fozard, J.L., Cermak, L.S., Arenberg, D., and Thompson, L.W. (eds.). Lawrence Erlbaum Associates, Hillsdale, New Jersey, 1980, pp. 47–65.

Salthouse, T. Speed of behavior and its implications for cognition. In *Handbook of the Psychology of Aging, Second edition.* Birren, J., and Schaie, K.W. (eds.). Van Nostrand Reinhold, New York, 1985, pp. 400–26.

Samuels, I., and Podbros, L.Z. And cognition in conceptual thinking during problem-solving: Effect of age. Paper presented at the 16th annual meeting of the International Neuropsychological Society, New Orleans, LA, 1988.

Sarpel, G., Chaudry, F., and Hindo, W. Magnetic resonance imaging of periventricular hyperintensity in a Veteran's Administration Hospital population. *Arch Neurol* 1987, 44: 725–8.

Schaie, K.W., and Hertzog, C. Measurement in the psychology of adulthood and aging. In *Handbook of the Psychology of Aging, Second edition.* Birren, J.E., and Schaie, K.W. (eds.). Van Nostrand Reinhold, New York, 1985, pp. 61–92.

Schaie, K.W., and Strother, C.R. Cognitive and personality variables in college graduates of advanced age. In *Human Behavior and Aging: Recent Advances in Research and Theory.* Talland, G.A. (ed.). Academic Press, New York, 1968, pp. 281–308.

Schaie, K.W., and Schaie, J.P. Clinical assessment and aging. In *Handbook of the Psychology of Aging.* Birren, J.E., and Schaie, K.W. (eds.). Van Nostrand Reinhold, New York, 1977, pp. 692–723.

Scheibel, A.B. Aging in human motor control systems. In *Sensory Systems and Communication in the Elderly.* Ordy, J.M., and Brizzee, (eds.). *Aging, Volume 10.* Raven Press, New York, 1979, pp. 297–310.

Scheibel, A.B. The gerohistology of the aging human forebrain: Some structuro-functional considerations. In *Brain Neurotransmitters and Receptors and Age-Related Disorders.* Enna, S.J. (ed.). *Aging Vol. 17.* Raven Press, New York, 1981, pp. 31–41.

Selkoe, D., and Kosik, K. Neurochemical changes with aging. In *Clinical Neurology of Aging.* Albert, M.L. (ed.). Oxford University Press, New York, 1984, pp. 53–75.

Shelton, M.D., Parsons, O.A., and Leber, W.R. Verbal and Visuospatial performance and aging: A neuropsychological approach. *J Gerontol* 1982; 37:336–41.

Steuer, J., and Jarvik, L.F. Cognitive functioning in the elderly: Influence of physical health. In *Aging: Biology and Behavior.* McGaugh, J.L. and Kiesler, S.B. (eds.). Academic Press, New York, 1981, pp. 231–53.

Strayer, D.L., Wickens, C.D., and Braune, R. Adult age difference in the speed and capacity of information processing: 2. An electrophysiological approach. *Psychol Aging* 1987; 2:99–110.

Tomlinson, B.E., Blessed, G., and Roth, M. Observations on the brains of non-demented old people. *J Neurol Sci* 1968; 7:331–56.

Tomlinson, B.E., and Kitchener, D. Granulovacuolar degeneration of hippocampal pyramidal cells. *J Pathol* 1972; 106:165–85.

Van Gorp, W., Satz, P., and Mitrushina, M. Neuropsychological processes associated with normal aging. *Dev Neuropsychol* (in press).

Van Gorp, W., Satz, P., Kiersch, M., and Henry, R. Normative data on the Boston Naming Test for a group of normal older adults. *J Clin Exp Neuropsychol* 1986; 8:702–5.

Van Gorp, W., Mitrushina, M., Cummings, J., Satz, P. and Modessitt, J. AIDS encephalopathy, Alzheimer's disease and normal aging: a comparison study. *Neuropsychiatry, Neuropsychology and Behavioral Neurology,* 1989; 2:5–20.

Veroff, A.E. The neuropsychology of aging. *Psychol Res* 1980; 41:259–68.

Vijayashankar, N., and Brody, H. A quantitative study of the pigmented neurons in the nuclei locus coeruleus and subcoeruleus in man as related to aging. *J Neuropathol Exp Neurol* 1979; 38:490–7.

Whelihan, W.M., and Lesher, E.L. Neuropsychological changes in frontal functions with aging. *Dev Neuropsychol* 1985; 1:371–80.

Whitehouse, P.J., Parhad, I.M., Hedreen, J.C., Clark, A.W., White, C.L. III, Struble, R.G., and Price, D.L. Integrity of the nucleus basalis of Meynert in normal aging. *Neurology* 1983; 33 (Suppl. 2):159.

Willis, L., Yeo, R.A., Thomas, P., and Garry, P.J. Differential declines in cognitive function with aging: The possible role of health status. *Dev Neuropsychol* 1988; 4(1):23–28.

Woodruff, D.S. Arousal, sleep and aging. In *Handbook of the Psychology of Aging, Second edition.* Birren, J.E., and Schaie, K.W. (eds.). Van Nostrand Reinhold, New York, 1985, pp. 261–95.

Yamamura, H., Ito, M., Kubota, K., and Matsuzawa, T. Brain atrophy during aging: A quantitative study with computed tomography. *J Gerontol* 1980; 35:492.

Zimmerman, R.D., Fleming, C.A., Lee, B.C.P., Saint-Louis, L.A., and Deck, M.D.F. Periventricular hyperintensity as seen by magnetic resonance: Prevalence and significance. *Am J Neuroradiol* 1986; 7:13–20.

17

Subcortical Mechanisms and Human Thought

JEFFREY L. CUMMINGS AND D. FRANK BENSON

A major neuroscientific discovery of the twentieth century is the recognition that alterations in the function of subcortical structures profoundly influence human thought and emotion. The preceding chapters of this book provide ample evidence that many degenerative processes, as well as vascular, inflammatory, demyelinating, and infectious diseases, have their principal impact on the striatum, thalamus, and subcortical white matter connections, and that damage to these structures leads to cognitive impairment (a dementia syndrome) as well as changes in the emotional state of the affected individual. The dementia syndromes produced by the different neuropathologic conditions have distinguishing neuropsychological characteristics, but they share several cardinal attributes such as psychomotor retardation, memory disturbances, alterations of executive control (strategic planning, set shifting, etc.), and emotional changes such as apathy and depression. Psychosis occurs with unusual frequency in several of the disorders.

The behavioral characteristics associated with subcortical dysfunction allow inferences to be drawn regarding the contribution of these structures to mental functions. This chapter will explore the application of the information gained from the study of subcortical dementia to these wider areas of brain–behavior relationships. The impact of emerging models of subcortical–cortical anatomic relationships (particularly those involving parallel circuits), the evolving information concerning the neurochemistry of the subcortical structures, and new theories stemming from cognitive science will be considered briefly in relation to the concept of subcortical dementia.

STRIATO-FRONTAL CIRCUITS AND SUBCORTICAL FUNCTION

Anatomical Organization

New anatomical information has become available that aids in understanding the links between subcortical structures and the frontal lobe and among the various subcortical structures themselves. A more comprehensive interpretation of the classic movement disorders and subcortical dementia can be constructed using these anatomical data. Alexander et al. (1986) identified five parallel circuits that link specific areas of the frontal lobe with subcortical structures and that receive reciprocal projections from the affiliated elements. They designated these processing loops as: (1) a motor circuit, (2)

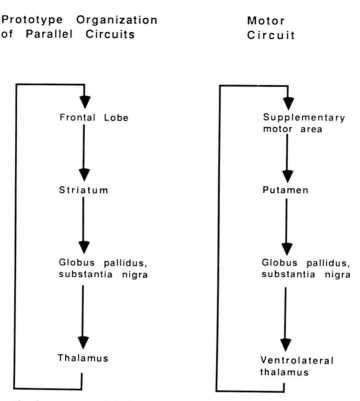

Figure 17-1   The figure on the left shows the prototypical anatomical arrangement applicable to all cortical–subcortical parallel circuits. The figure on the right shows the specific anatomic organization of the motor circuit (modified from Alexander et al., 1986).

an oculomotor circuit, (3) a dorsolateral prefrontal circuit, (4) a lateral orbitofrontal circuit, and (5) an anterior cingulate circuit. Each circuit incorporates projections from the frontal lobe to the striatum, from striatum to globus pallidus and substantia nigra, from these structures to thalamus, and from thalamus back to specific regions of the frontal lobe (Figure 17-1). While sharing the same gross anatomic structures, utilizing the same chemical transmitters, and having a common regional neurophysiology and cytoarchitectonic organization, the parallel circuits remain segregated throughout their courses.

The motor circuit (Figure 17-1) originates in the supplementary motor area and projects in a somatotopically organized manner to the putamen. From the putamen efferents project to the ventral globus pallidus and the lateral substantia nigra. In turn, the globus pallidus has projections to the ventrolateral thalamus, and the substantia nigra projects to the ventromedial thalamus. Both thalamic nuclei send efferent connections back to the supplementary motor area, completing a circuit rich in motor system input (Alexander et al., 1986). The supplementary motor area has projections to the motor cortex, allowing the cortiocostriatal circuit to influence the descending pyramidal output to the spinal cord (Botez and Barbeau, 1971). The oculomotor circuit

Dorsolateral
Prefrontal

Lateral
Orbitofrontal

Anterior
Cingulate

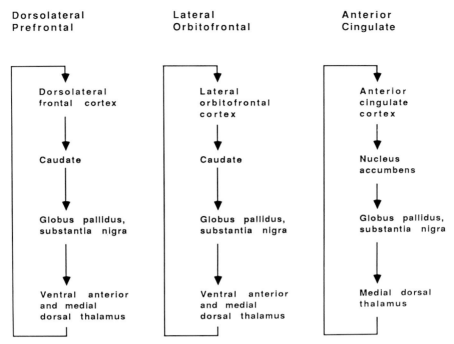

Figure 17-2 Three cortical–subcortical circuits relevant to intellectual function (modified from Alexander et al., 1986).

originates in the frontal eye field (area 8) and projects through specific regions of putamen and globus pallidus to the thalamus and back to the frontal cortex.

The pattern of organization evident within the motor and oculomotor circuits is recapitulated in the three parallel circuits relevant to higher cognitive functions (Figure 17-2). Dorsal prefrontal circuit neurons project to the dorsolateral portions of the caudate nucleus; these in turn project to the dorsomedial globus pallidus and rostral substantia nigra. These nuclei connect with the ventral anterior and medial dorsal thalamic regions, respectively. The thalamic nuclei complete the circuit by projecting back to the prefrontal cortex. The principal structures of the lateral orbitofrontal circuit include the lateral orbitofrontal cortex, the ventromedial caudate nucleus, the dorsomedial globus pallidus and rostromedial substantia nigra, and the ventral anterior and dorsomedial thalamic nuclei, with projections back to the orbitofrontal areas. The anterior cingulate circuit originates in the anterior cingulate gyrus of the medial frontal lobe. These neurons project (with others from the hippocampus, amygdala, and temporal cortex) to the nucleus accumbens and the olfactory tubercle (the limbic striatum). These ventral striatal structures project to the anterior globus pallidus and substantia nigra, which connect to the paramedian portion of the medial dorsal nucleus of the thalamus. The latter has prominent efferent connections with the anterior cingulate gyrus (Alexander et al., 1986). Each of the stations of these circuits receives input from other sources, and each has efferent connections in addition to those described in the parallel circuits. Nonetheless, the anatomical connections of each circuit create integrated loops that act as cohesive functional units.

Functional Implications

There are many important implications of the striato-frontal parallel circuits. The three frontal regions anchoring the circuits—dorsal frontal, orbitofrontal, and cingulate cortices—correspond to the sites of three postulated frontal lobe behavioral syndromes (Cummings, 1985). Lesions involving the dorsal convexity of the frontal lobe produce disturbances of executive control functions such as motor programming, set maintenance and shifting, and self-monitoring (Lezak, 1983; Lhermitte et al., 1972; Shallice, 1982). Injury to the orbitofrontal cortex leads to behavioral disinhibition, impulsiveness, and disregard for customary social constraints on behavior—the "pseudopsychopathic" behavior pattern described by Blumer and Benson (1975). Damage to the medial frontal-cingulate area leads to akinesia and apathy (Damasio and Van Hoesen, 1983; Blumer and Benson, 1975; Stuss and Benson, 1986). While involvement of these three cortical regions can lead to relatively specific behavioral syndromes, involvement of other areas within their respective circuits can produce many of the same behavioral phenomena, accounting for the similarity of the features of subcortical dementia to those of frontal lobe syndromes. With lesions of either the frontal lobe or the related subcortical structures, similar alterations in intellectual performance and demeanor may occur. Indeed, the similarity of subcortical dementia syndromes and frontal lobe disorders is a necessary correlate of the parallel circuits. Certain behavioral changes may be unique to frontal lobe damage or subcortical dysfunction, but these have not been delineated.

The organization and anatomic specificity of the motor and fronto-striatal parallel circuits also provides an explanation for the recognized relationship of the subcortical dementias to extrapyramidal motor disorders. Diseases that involve the cortico-striatal circuits containing the caudate, putamen, globus pallidus, or substantia nigra disrupt motor function and simultaneously affect cognitive activity through disturbances of the parallel loops mediating cognitive function. Pathology involving either the frontal cortex or the thalamus will affect circuits encompassing the basal ganglia. Primary basal ganglia disorders tend to produce more marked motor problems than are evidenced in frontal lobe and thalamic disorders, but pathology anywhere within the circuits tends to affect both motor and cognitive functions.

The structures involved in the different parallel circuits also provide a basis for understanding the differences in symptomatology among the disorders producing subcortical dementia. For example, the dementia of Huntington's disease appears early in the illness course and becomes pervasive, whereas the dementias of Parkinson's disease and of Wilson's disease may remain mild throughout most of the course of these conditions. Huntington's disease produces marked involvement of the caudate, the structure receiving most of the prefrontal input from circuits arising in the dorsolateral cortex. Wilson's disease, on the other hand, has its greatest impact on the putamen, which receives most of its input from the supplementary motor area and the substantia nigra and plays a greater role in the motor circuit. Similarly, nigral degeneration in Parkinson's disease results in preferential depletion of dopamine from the putamen; there are less marked alterations in the caudate. Thus, diseases affecting the caudate have greater impact on the systems mediating prefrontal connections and produce greater cognitive disturbances. Disorders affecting the putamen spare the prefrontal connections and produce less severe intellectual compromise.

Parallel circuits offer a potential explanation for many heretofore enigmatic aspects of subcortical dementia and provide an anatomical model on which to develop further studies of the structures mediating aspects of impaired intellectual function and disturbed behavior in the subcortical dementia syndromes.

NEUROCHEMICAL ASPECTS OF SUBCORTICAL FUNCTION

Many of the principal neurotransmitters of the brain share a common anatomical organization characterized by production in nuclei located in the brain stem or basal forebrain and transport rostrally to target areas in the basal ganglia or cortex (Nieuwenhuys, 1985). The locus ceruleus manufactures norepinephrine and sends ascending axons to the septum, amygdala, hippocampus, cerebellum, and the entire neocortex. Dopamine is synthesized in the substantia nigra and ventral tegmental area of the mesencephalon and is transported to the striatum, medial frontal cortex, cingulate cortex, septum, and amygdala. The nucleus basalis, a corticoid basal forebrain nucleus, produces acetylcholine for export to the hippocampus and neocortex. Serotonin-synthesizing neurons are located in the median and paramedian areas of the mesencephalon, pons, and medulla an project locally to the central raphe nuclei. These imported neurotransmitters interact with intrinsic neurons utilizing acetylcholine, amino acid transmitters, or neuropeptides.

Over the past 30 years, in concert with advances in understanding the anatomical organization of the cerebral structures, the functional roles of the transmitters have been actively studied, and the means by which they account for clinical symptoms are beginning to be understood (Di Chiara and Gessa, 1981; Nieuwenhuys, 1985; Sandler et al., 1985).

Penny and Young (1983) have proposed a biochemical organization utilizing a parallel circuit scheme similar to that discussed above. Based on mutually confirmatory anatomic, biochemical, and physiological observations, they proposed an excitatory positive feedback loop connecting the cortex to the thalamus and back to the cortex. They speculated that the main cortico-thalamic transmitter is the excitatory substance glutamate. They further hypothesized that this excitatory loop is modulated by the type of cortico-striato-pallido/nigro-thalamo-cortical circuits later elaborated in more detail by Alexander et al. (1986). Cortico-striatal cells utilize inhibitory glutamate; striato-pallidal and striato-nigral cells have inhibitory GABA-ergic (gamma-aminobutyric acid) connections; pallidal and nigral cells make inhibitory GABA-ergic projections to the thalamus (Figure 17-3). The globus pallidus and substantia nigra function to inhibit and modulate the excitatory thalamocortical loop. Striatal cells also establish inhibitory interconnections (using GABA or glycine) with inhibitory dopaminergic cells projecting back to the striatum via the nigrostriatal tract. Thus, in conditions such as Huntington's disease, loss of GABA-ergic cells of the striatum lead to disinhibition of the thalamocortical loop and of the striatal cells (via the negative feedback loop with the substantia nigra), resulting in an inability to select and maintain appropriate movements and an aberrant generation of inappropriate movements (e.g., chorea). In Parkinson's disease, loss of nigral modulatory influences results in a failure to modify ongoing behavioral activity. Thus, if there is movement, it will continue (festination); and if there is no movement, the person will remain inert (akinesia).

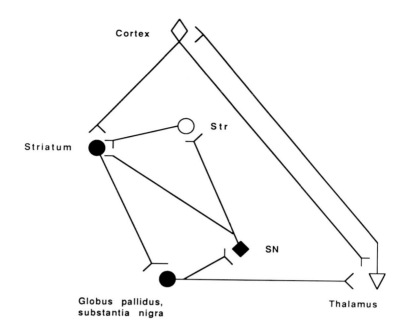

Cortex

Str

Striatum

SN

Globus pallidus,
substantia nigra

Thalamus

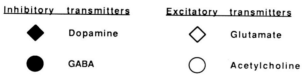

Inhibitory transmitters   Excitatory transmitters

Dopamine   Glutamate

GABA   Acetylcholine

Figure 17-3   Transmitters of the cortical–subcortical circuits (SN, substantia nigra; Str, striatum; filled nuclei use inhibitory transmitters; open nuclei use excitatory transmitters (modified from Penny and Young, 1983).

This elementary model of transmitter function leaves many clinical phenomena unexplained and ignores the other pathologic changes of basal ganglia diseases that inevitably complicate any attempt to establish parsimonious explanations for clinical observations. For example, the dopamine deficiency of Parkinson's disease is accompanied by deficits of norepinephrine, serotonin, and several neuropeptides. Each of these substances probably plays a role in the behavioral alterations seen in the disease. Nevertheless, the proposed excitatory and inhibitory loops are consistent with the parallel circuits proposed from anatomical studies, and the serial arrangement of inhibitory and excitatory transmitters provides plausible explanations for a number of clinical observations.

Extension of this preliminary model holds considerable promise for better understanding of the behavioral alterations seen in the subcortical dementias. For example, disinhibition of the thalamocortical loop involving the dorsolateral prefrontal circuit could explain the impairment in achieving and maintaining set that characterizes subcortical dementia syndromes. Persistent thalamocortical excitation could result in the continuation of ongoing behavioral sets (perseveration), as well as failure to initiate or change sets when appropriate. Within the lateral orbitofrontal circuit, unmodulated corticothalamic excitation could account for the uninhibited impulsiveness of some patients with subcortical dementias. While both conjectural and incomplete, tentative hypotheses of this type may lead to an improved understanding of the cerebral basis of behavior and thought. Subcortical behavioral syndromes provide an important opportunity to test hypotheses generated from experimental models of transmitter organization and function.

COGNITIVE SCIENCE AND SUBCORTICAL FUNCTION

Concepts such as subcortical dementia are most stimulating and useful when they interact with and enhance other models of brain function. The past few decades have seen the emergence of a new brand of psychology—cognitive science—aimed at probing the mental structures that provide order to cognition (Gardner, 1985). Unlike behaviorism, in which the processes linking stimulus and response were relegated to an unknowable and therefore irrelevant "black box," cognitive science seriously probes the mental mechanisms underlying human experience and thought (Kihlstrom, 1987; Stillings et al., 1987). Processing models based on information theory and computer research (artificial intelligence) are used to inform the approach of cognitive psychology to the study of memory, perception, and language. The combination of cognitive science with another relatively young discipline, neuropsychology, holds tremendous promise for outlining and exploring the brain functions associated with specific mental processes.

Modularity theory is one approach in cognitive psychology (Gardner, 1983; Fodor, 1983) that provides a conceptual framework for the study of the neurologic basis of intellectual activity. One proponent, Fodor (1983), hypothesized that mental processes (modules) are organized vertically into self-contained units mediating domain-specific information. Language and visual perception are two examples of such vertically organized processes. Horizontally organized functions, in contrast, entail operations that cut across domains. Examples of horizontal faculties include attention, memory, and judgment. These concepts map relatively well onto the instrumental–fundamental distinction discussed in Chapter 1 of this volume, in which it was noted that some major functions such as language and perception are instrumental activities mediated by the cerebral cortex, whereas attention, motivation, and mood represent more fundamental functions mediated largely by subcortical structures (Albert, 1978). Fundamental functions would be regarded as domain-nonspecific horizontally organized faculties; instrumental functions would be viewed as domain-specific vertically organized faculties.

A similar but more anatomically oriented model emanated from the neuropsychological studies of Luria (1973). He conceptualized three major functional compartments: basal, posterior cortical, and frontal. The basal (subcortical) structures acted to provide *cerebral tone*, a term borrowed from the earlier Pavlovian approach. The posterior cortical functions included the processing of all sensory–motor activities; the frontal segment acted to analyze, monitor, and control the other functions. Luria posited a close reciprocal relationship between the basal (subcortical) and frontal activities, with both participating in the control of the posterior cortical functions.

Further investigation of the subcortical dementias using one of the cognitive science or neuropsychological models may provide new insights into patterns of brain function; reciprocally, future advances in theories of brain control may guide experimental investigation of patients with subcortical dementia syndromes. Clinical studies of dementia syndromes have already demonstrated convincing relationships between pathologic changes in specific cortical or subcortical areas and specific patterns of behavioral alteration. These data, however, must be buttressed by other approaches to advance the understanding of normal thinking or of such complex processes as the experience of self-consciousness. Synergistic interactions between cognitive psychology, artificial intelligence, anthropology, and linguistics are currently occurring in the new field of cognitive science. The addition of this information to the rapidly expanding knowledge of neuroscience and the clinical insights available from neuropsychology, neurology, and neuropsychiatry will eventually produce a far richer view of human mental activities.

REFERENCES

Albert, M.L. Subcortical dementia. In *Alzheimer's Disease: Senile Dementia and Related Disorders*. Katzman, R., Terry, R.D., and Bick, K.L. (eds.). Raven Press, New York, 1978, pp. 173–9.

Alexander, G.E., DeLong, M.R., and Strick, P.L. Parallel organization of functionally segregated circuits linking basal ganglia and cortex. *Annu Rev Neurosci* 1986; 9:357–81.

Botez, M.I., and Barbeau, A. Role of subcortical structures and particularly of the thalamus in the mechanisms of speech and language. *Int J Neurol* 1971; 8:300–20.

Blumer, D., and Benson, D.F. Personality changes with frontal and temporal lobe lesions. In *Psychiatric Aspects of Neurologic Disease*. Benson, D.F., and Blumer, D. (eds.). Grune and Stratton, New York, 1975, pp. 151–70.

Cummings, J.L. *Clinical Neuropsychiatry*. Grune and Stratton, New York, 1985.

Damasio, A.R., and Van Hoesen, G.W. Emotional disturbances associated with focal lesions of the limbic frontal lobe. In *Neuropsychology of Human Emotion*. Heilman, K.M., and Satz, P. (eds.). Guilford Press, New York, 1983, pp. 85–110.

Di Chiara, G., and Gessa, G.L. (eds.). *GABA and the Basal Ganglia*. Raven Press, New York, 1981.

Fodor, J.A. *The Modularity of Mind*. MIT Press, Cambridge, Massachusetts, 1983.

Gardner, H. *Frames of Mind. The Theory of Multiple Intelligences*. Basic Books, New York, 1983.

Gardner, H. *The Mind's New Science: A History of the Cognitive Revolution*. Basic Books, New York, 1985.

Kihlstrom, J.F. The cognitive unconscious. *Science* 1987; 237:1145–52.

Lezak, M.D. *Neuropsychological Assessment, Second edition*. Oxford University Press, New York, 1983.

Lhermitte, F., Derouesne, J., and Signoret, J.-L. Analyse neuropsychologigue du syndrome frontal. *Rev Neurol (Paris)* 1972; 127:415–40.

Luria, A.R. *The Working Brain. An Introduction to Neuropsychology*. (Haigh, B., translator). Basic Books, New York, 1973.

Nieuwenhuys, R. *Chemoarchitecture of the Brain*. Springer-Verlag, New York, 1985.

Penny, J.B., Jr., and Young, A.B. Speculations on the functional anatomy of basal ganglia disorders. *Annu Rev Neurosci* 1983; 6:73–94.

Sandler, M., Feuerstein, C., and Scatton, B. (eds.). *Neurotransmitter Interactions in the Basal Ganglia*. Raven Press, New York, 1985.

Shallice, T. Specific impairments of planning. In *The Neuropsychology of Cognitive Function*. Broadbent, D.E., and Weiskrantz, L. (eds.). Royal Society, London, 1982, pp. 199–209.

Stillings, N.A., Feinstein, M.H., Garfield, J.L., Rissland, E.L., Rosenbaum, D.A., Weisler, S.E., and Baker-Ward, L. *Cognitive Science. An Introduction*. MIT Press, Cambridge, Massachusetts, 1987.

Stuss, D.T., and Benson, D.F. *The Frontal Lobes*. Raven Press, New York, 1986.

Index